THE 12-LEAD ECG

IN ACUTE CORONARY SYNDROMES

THE 12-LEAD ECG
IN ACUTE CORONARY SYNDROMES

Tim Phalen • President, ECG Solutions, Inc.
Barbara Aehlert, MSEd, BSPA, RN • President, Southwest EMS Education, Inc.

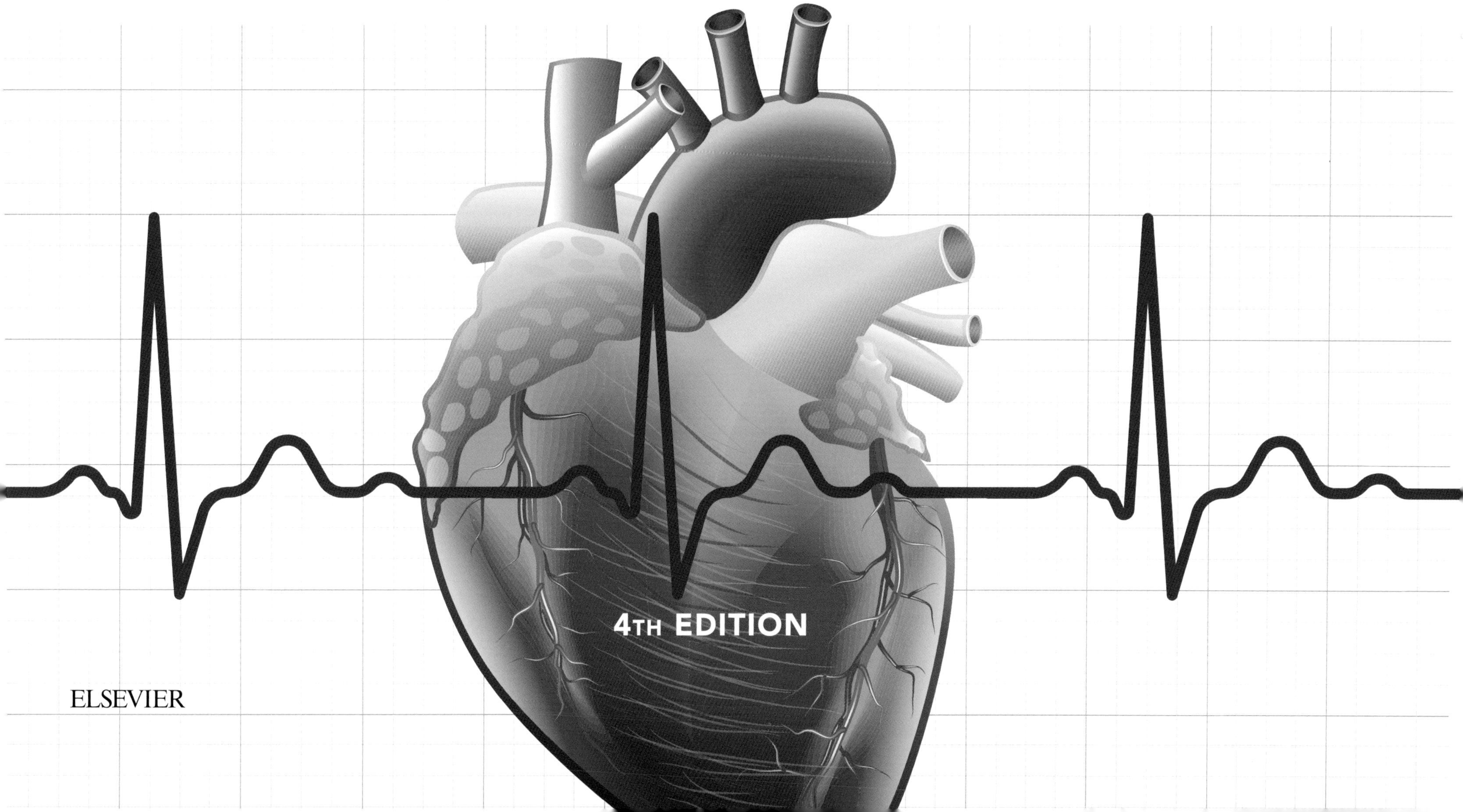

ELSEVIER

3251 Riverport Lane
St. Louis, Missouri 63043

THE 12-LEAD ECG IN ACUTE CORONARY SYNDROMES ISBN: 978-0-323-49789-3

Library of Congress Control Number: 2018941262

Senior Content Strategist: Sandra Clark
Content Development Manager: Melissa Jayne Kinsey
Content Development Specialist: Danielle Frazier
Publishing Services Manager: Deepthi Unni
Project Manager: Janish Ashwin Paul
Design Direction: Amy Buxton

Printed in India

Last digit is the print number: 9 8 7 6

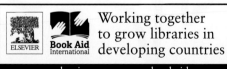

Preface

The challenge in providing a simplified method of 12-lead ECG acquisition and infarct recognition lies in determining which information is absolutely necessary for effective identification and treatment of acute coronary syndromes. If a text provides too much information, you are quickly overwhelmed. If it supplies inadequate information, it's of little benefit to your clinical practice. In writing this book, I attempted to walk that fine line and avoid both of these outcomes.

We've assumed that the reader has successfully completed a basic ECG recognition course before undertaking 12-lead ECG interpretation. As a result, we've chosen to provide only a brief review of waveform identification and measurement, and rate and rhythm determination. We assume that the reader is proficient in basic dysrhythmia recognition.

We know that the transition from interpreting ECGs in a textbook to actually using 12-lead ECG interpretive skills in clinical practice is a big step. To help you make the leap, we present information in an easy-to-understand format. Using tables, illustrations, and a large number of practice 12-lead ECGs, you'll learn to recognize ST-elevation myocardial infarction (STEMI), non–ST-elevation myocardial infarction (NSTEMI), and common ST-elevation variants.

With this edition, we feel it's important to recognize the increasing presence of nonphysician practitioners (NPPs)—that is, physician assistants and advanced-practice nurses in prehospital and hospital settings. NPPs play a key role in caring for patients with ischemic heart disease, both during and after an acute ischemic event. With this in mind, and where appropriate, the word "physician" has been changed to "provider" throughout this text.

We've made every effort to offer information that's consistent with current literature; however, we encourage you to learn and follow local protocols as defined by your medical advisors. We hope this text gives you a practical jumpstart toward infarct recognition, convinces you that 12-leads don't have to be intimidating, and encourages you to learn even more advanced electrocardiography.

Tim Phalen
Barbara Aehlert

Acknowledgments

Our thanks to the manuscript reviewers, who provided insightful comments and suggestions. A special thanks to Melissa Kinsey for her assistance with this project, and to Dr. Greg Lachar, Andrew Baird, Andrea Lowrey, Paul Honeywell, and Jay Wood for providing many of the 12-lead ECGs used in this text.

Tim Phalen
Barbara Aehlert

About the Authors

Since 1994, Tim Phalen has led ECG workshops for more than 75,000 participants in a dozen countries. Before he became a full-time speaker, Tim was a paramedic for 14 years. He began integrating 12-lead ECGs into patient care in the 1980s. Tim feels fortunate to have learned from many great instructors along the way, of whom the most helpful and influential was Dr. Henry Marriott.

Barbara Aehlert has been a registered nurse for more than 40 years, with clinical experience in medical/surgical nursing, critical care nursing, prehospital education, and nursing education. Barbara is an active CPR and ACLS instructor.

Reviewers for the Fourth Edition

Alyson Dingler, RN
Adjunct Clinical Professor/RN CVICU
Yuba Community College/Rideout Regional Medical Center
Marysville, California

Steve Vandeventer, EMT-P
Education & Quality Specialist
Mecklenburg EMS Agency
Charlotte, North Carolina

Joshua Borkosky, BS, FP-C, EMSI
EMS Education Manager
University of Cincinnati College of Medicine
Division of Emergency Medical Services
Cincinnati, Ohio

Bernadette Henrichs, PhD, CRNA, CCRN
Professor and Director, Nurse Anesthesia Program
Goldfarb School of Nursing at Barnes-Jewish College
St. Louis, Missouri

Angela McConachie, RN, MSN-FNP, DNP
Assistant Professor
Goldfarb School of Nursing at Barnes-Jewish Hospital
St. Louis, Missouri

Hannah C. Muthersbaugh, MMS, NRP, PA-C
Emergency Medicine PA/EMS Assistant Medical Director
Wake Forest Baptist Health/Guilford County Emergency Services
Greensboro, North Carolina

Steven R. Ward, MMS/MHS, NRP, PA-C
Principal Faculty/Emergency Medicine PA
Mount St. Joseph University/University of Cincinnati Emergency Medicine
Cincinnati, Ohio

Contents

1 REVIEWING THE BASICS

2 LEADS, AXIS, AND ACQUISITION OF THE 12-LEAD ECG

3 ACUTE CORONARY SYNDROMES

4 ST-ELEVATION VARIANTS

5 PRACTICE ECGs

Reviewing the Basics

1

CHAPTER

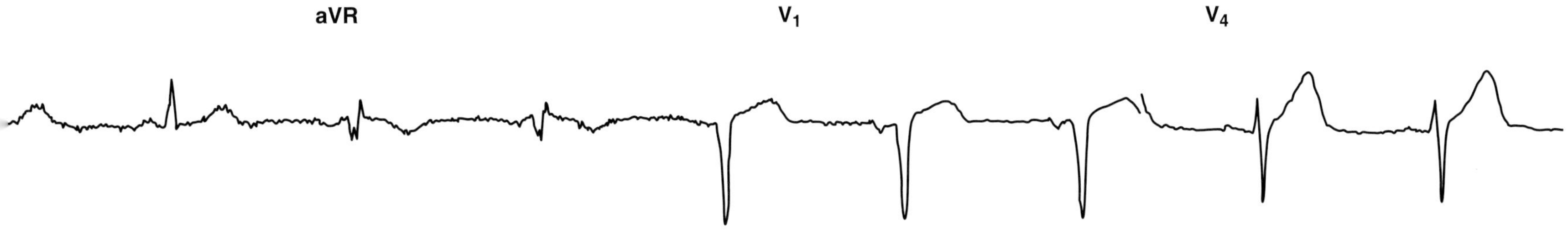

LEARNING OBJECTIVES

After reading this chapter, you should be able to:

1. Identify and describe the heart's layers, chambers, valves, and surfaces.
2. Describe the flow of blood through the normal heart and lungs to the systemic circulation.
3. Name the primary branches and areas of the heart supplied by the right and left coronary arteries.
4. Appreciate the variance in normal coronary artery distribution.
5. Describe the normal sequence of electrical conduction through the heart.
6. Define and describe each of the waveforms, segments, complexes, and intervals as they relate to electrical activity in the heart.

KEY TERMS

accessory pathway: An extra bundle of working myocardial tissue that forms a connection between the atria and ventricles outside the normal conduction system

acute coronary syndromes: Distinct conditions caused by a similar sequence of pathologic events involving abruptly reduced coronary artery blood flow

automaticity: Ability of cardiac pacemaker cells to spontaneously initiate an electrical impulse without being stimulated from another source (such as a nerve)

baseline: Straight line recorded on electrocardiographic graph paper when no electrical activity is detected

biphasic: Waveform that is partly positive and partly negative
complex: Several waveforms
depolarization: Movement of ions across a cell membrane, causing the inside of the cell to become more positive; an electrical event expected to result in contraction
interval: A waveform and a segment.
ischemia: Decreased supply of oxygenated blood to a body part or organ
isoelectric line: Absence of electrical activity; observed on the electrocardiogram as a straight line
membrane potential: Difference in electrical charge across the cell membrane
repolarization: Movement of ions across a cell membrane in which the inside of the cell is restored to its negative charge
segment: Line between waveforms; named by the waveform that precedes and follows it

STRUCTURE OF THE HEART

The human heart is a hollow muscular organ that is about the size of the individual's fist. It lies between the lungs in the mediastinum. The heart is protected anteriorly by the sternum and ribs and posteriorly by the ribs and vertebral column. About two-thirds of the heart lies to the left of the midline of the sternum.

The walls of the heart are made up of three tissue layers: the endocardium, myocardium, and epicardium. The heart's layers are summarized in Table 1.1.

TABLE 1.1 Layers of the Heart Wall

Heart Layer	Location	Description
Endocardium	Innermost layer	Thin layer that lines the heart's inner chambers, valves, chordae tendineae, and papillary muscles; continuous with the innermost layer of the body's arteries, veins, and capillaries
Myocardium	Middle layer	Thick, muscular layer consisting of cardiac muscle cells that contract and relax; the *subendocardial area* is the innermost half of the myocardium and the outermost half is the *subepicardial area*
Epicardium (visceral pericardium)	Outermost layer	Thin layer that contains blood capillaries, lymph capillaries, nerve fibers, and fat; this layer is enveloped by the pericardial sac, which anchors the heart within the chest

Heart Chambers

The heart is divided into four chambers. The two upper chambers are the right and left atria, and the two lower chambers are the right and left ventricles (Fig. 1.1).

The atria are thin-walled chambers that store blood during ventricular contraction (systole) and then fill the ventricles with blood during ventricular relaxation (diastole) (Lohr & Benjamin, 2016). The left atrium receives freshly oxygenated blood from the lungs via the right and left pulmonary veins. Blood is pumped from the atria through an atrioventricular (AV) valve (tricuspid or mitral) and into the ventricles. The heart's two lower chambers, the right and left ventricles, are responsible for pumping blood.

The right and left sides of the heart are separated by a *septum*, which is an internal wall of connective tissue. The *interatrial septum* separates the right and left atria. The *interventricular septum* separates the right and left ventricles (Fig. 1.2). The septa separate the heart into two functional pumps. The right atrium and right ventricle make up one pump. The left atrium and left ventricle make up the other.

The right side of the heart is a low-pressure system (i.e., the pulmonary circuit). The right atrium receives blood from the superior vena cava, the inferior vena cava, and the coronary sinus. The superior vena cava returns blood to the heart from the head, neck, and arms. The inferior vena cava returns blood to the heart from the thorax, abdomen, pelvis, and legs. The coronary sinus drains the blood from most of the vessels that supply the walls of the heart with blood. Blood entering the right ventricle flows through the tricuspid valve to the right ventricle. The right ventricle pumps the blood through the pulmonic semilunar valve to the pulmonary trunk, which divides into right and left pulmonary arteries. The pulmonary arteries enter the right and left lungs, where the exchange of oxygen and carbon dioxide occurs. Oxygenated blood is returned to the left atrium of the heart through four pulmonary veins, two from each lung.

The left ventricle is larger and its walls are nearly twice as thick as the right ventricle (Netter, 2014). This is because the left side of the heart is a high-pressure pump (i.e., the systemic circuit) and the left ventricle must overcome a lot of pressure and resistance

Consider This

Each ventricle holds about 150 mL of blood when it is full. They normally eject about half this volume (70–80 mL) with each contraction. Stroke volume is the amount of blood ejected from a ventricle with each heartbeat. The ejection fraction is the percentage of blood pumped out of a ventricle with each contraction. Ejection fraction is used as a measure of ventricular function. A normal ejection fraction is between 50% and 65%. A person is said to have impaired ventricular function when the ejection fraction is less than 40%. Examples of patients who may have a poor ejection fraction include those with heart failure, severe cardiomyopathy, or myocardial damage from a previous heart attack.

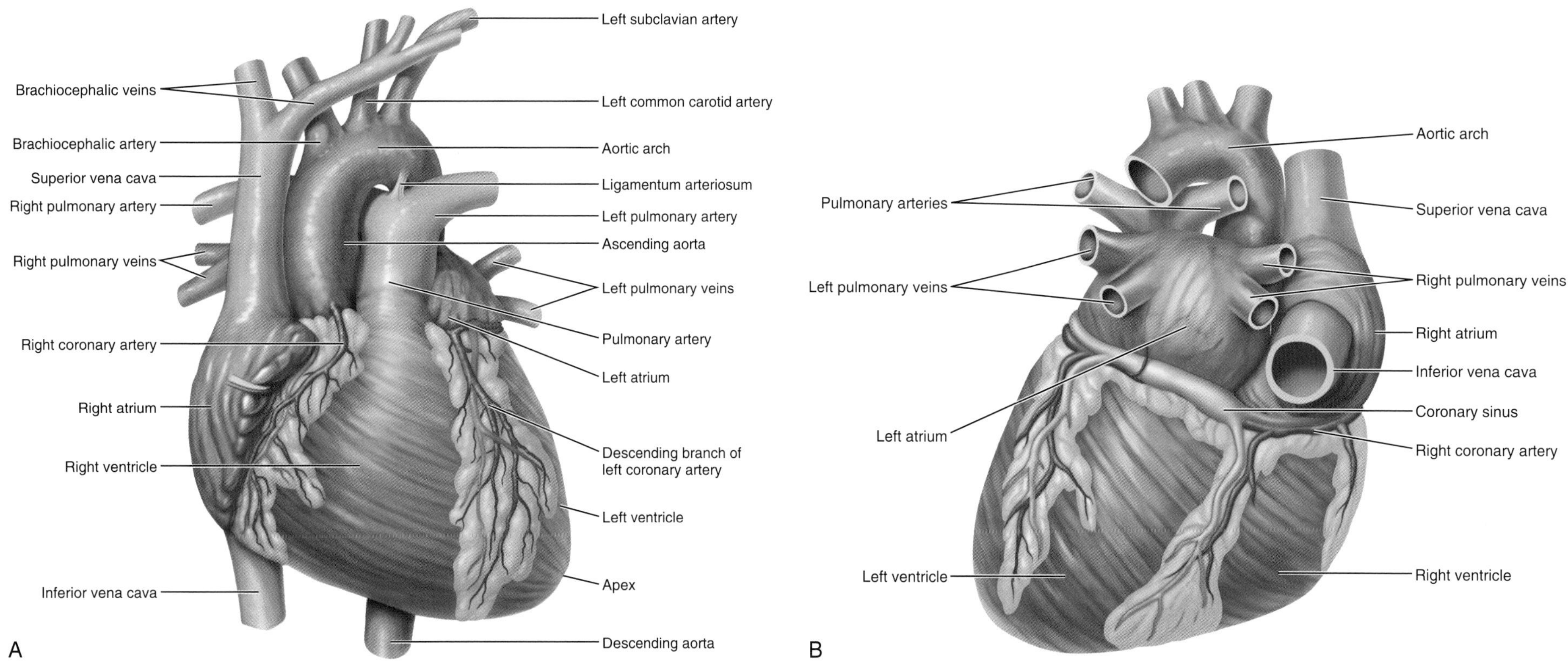

Fig. **1.1** The heart. **A,** Anterior view. **B,** Posterior view. (From Solomon, E. P. [2016]. *Introduction to human anatomy and physiology* [4th ed.]. Maryland Heights, MO: Saunders.)

from the arteries and contract forcefully to pump blood out to the body. Blood entering the left atrium flows through the mitral valve to the left ventricle. When the left ventricle contracts, blood is pumped through the aortic semilunar valve into the ascending aorta, the coronary arteries, the aortic arch, and the descending aorta. Branches of the aorta transport blood from the heart to the tissues and organs of the body.

Heart Valves

The four valves in the heart are responsible for ensuring the forward flow of blood through the heart's chambers. There are two types of cardiac valves: atrioventricular (AV) valves and semilunar (SL) valves (Fig. 1.3).

The AV valves separate the atria from the ventricles. The tricuspid valve is the AV valve that lies between the right atrium and right ventricle. It consists of three separate cusps or flaps. The mitral (or bicuspid) valve has only two cusps. It lies between the left atrium and left ventricle. Chordae tendineae, which are thin strands of connective tissue, are attached to the underside of the AV valves on one end. On the other end, they are attached to papillary muscles, which are small mounds of myocardium. Papillary muscles project inward from the lower portion of the ventricular walls. The chordae tendineae and papillary muscles serve as anchors. When the ventricles contract and relax, the papillary muscles adjust their tension on the chordae tendineae, preventing them from bulging too far into the atria.

The pulmonic and aortic valves are SL valves**.** These valves prevent backflow of blood from the aorta and pulmonary arteries into the left and right ventricles, respectively. The SL valves have three cusps shaped like half moons, hence the name "semilunar." Unlike the AV valves, the SL valves are not attached to chordae tendineae. Blood flow through the normal heart and pulmonary circulation is summarized in Box 1.1.

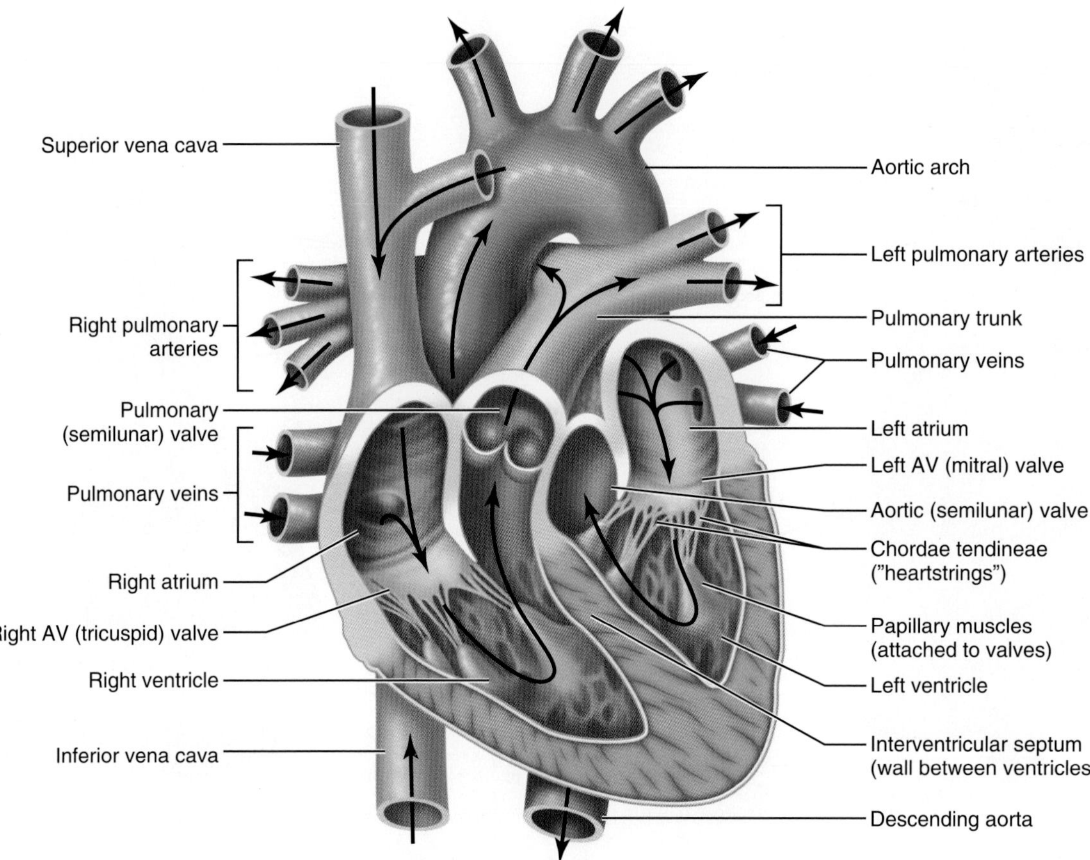

Fig. **1.2** Internal view of the heart showing chambers, valves, and connecting blood vessels. Arrows indicate the direction of blood flow. *AV,* Atrioventricular. (From Solomon, E. P. [2016]. *Introduction to human anatomy and physiology* [4th ed.]. Maryland Heights, MO: Saunders.)

Consider This

Valvular heart disease is the term used to describe a malfunctioning heart valve. Types of valvular heart disease include the following:

- *Valvular stenosis*. If a valve narrows, stiffens, or thickens, the valve is said to be stenosed. The heart must work harder to pump blood through a stenosed valve.
- *Valvular prolapse*. If a valve flap inverts, it is said to prolapse. Prolapse can occur if one valve flap is larger than the other. It can also occur if the chordae tendineae stretch markedly or rupture.
- *Valvular regurgitation*. Blood can flow backward, or regurgitate, if one or more of the heart's valves doesn't close properly. Valvular regurgitation is also known as valvular incompetence or valvular insufficiency.

Heart Surfaces

The anterior surface of the heart is formed by portions of the right atrium and the left and right ventricles. However, because the heart is tilted slightly toward the left in the chest, the right ventricle is the area of the heart that lies most directly behind the sternum. The heart's left side (i.e., left lateral surface) is made up mostly of the left ventricle. The heart's inferior surface, also called the *diaphragmatic surface*, is formed primarily by the left ventricle with a small portion of the right ventricle.

Coronary Arteries

The work of the heart is important. To ensure that it has an adequate blood supply, the heart makes sure to provide itself with a fresh supply of oxygenated blood before supplying the rest of the body. This freshly oxygenated blood is supplied mainly by the

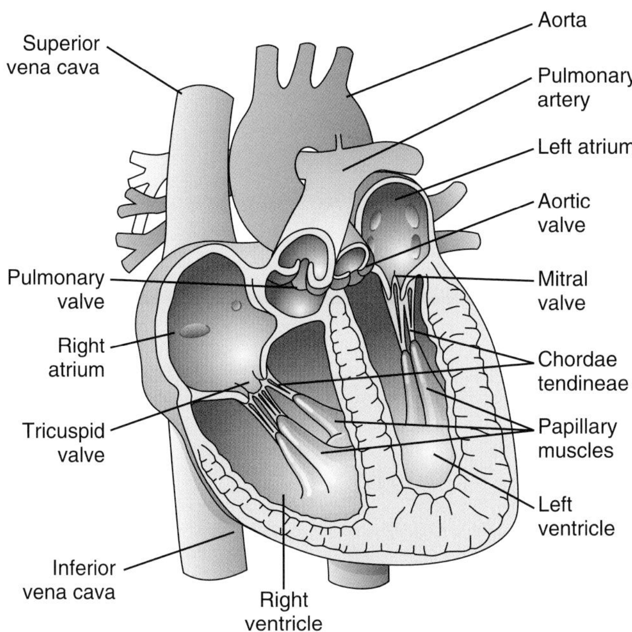

Fig. **1.3** Chambers and valves of the heart. Chordae tendineae and papillary muscles attach the leaflets of the atrioventricular valves to the ventricular myocardium. (From Copstead-Kirkhorn, L., & Banasik, J. L. [2013]. *Pathophysiology* [5th ed.]. Philadelphia, PA: Elsevier.)

Box 1.1 Blood Flow Through the Normal Heart and Pulmonary Circulation

Blood from the superior and inferior vena cavae and the coronary sinus enters the right atrium → tricuspid valve → right ventricle → pulmonic semilunar valve → pulmonary trunk → right and left pulmonary arteries → pulmonary capillaries (within the lungs) → four pulmonary veins → left atrium → mitral valve → left ventricle → aortic semilunar valve → ascending aorta

branches of two vessels—the right and left coronary arteries. The openings to these vessels lie just beyond the cusps of the aortic SL valve.

The right and left coronary arteries are found on the epicardial surface of the heart and feed this area first before their branches penetrate the myocardium to supply the subendocardium with blood (Fig. 1.4). The diameter of these "feeder branches" (i.e., collateral circulation) is much narrower.

When a temporary or permanent blockage occurs in a coronary artery, the blood supply to the heart muscle is impaired, and myocardial cells distal to the site of the blockage are starved for oxygen and other nutrients. Acute coronary syndrome (ACS) is a term that refers to distinct conditions caused by a similar sequence of pathologic events involving

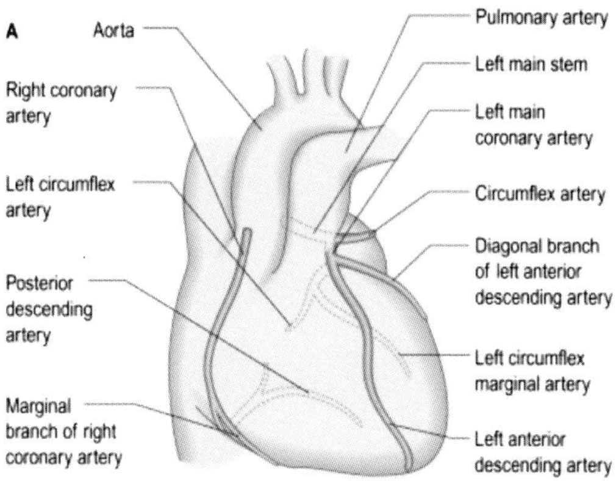

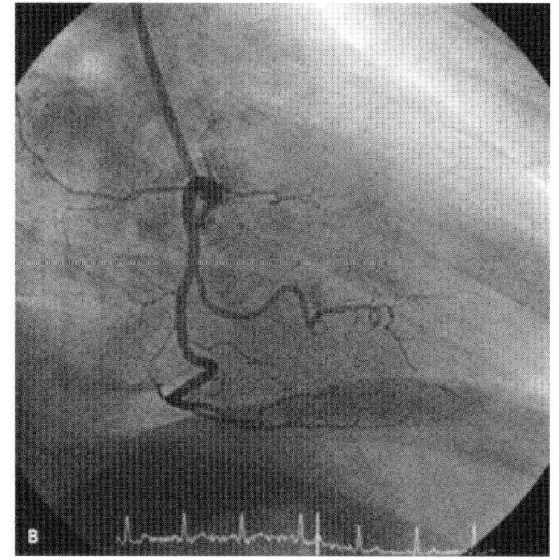

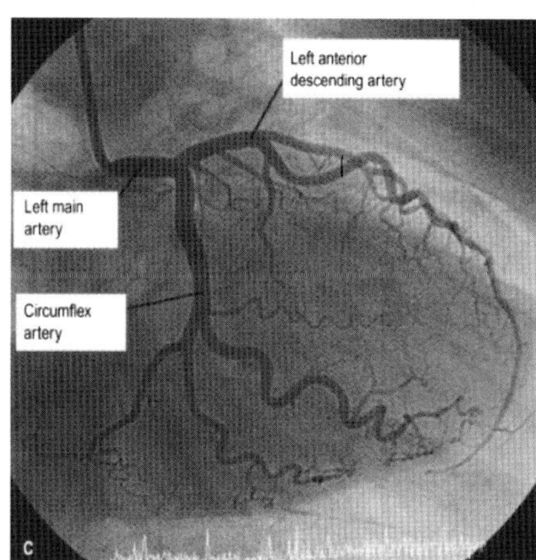

Fig. **1.4** The coronary circulation. **A,** The normal coronary arterial anatomy. **B,** Angiogram of the dominant right coronary system. **C,** Angiogram of the left coronary system from the same patient (right anterior oblique projection). (From Kumar, P., & Clark, M. [2017]. *Kumar and Clark's clinical medicine* [9th ed.]. The Netherlands: Elsevier.)

abruptly reduced coronary artery blood flow (Amsterdam et al., 2014). This sequence of events results in conditions that range from myocardial ischemia (i.e., a decreased supply of oxygenated blood to a body part or organ) to death (i.e., necrosis) of the heart muscle. An understanding of coronary artery anatomy and the areas of the heart that each vessel supplies can help you predict which coronary artery is blocked and anticipate problems associated with blockage of that vessel.

Right Coronary Artery

The right coronary artery (RCA) originates from the right side of the aorta and travels along the groove between the right atrium and right ventricle. Branches of the RCA supply blood to the right atrium, right ventricle, and the inferior and posterior walls of the left ventricle in most individuals.

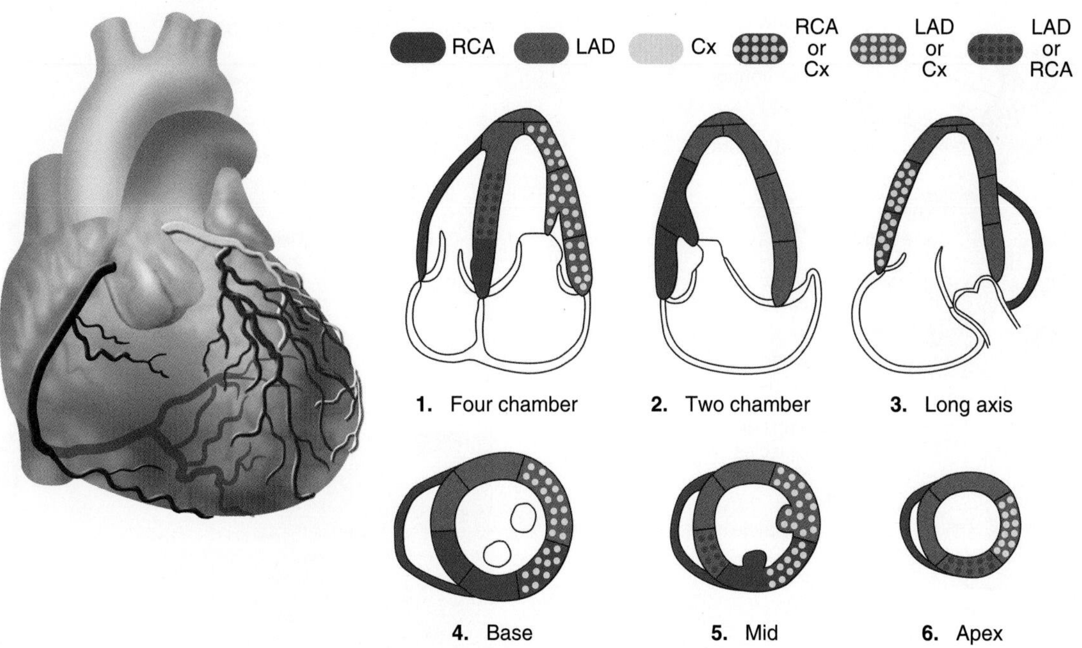

Fig. 1.5 Typical myocardial segments supplied by the right coronary artery (RCA), left anterior descending artery (LAD), and circumflex (Cx) coronary arteries. The coronary anatomy is shown on the left with the corresponding wall segments in standard echocardiographic views on the right. The arterial distribution varies between patients. Some segments have variable coronary perfusion as indicated by the hatched regions. (From Lang, R. M., Bierig, M., Devereux, R. B., Flachskampf, F. A., Foster, E., . . . Chamber Quantification Writing Group; American Society of Echocardiography's Guidelines and Standards Committee; European Association of Echocardiography [2005]. Recommendations for chamber quantification: A report from the American Society of Echocardiography's Guidelines and Standards Committee and the Chamber Quantification Writing Group, developed in conjunction with the European Association of Echocardiography, a branch of the European Society of Cardiology. *Journal of the American Society of Echocardiography, 18* (12), 1440–1463.)

Left Coronary Artery

The left coronary artery (LCA) originates from the left side of the aorta. The first segment of the LCA is the left main coronary artery, also called the *left main trunk*. It supplies oxygenated blood to its two primary branches: the left anterior descending (LAD), also called the *anterior interventricular* artery, and the circumflex artery (Cx). These vessels are slightly smaller than the left main coronary artery.

In most people, the LAD travels along the groove that lies between the right and left ventricles, courses along the heart's apex, and ends along the left ventricle's inferior surface. In the remaining individuals, the LAD doesn't reach the inferior surface. Instead, it stops at or before the heart's apex. The major branches of the LAD are the septal and diagonal arteries. The septal branches of the LAD supply blood to the interventricular septum. The diagonal branches supply the anterior and lateral walls of the left ventricle. The Cx circles around the left side of the heart and supplies blood to the left atrium and the posterior and lateral walls of the left ventricle.

Coronary Artery Dominance

The blood supply to the inferior and posterior areas of the left ventricle varies. In about 85% of people, the RCA forms the posterior descending artery, and in about 10% of people, the circumflex artery forms the posterior descending artery (Lohr & Benjamin, 2016). The coronary artery that forms the posterior descending artery is considered the *dominant* coronary artery. If a branch of the RCA becomes the posterior descending artery, the coronary artery arrangement is described as a *right-dominant system*. If the Cx branches and ends at the posterior descending artery, the coronary artery arrangement is described as a *left-dominant system*. In some people, neither coronary artery is dominant. If damage to the posterior wall of the left ventricle is suspected, a cardiac catheterization is usually necessary to determine which coronary artery is involved. The areas of the heart supplied by the major coronary arteries are shown in Fig. 1.5.

Coronary Veins

Blood that has passed through the myocardial capillaries is drained by branches of the cardiac veins that join the coronary sinus, which lies in the groove (sulcus) that separates the atria from the ventricles. The coronary sinus drains into the right atrium.

CARDIAC CYCLE

The cardiac cycle has two phases for each heart chamber: systole and diastole. Systole is the period during which the chamber is contracting and blood is being ejected. Diastole is the period of relaxation during which the chambers are allowed to fill. The myocardium receives its fresh supply of oxygenated blood from the coronary arteries during ventricular diastole. The cardiac cycle depends on the ability of the cardiac muscle to contract and on the condition of the heart's conduction system. The efficiency of the heart as a pump may be affected by abnormalities of the cardiac muscle, the valves, or the conduction system.

During the cardiac cycle, the pressure within each chamber of the heart rises in systole and falls in diastole. The heart's valves ensure that blood flows in the proper direction. Blood flows from one heart chamber to another from higher to lower pressure. These pressure relationships depend on the careful timing of contractions. The heart's conduction system provides the necessary timing of events between atrial and ventricular systole.

Atrial Systole and Diastole

During atrial diastole, blood from the superior and inferior vena cavae and the coronary sinus enters the right atrium. The right atrium fills and distends. This pushes the tricuspid valve open and the right ventricle fills. The left atrium receives blood from the four pulmonary veins (two from the right lung and two from the left lung). The flaps of the mitral valve open as the left atrium fills. This allows blood to flow into the left ventricle.

The ventricles are 70% filled before the atria contract. Contraction of the atria forces additional blood (about 10% to 30% of the ventricular capacity) into the ventricles. This is called the atrial kick. Thus the ventricles become completely filled with blood during atrial systole. The atria then enter a period of atrial diastole, which continues until the start of the next cardiac cycle.

Ventricular Systole and Diastole

Ventricular systole occurs as atrial diastole begins. As the ventricles contract, blood is propelled through the systemic and pulmonary circulation and toward the atria. The SL valves close and the heart then begins a period of ventricular diastole. During ventricular diastole, the ventricles begin to passively fill with blood, and both the atria and ventricles are relaxed. The cardiac cycle begins again with atrial systole and the completion of ventricular filling.

ELECTROPHYSIOLOGY REVIEW

Human body fluids contain electrolytes, which are elements or compounds that break into charged particles (i.e., ions) when melted or dissolved in water or another solvent. Differences in the composition of ions between the intracellular and extracellular fluid compartments are important for normal body function, including the activity of the heart. Body fluids that contain electrolytes conduct an electric current. Electrolytes move about in body fluids and carry a charge.

A slight difference in the concentrations of charged particles across the membranes of cells is normal; thus, potential energy (i.e., voltage) exists because of the imbalance of charged particles, and this imbalance makes the cells excitable. The voltage (i.e., the difference in electrical charges) across the cell membrane is the membrane potential. The energy expended by the cells to move electrolytes across the cell membrane creates a flow of current, which is expressed in volts. Voltage appears on an electrocardiogram (ECG) as spikes or waveforms.

Depolarization

When a cell is at rest (i.e., polarized), the inside of the cell is more negative than the outside. When a cell is stimulated, the cell membrane becomes permeable to Na^+ and K^+, allowing the passage of electrolytes after it is open. Na^+ rushes into the cell through Na^+ channels. This causes the inside of the cell to become more positive relative to the outside. The movement of charged particles across a cell membrane that causes the inside of the cell to become positive is called depolarization. A spike (i.e., a waveform) is then recorded on the ECG. Depolarization proceeds from the endocardium to the epicardium.

Consider This

Depolarization is an electrical event that must take place before the heart can contract and pump blood, which is a mechanical event.

An impulse normally begins in the pacemaker cells found in the sinoatrial (SA) node of the heart. A chain reaction occurs from cell to cell in the heart's electrical conduction system until all the cells have been stimulated and depolarized. Eventually, the impulse is spread from the pacemaker cells to the working myocardial cells, which contract when they are stimulated.

Consider This

The ability of cardiac pacemaker cells to create an electrical impulse without being stimulated from another source, such as a nerve, is called automaticity. Increased blood concentrations of calcium (Ca^{++}) increases automaticity. Decreased concentrations of potassium (K^+) in the blood decreases automaticity.

Repolarization

After the cell depolarizes, it quickly begins to recover and restore its electrical charges to normal. The movement of charged particles across a cell membrane in which the inside of the cell is restored to its negative charge is called repolarization. The cell membrane stops the flow of Na^+ into the cell and allows K^+ to leave it. Negatively charged particles are left inside the cell; thus, the cell is returned to its resting state. This causes contractile proteins in the working myocardial cells to separate (i.e., relax). Repolarization proceeds from the epicardium to the endocardium.

Consider This

When the atria are stimulated, a P wave is recorded on the ECG; thus, the P wave represents atrial depolarization. When the ventricles are stimulated, a QRS complex is recorded on the ECG; thus, the QRS complex represents ventricular depolarization. On the ECG, the ST segment and T wave represent ventricular repolarization. A waveform representing atrial repolarization is usually not seen on the ECG because it is small and buried in the QRS complex.

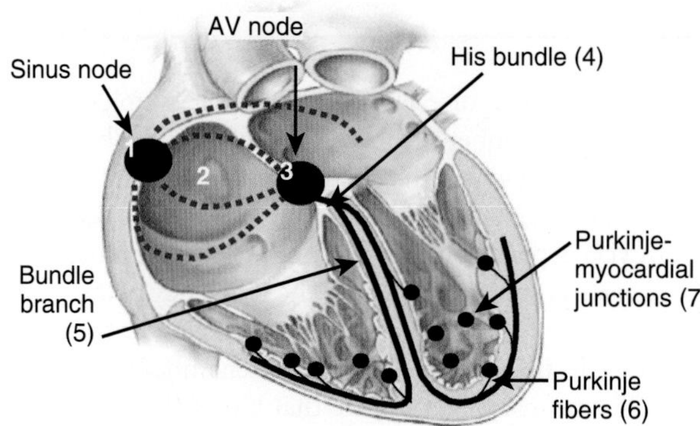

Fig. **1.6** The cardiac action potential originates in the sinoatrial (SA) node (1), continues in the atrial wall (2), and is delayed in the atrioventricular (AV) node (3). Conduction within the ventricles is initially rapid within the rapid conduction system: His bundle (4), right and left bundle branches (5), and Purkinje fibers (6). The impulse is transferred from the rapid conduction system to the working myocardium in the Purkinje-myocardial junctions (7), which are located in the endocardium. Within the slowly conducting working myocardium, the impulse is conducted from endocardium to epicardium. (From Ellenbogen, K. A., Wilkoff, B. L., Kay, G. N., Lau, C. P., & Auricchio, A. [2017]. *Clinical cardiac pacing, defibrillation and resynchronization therapy* [5th ed.]. Philadelphia, PA: Elsevier.)

The Cardiac Action Potential

The action potential of a cardiac cell reflects the rapid sequence of voltage changes that occur across the cell membrane during the electrical cardiac cycle. The configuration of the action potential varies depending on the location, size, and function of the cardiac cell.

CONDUCTION SYSTEM

The heart's conduction system is a collection of specialized pacemaker cells that are arranged in a system of interconnected pathways (Fig. 1.6). The normal heartbeat is the result of an electrical impulse that begins in the SA node, which is specialized conducting tissue located in the upper posterior part of the right atrium where the superior vena cava and the right atrium meet. The SA node is supplied by a branch of the RCA in about 60% of the population and a branch of the Cx in about 40% (Lohr & Benjamin, 2016).

As the impulse leaves the SA node, a chain reaction occurs from cell to cell in the heart's electrical conduction system until all the cells have been stimulated and depolarized (i.e., the inside of the cell becomes more positive). This chain reaction is a *wave of depolarization.* As the impulse that began in the SA node spreads, it stimulates the right atrium and the interatrial septum, and it travels along a special pathway called *Bachmann's bundle* to stimulate the left atrium. This results in contraction of the right and left atria at almost the same time.

The electrical impulse is conducted from the atria to the AV node, which is a group of specialized conducting cells located in the floor of the right atrium immediately behind the tricuspid valve. As the impulse enters the AV node through internodal pathways, conduction is markedly slowed. This delay in conduction allows both atrial chambers to contract and empty blood into the ventricles before the next ventricular contraction begins. The bundle of His, also called the *common bundle* or the *AV bundle*, is a continuation of the AV node and connects the AV node with the bundle branches. The AV node and the bundle of His are called the *AV junction.* Some people have two or more conduction pathways in the area of the AV node that conduct impulses at different speeds and recover at different rates (Zimetbaum, 2016). The pathways join into a final common pathway before impulses exiting the AV node continue to the bundle of His.

Normally, the atria and ventricles are separated by a continuous barrier of fibrous tissue, which acts as an insulator to prevent passage of an electrical impulse through any route other than the AV node and bundle. When the AV node and bundle are bypassed by an abnormal pathway, the abnormal route is called an accessory pathway.

The bundle of His divides into the right and left bundle branches. The right bundle branch innervates the right ventricle. The left bundle branch divides into *fascicles*, which are small bundles of nerve fibers that allow electrical innervation of the larger, more muscular left ventricle.

The right and left bundle branches divide into smaller and smaller branches and then into a special network of fibers called the *Purkinje fibers*. The Purkinje fibers have pacemaker cells that have an intrinsic rate of 20 to 40 beats/min. The electrical impulse spreads rapidly through the right and left bundle branches and the Purkinje fibers to

TABLE 1.2 Summary of the Conduction System

Structure	Function
SA node	• Primary pacemaker; intrinsic pacemaker rate: 60 to 100 beats/min • Initiates impulse that is normally conducted throughout the left and right atria • Supplied by a branch of the RCA in about 60% of individuals
AV node	• Receives impulse from SA node and delays relay of the impulse to the bundle of His, allowing time for ventricular filling before the onset of ventricular contraction
Bundle of His (AV bundle)	• Receives impulse from AV node and relays it to right and left bundle branches • The AV node and the bundle of His make up the *AV junction*, which has an intrinsic pacemaker rate of 40 to 60 beats/min • Supplied by a branch of the RCA in 85% to 90% of individuals
Right and left bundle branches	• Receives impulse from bundle of His and relays it to Purkinje fibers
Purkinje fibers	• Receives impulse from bundle branches and relays it to ventricular myocardium • Intrinsic pacemaker rate: 20 to 40 beats/min

AV, Atrioventricular; *SA*, sinoatrial.

reach the ventricular muscle. The electrical impulse spreads from the endocardium to the myocardium, finally reaching the epicardial surface. The ventricular walls are stimulated to contract in a twisting motion that wrings blood out of the ventricular chambers and forces it into arteries. The term *His-Purkinje system*, or *His-Purkinje network*, refers to the bundle of His, bundle branches, and Purkinje fibers. The conduction system is summarized in Table 1.2.

Ectopic Pacemakers

Areas of the heart other than the SA node can initiate beats (i.e., intrinsic automaticity) and assume pacemaker responsibility under special circumstances. The terms *ectopic*, which means "out of place," and *latent* are used to describe an impulse that originates from a source other than the SA node. Ectopic pacemaker sites include the cells of the AV junction and Purkinje fibers, although their intrinsic rates are slower than that of the SA node. An ectopic pacemaker is normally prevented from discharging because of the dominance of the SA node's rapidly firing pacemaker cells.

Although ectopic pacemakers supply a backup or safety mechanism in the event of SA node failure, such sites can be problematic if they fire while the SA node is still functioning. For example, ectopic sites may cause early (i.e., premature) beats or sustained rhythm disturbances.

WAVEFORMS, COMPLEXES, SEGMENTS, AND INTERVALS

ECG paper is used to record the speed and magnitude of the heart's electrical impulses. This graph paper consists of small and large boxes measured in millimeters. The smallest boxes are 1 mm wide and 1 mm high (Fig. 1.7). Each large box, which is the width of five small boxes, represents 0.20 second. The horizontal axis of the paper corresponds to time. Time is used to measure the interval between or duration of specific cardiac events, which is stated in seconds.

Consider This

When reviewing a 12-lead ECG, intervals and duration are usually expressed in milliseconds. There are 1000 milliseconds (msec) in 1 second. Move the decimal point three places to the right when converting from seconds to milliseconds.

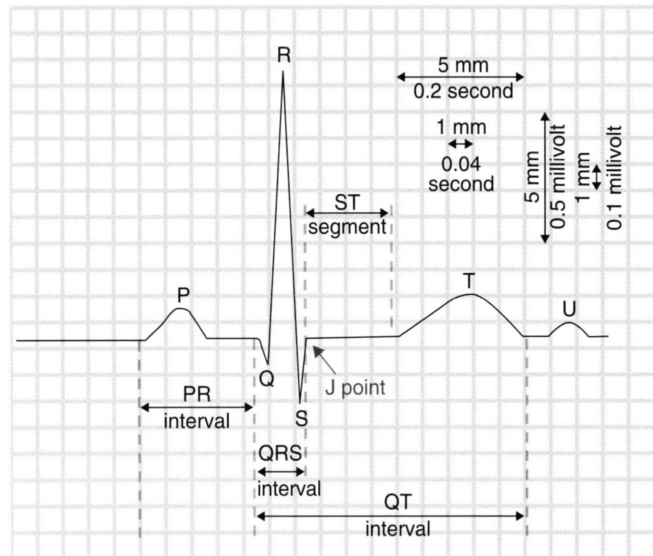

Fig. 1.7 Inscription of a normal electrocardiogram (ECG). Sinoatrial nodal depolarization is not visible on the surface ECG; the P wave corresponds to atrial muscle depolarization. The PR interval denotes conduction through the atrial muscle, atrioventricular node, and His-Purkinje system. The QRS complex reflects ventricular muscle depolarization. The ST segment and T wave (and U wave, if present) represent ventricular repolarization. The J point lies at the junction of the end of the QRS complex and beginning of the ST segment. The QT interval is measured from the onset of the QRS to the end of the T wave. Note the gridlines. On the horizontal axis, each 1-mm line ("small" box) denotes 0.04 second (40 msec); a "big" box denotes 0.20 second (200 msec). On the vertical axis, 1 mm (small box) corresponds to 0.1 mV; 10 mm (two big boxes) therefore denotes 1 mV. (From Goldman, L., & Schafer, A. I. [2016]. *Goldman's Cecil medicine* [25th ed.]. Philadelphia, PA: Saunders.)

The rate at which ECG paper goes through the printer is adjustable and is designated on the 12-lead ECG printout. Standard paper speed is 25 mm/sec. At this speed, each 1-mm box represents 0.04 second (40 msec) and each 5-mm gridline, a large box, represents 0.20 second (200 msec). The rate at which ECG paper goes through the printer is adjustable. A faster paper speed makes the rhythm appear slower and the QRS complex wider. Thus in cases of rapid heart rates, a faster paper speed makes it easier to see the waveforms and analyze the rhythm. A slower paper speed makes the rhythm appear faster and the QRS narrower.

The vertical axis of the graph paper represents the voltage or amplitude of the ECG waveforms or deflections. Voltage is measured in millivolts (mV). Voltage may appear as a positive or negative value because voltage is a force with direction as well as amplitude. Amplitude is measured in millimeters. The cardiac monitor's sensitivity to electrical current is variable. The button or control that adjusts the monitor's sensitivity can be labeled with a variety of names, some of which are ECG *size*, *sensitivity*, *gain*, and *calibration*. When the sensitivity is increased, a larger complex is produced. Likewise, a smaller complex is the result of decreased sensitivity. The default value for ECG machine calibration is 10 mm/mV. This means that when the ECG machine is properly calibrated, a 1-mV electrical signal produces a deflection that measures exactly 10 mm tall (i.e., the height of 10 small boxes). When a calibration marker is present, it appears at the extreme left side of the ECG tracing, before the first waveform. Clinically, the height of a waveform is usually stated in millimeters rather than in millivolts. The significance of standard calibration is moot when the monitor is used only to determine rate and rhythm. However, proper calibration is critical when analyzing ST segments.

Consider This

Certain instances may warrant the use of a nonstandard calibration. If the ECG waveforms are too large to fit the page, the calibration should be reduced. Likewise, if the waveforms are too small to read, then the calibration should be increased. When changes in calibration are necessary, choose a calibration that will make interpretation easier. Therefore, if an increase in QRS size is needed, double the calibration. Likewise, if a reduction in ECG size in necessary, halve the calibration. Always include a calibration pulse and note the change in calibration on the ECG printout.

A waveform (i.e., a deflection) is movement away from the baseline in a positive (i.e., upward) or negative (i.e., downward) direction. Each waveform that you see on an ECG is related to a specific electrical event in the heart. Waveforms are named alphabetically, beginning with P, QRS, T, and occasionally U. When electrical activity is not detected, a straight line is recorded. This line is called the baseline or isoelectric line. If the wave of depolarization (i.e., the electrical impulse) moves toward the positive electrode, the waveform recorded on ECG graph paper will be upright (i.e., a positive deflection). If the wave of depolarization moves away from the positive electrode, the waveform recorded will be inverted (i.e., a downward or negative deflection). A biphasic (i.e., partly positive, partly negative) waveform or a straight line is recorded when the wave of depolarization moves perpendicularly to the positive electrode. The term *equiphasic* may be used instead of *biphasic* to describe a waveform that has no net positive or negative deflection.

A complex consists of several waveforms. A segment is a line between waveforms. It is named by the waveform that precedes or follows it. An interval is made up of a waveform and a segment. Normal waveforms, segments, and intervals are summarized in Tables 1.3 and 1.4.

TABLE 1.3 Waveforms and Complexes

ECG Component	Physiology
P wave	• Atrial depolarization • Normally 0.12 second (120 msec) or less
QRS complex	• Ventricular depolarization • Q wave is the first negative deflection, R wave is the first positive deflection, S wave is the first negative deflection after an R wave • With the exception of leads III and aVR, a normal Q wave in the limb leads is less than 0.03 second (30 msec) in duration. A pathologic Q wave is more than 0.03 second (30 msec) in duration or more than 30% of the height of the following R wave in that lead, or both (Anderson, 2016). • Normally 0.075 to 0.11 second (75 to 110 msec)
T wave	• Ventricular repolarization • Normally slightly asymmetric

ECG, Electrocardiogram.

TABLE 1.4 Segments and Intervals

ECG Component	Physiology
PR interval	• Conduction through atrial tissue, the AV junction, and the His-Purkinje system • 0.12 to 0.20 second (120 to 200 msec)
ST segment	• Early ventricular repolarization • Normally isoelectric (i.e., flat) • Displacement (e.g., elevation, depression) is measured at the J point, which is the point where the QRS complex and ST segment meet

TABLE 1.4 Segments and Intervals—cont'd

ECG Component	Physiology
TP segment	• Represents the period of no electrical activity between the end of a PQRST cycle and the onset of the next • Normally isoelectric • Used as the reference point from which to estimate the position of the isoelectric line and determine ST-segment displacement • Often unrecognizable with rapid heart rates
QT interval	• Onset of ventricular depolarization and end of ventricular repolarization • Varies with age, gender, and heart rate • Considered short if it is 0.39 second (390 msec) or less; considered prolonged if it is 0.46 second (460 msec) or longer in women or 0.45 second (450 msec) or longer in men (Rautaharju, Surawicz, & Gettes, 2009)

AV, Atrioventricular; *ECG*, electrocardiogram.

ASSESSING REGULARITY

The R-R (R wave-to-R wave) and P-P (P wave-to-P wave) intervals are used to determine the rate and regularity of a cardiac rhythm. To evaluate the regularity of the ventricular rhythm on a rhythm strip, the interval between two consecutive R waves is measured. The distance between succeeding R-R intervals is measured and compared. If the ventricular rhythm is regular, the R-R intervals will measure the same. To evaluate the regularity of the atrial rhythm, the same procedure is used but the interval between two consecutive P waves is measured and compared with succeeding P-P intervals.

DETERMINING RATE

Calculating the heart rate is important because deviations from normal can affect the patient's ability to maintain an adequate blood pressure and cardiac output. A 12-lead ECG machine is usually very accurate in calculating heart rate. This value, in addition to intervals and durations, is documented on the 12-lead ECG printout.

Several methods can be used to calculate heart rate. To use the 6-second method, count the number of complete QRS complexes within a period of 6 seconds and multiply that number by 10 to find the number of complexes in 1 minute. To use the large box method of rate determination, also called the *rule of 300*, count the number of large boxes between an R-R interval and divide into 300. To use the small box method of rate determination, also called *the rule of 1500*, count the number of small boxes between the R-R interval and divide into 1500.

REFERENCES

Amsterdam, E. A., Wenger, N. K., Brindis, R. G., Casey Jr, D. E., Ganiats, T. G. Holmes Jr, D. R., et al. (2014). 2014 AHA/ACC guideline for the management of patients with non-ST-elevation acute coronary syndromes. *Journal of the American College of Cardiology, 64* (24), 1–150.

Anderson, J. L. (2016). ST segment elevation acute myocardial infarction and complications of myocardial infarction. In L. Goldman & A. I. Schafer (Eds.), *Goldman-Cecil medicine* (25th ed., pp. 441–456). Philadelphia, PA: Saunders.

Lohr, N. L., & Benjamin, I. J. (2016). Structure and function of the normal heart and blood vessels. In I. J. Benjamin, R. C. Griggs, E. J. Wing, & J. G. Fitz (Eds.), *Andreoli and Carpenter's Cecil essentials of medicine* (9th ed., pp. 16–21). Philadelphia, PA: Saunders.

Netter, F. H. (2014). Thorax study guide. In *Atlas of Human Anatomy* (6 ed., pp. e49–61). Philadelphia, PA: Saunders.

Rautaharju, P. M., Surawicz, B., & Gettes, L. S. (2009). AHA/ACCF/HRS Recommendations for the standardization and interpretation of the electrocardiogram. Part IV: The ST segment, T and U waves, and the QT interval: A scientific statement from the American Heart Association Electrocardiography and Arrhythmias. *Journal of the American College of Cardiology, 53* (11), 982–991.

Zimetbaum, P. (2016). Cardiac arrhythmias with supraventricular origin. In L. Goldman & A. I. Schafer (Eds.), *Goldman's Cecil medicine.* (25th ed., pp. 356–366). Philadelphia, PA: Saunders.

QUICK REVIEW

1. The heart is divided into _____ chambers but functions as a _____-sided pump.
   a. two; four
   b. three; two
   c. four; two
   d. four; three

2. The myocardium is thickest in the
   a. right atrium.
   b. right ventricle.
   c. left atrium.
   d. left ventricle.

3. The tricuspid valve lies between the
   a. right atrium and right ventricle.
   b. left atrium and left ventricle.
   c. right ventricle and pulmonary artery.
   d. left ventricle and aorta.

4. In most individuals, the SA node and AV bundle are supplied by a branch of the _____ coronary artery.
   a. right
   b. left main
   c. circumflex
   d. left anterior descending

5. In the heart's conduction system, the _____ receive(s) an electrical impulse from the bundle of His and relay(s) it to the Purkinje fibers in the ventricular myocardium.
   a. AV node
   b. AV junction
   c. SA node
   d. right and left bundle branches

6. The portion of the ECG tracing between the QRS complex and the T wave is called the
   a. PR segment.
   b. ST segment.
   c. TP segment.
   d. QT interval.

7. On the ECG, the P wave represents atrial _____, and the QRS complex represents ventricular _____.
   a. depolarization; depolarization
   b. repolarization; repolarization
   c. repolarization; depolarization
   d. depolarization; repolarization

8. Which of the following correctly reflects examples of ectopic (i.e., latent) pacemakers?
   a. The SA node and AV junction
   b. The SA node and Purkinje fibers
   c. The AV junction and Purkinje fibers
   d. The AV junction and left bundle branch

ANSWERS

1. **C**. The heart has four chambers—two atria and two ventricles. The right and left sides of the heart are separated by an internal wall of connective tissue called a septum. The interatrial septum separates the right and left atria. The interventricular septum separates the right and left ventricles. The septa separate the heart into two functional pumps. The right atrium and right ventricle make up one pump. The left atrium and left ventricle make up the other.

2. **D**. The thickness of the myocardium varies from one heart chamber to another. This variation in thickness is related to the amount of resistance that must be overcome to pump blood out of the different chambers. For example, the atria encounter little resistance when pumping blood to the ventricles. As a result, the atria have a thin myocardial layer. On the other hand, the ventricles must pump blood to either the lungs (the right ventricle) or the rest of the body (the left ventricle). So the ventricles have a much thicker myocardial layer than the atria. The wall of the left ventricle is thicker than that of the right because the left ventricle propels blood to most vessels of the body. The right ventricle moves blood only through the blood vessels of the lungs and then into the left atrium.

3. **A**. The tricuspid valve is the atrioventricular valve that lies between the right atrium and right ventricle. It consists of three separate cusps or flaps.

4. **A**. The SA node receives its blood supply from the SA node artery that runs lengthwise through the center of the node. The SA node artery originates from the right coronary artery in about 60% of people. The AV bundle is supplied by the right coronary artery in 85% to 90% of the population. In the remainder, the circumflex artery provides the blood supply.

5. **D**. The right bundle branch innervates the right ventricle. The left bundle branch spreads the electrical impulse to the interventricular septum and left ventricle.

6. **B**. The ST segment is the portion of the ECG tracing between the QRS complex and the T wave.

7. **A**. On the ECG, the P wave represents atrial depolarization, and the QRS complex represents ventricular depolarization.

8. **C**. Ectopic pacemaker sites include the cells of the AV junction and Purkinje fibers, although their intrinsic rates are slower than that of the SA node. Although an ectopic pacemaker is normally prevented from discharging because of the dominance of the SA node's rapidly firing pacemaker cells, an ectopic site may assume pacemaker responsibility in the following circumstances: (1) the SA node fires too slowly because of vagal stimulation or suppression by medications; (2) the SA node fails to generate an impulse because of disease or suppression by medications; (3) the SA node action potential is blocked because of disease in conducting pathways, failing to activate the surrounding atrial myocardium; or (4) the firing rate of the ectopic site becomes faster than that of the SA node.

Leads, Axis, and Acquisition of the 12-Lead ECG

2

CHAPTER

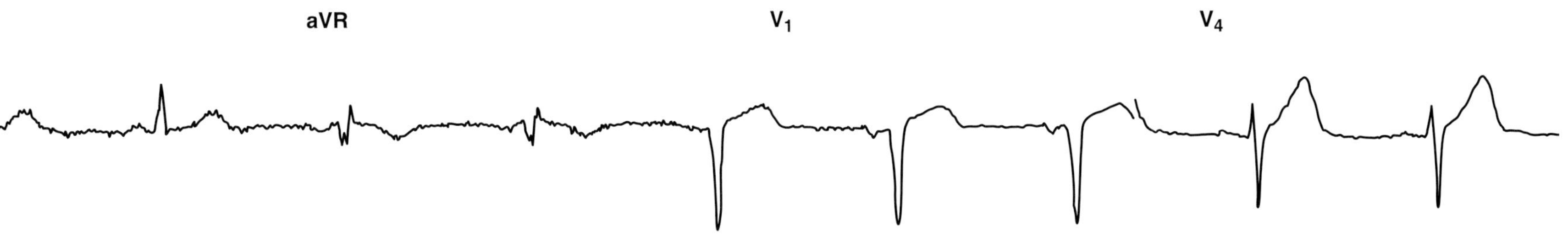

LEARNING OBJECTIVES

After reading this chapter, you should be able to:

1. Give examples of indications for using a 12-lead electrocardiogram (ECG).
2. Describe correct anatomic placement of the standard limb leads, the augmented leads, and the chest leads.
3. Discuss the determination of electrical axis using leads I and aVF.
4. Relate the cardiac surfaces or areas represented by the ECG leads.
5. Develop a reliable approach to quickly acquire a clear and accurate 12-lead ECG.
6. Explain the methods used to minimize the occurrence of artifact.
7. Recognize the importance of accurate lead placement before obtaining the ECG.
8. Understand the significance of frequency response in producing a reliable tracing.

KEY TERMS

artifact: Distortion of an ECG tracing by electrical activity that is noncardiac in origin

electrical axis: Net direction, or angle in degrees, in which the main vector of depolarization is pointed

electrode: An adhesive pad containing a conductive substance in the center that is applied to the patient's skin

frequency response: The spectrum in which an ECG can accurately reproduce the signals it is sensing

lead: A record (i.e., tracing) of electrical activity, specifically the fluctuation in voltage differences, between positive and negative electrodes
vector: Quantity having direction and magnitude, usually depicted by a straight arrow whose length represents magnitude and whose head represents direction

THE ELECTROCARDIOGRAM

The basic function of the electrocardiogram (ECG) is to detect and record current flow within the heart as measured on the body's surface. An **electrode** is an adhesive pad containing a conductive substance in the center that is applied to the patient's skin. The conductive media of the electrode conducts skin surface voltage changes through wires to a cardiac monitor. Electrodes are applied at specific locations on the patient's chest wall and extremities to view the heart's electrical activity from different angles and planes. One end of a monitoring cable, also called a *lead wire*, is attached to the electrode and the other to an ECG machine. The cable conducts current back to the cardiac monitor.

A **lead** is a record (i.e., tracing) of electrical activity, specifically the fluctuation in voltage differences, between positive and negative electrodes (Lederer, 2017). A standard 12-lead ECG uses 10 electrodes, 4 on the limbs and 6 on the chest wall, to record the heart's electrical activity from 12 angles. Each lead records the *average* current flow at a specific time in a portion of the heart. Box 2.1 lists examples of indications for obtaining a 12-lead ECG.

Frontal Plane Leads

Frontal plane leads view the heart from the front of the body as if it were flat. Six leads (leads I, II, III, aVR, aVL, and aVF) view the heart in the frontal plane (Fig. 2.1). Leads I, II, and III are called *standard limb leads*. A bipolar lead is an ECG lead that has a positive and negative electrode. Each lead records the difference in electrical potential (voltage) between two selected electrodes. Although all ECG leads are technically bipolar, leads I, II, and III use two distinct electrodes, one of which is connected to the positive input of the ECG machine and the other to the negative input (Surawicz et al., 2009).

Box 2.1 Indications for Obtaining a 12-Lead Electrocardiogram

- Abdominal or epigastric pain
- Assisting in dysrhythmia interpretation
- Chest pain or discomfort
- Diabetic ketoacidosis
- Dizziness
- Dyspnea
- Electrical injuries
- Known or suspected electrolyte imbalances
- Known or suspected medication overdoses
- Right or left ventricular failure
- Status before and after electrical therapy (e.g., defibrillation, cardioversion, pacing)
- Stroke
- Syncope or near syncope
- Unstable patient, unknown etiology

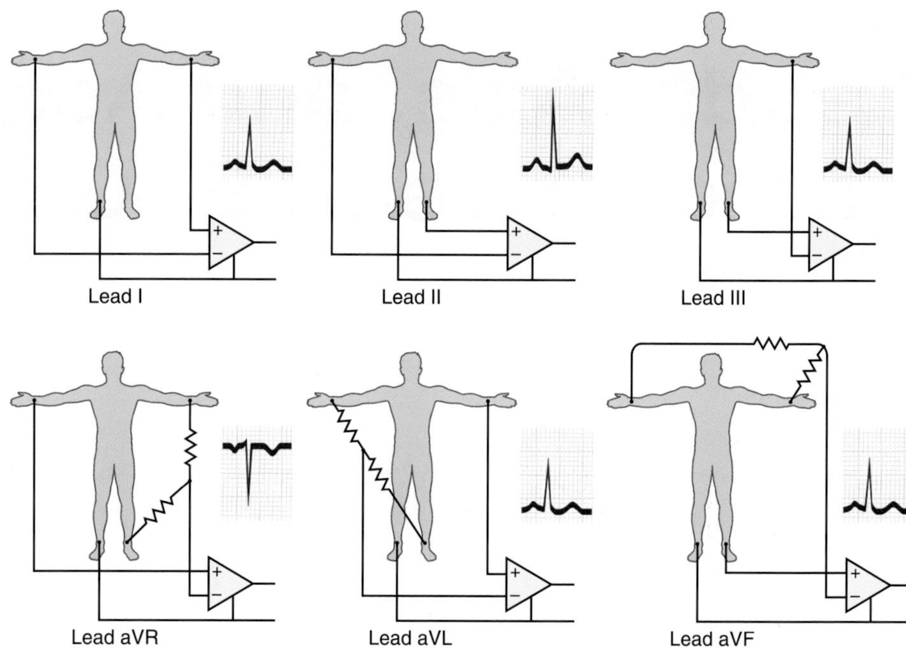

Fig. 2.1 Normal cardiac activation as shown in the limb leads. Under normal circumstances, P waves and QRS complex are typically upright in leads I, II, III, and aVF and inverted in aVR. In lead aVL, P waves are usually upright, although QRS complexes may be either upright or inverted. The right leg electrode serves to ground the system. (From Goldman, L., & Schafer, A. I. [2016]. *Goldman's Cecil medicine* [25th ed.]. Philadelphia, PA: Saunders.)

Lead I compares the difference in electrical potential between the left arm (+) and right arm (−) electrodes. It views the lateral surface of the left ventricle. Lead II compares the difference in electrical potential between the left leg (+) and right arm (−) electrodes. It views the inferior surface of the left ventricle. Lead III compares the difference in electrical potential between the left leg (+) and left arm (−) electrodes and views the left ventricle's inferior surface. Waveforms are usually positive in leads I, II, and III.

Leads aVR, aVL, and aVF are *augmented limb leads* that record measurements at a specific electrode with respect to a reference electrode. Frank Norman Wilson and colleagues used the term *central terminal* to describe a reference point that is the average of the limb lead electrical potentials. In the augmented leads, the Wilson central terminal (WCT) is calculated by the ECG machine's computer as an average potential of the electrical currents from the two electrodes other than the one being used as the positive electrode. For example, in lead aVL, the positive electrode is located on the patient's left arm. The ECG machine's computer calculates the central terminal by joining the electrical currents obtained from the electrodes on the patient's right arm and left leg. Lead aVL therefore represents the difference in electrical potential between the left arm and the central terminal. The electrical potential of the central terminal is essentially zero.

The electrical potential produced by the augmented leads is normally relatively small. The ECG machine augments (magnifies) the amplitude of the electrical potentials detected at each extremity by about 50% over those recorded at the standard limb leads. The "a" in aVR, aVL, and aVF refers to "augmented." The "V" refers to voltage, and the last letter refers to the position of the positive electrode. The "R" refers to the right arm, the "L" to left arm, and the "F" to left foot (i.e., leg).

Lead aVR views the heart from the right shoulder, which is the positive electrode. Because the wave of depolarization is moving away from lead aVR, waveforms in this lead are typically negative. Until recently, lead aVR was thought to have little diagnostic value because it views current flow away from the normal direction of left ventricular depolarization (Ching & Ting, 2015). Studies suggest than ST-segment elevation (STE) that is 1 mm or greater in lead aVR may be a significant indicator of left main coronary artery disease, proximal left anterior descending disease, or at least multivessel coronary artery disease (Omar & Camporesi, 2014; Vorobiof & Ellestad, 2011).

Lead aVL combines views from the right arm and the left leg, with the view being from the left arm and oriented to the lateral wall of the left ventricle. Waveforms observed in this lead are usually positive but may be biphasic (i.e., partly positive, partly negative). Lead aVF combines views from the right arm and the left arm toward the left leg; it views the inferior surface of the left ventricle from the left leg. Waveforms observed in this lead are usually positive but may be biphasic.

Horizontal Plane Leads

Six chest (precordial or "V") leads view the heart in the horizontal plane. This allows a view of the front and left side of the heart. The chest leads are identified as V_1, V_2, V_3, V_4, V_5, and V_6. Each electrode placed in a "V" position is a positive electrode, measuring electrical potential with respect to the WCT (Fig. 2.2). The chest leads are summarized in Table 2.1.

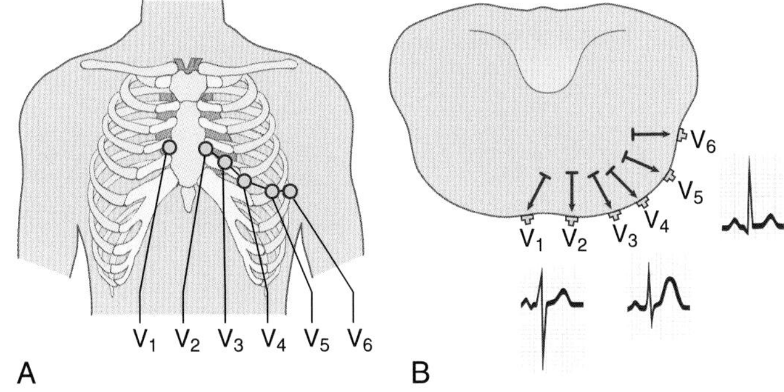

Fig. 2.2 Chest leads. **A,** Positioning of the chest leads on the chest wall. **B,** Normal cardiac activation as seen in the chest leads. (From Goldman, L., & Schafer, A. I. [2016]. *Goldman's Cecil medicine* [25th ed.]. Philadelphia, PA: Saunders.)

TABLE 2.1 Chest Leads

Lead	Positive Electrode Position	Heart Area Viewed
V_1	Right side of sternum, fourth intercostal space	Interventricular septum
V_2	Left side of sternum, fourth intercostal space	Interventricular septum
V_3	Midway between V_2 and V_4	Anterior surface
V_4	Left midclavicular line, fifth intercostal space	Anterior surface
V_5	Left anterior axillary line, fifth intercostal space	Lateral surface
V_6	Left midaxillary line, fifth intercostal space	Lateral surface

When viewing the chest leads in a normal heart, the R wave becomes taller (i.e., increases in amplitude) and the S wave becomes smaller as the electrode is moved from right to left. This pattern is called *R-wave progression*. The *transition zone* is the area at which the amplitude of the R wave begins to exceed the amplitude of the S wave (Ganz, 2016). This usually occurs in the area of leads V_3 and V_4. Electrode placement in the correct intercostal space is critical when evaluating R-wave progression.

LAYOUT OF THE 12-LEAD ECG

Look at the 12-lead ECG in Fig. 2.3. Notice that the standard limb leads are recorded in the first column, the augmented limb leads in the second column, and the chest leads in the third and fourth columns. The 12-lead ECG provides a 2.5-second view of each lead because it is assumed that 2.5 seconds is long enough to capture at least one representative complex. Although most 12-lead ECG machines obtain the signals for all leads at the same time, other machines obtain the signals sequentially (i.e., all limb leads, then the augmented limb leads, followed by leads V_1 through V_3, and finally leads V_4 through V_6). The 12-lead ECG machines used in the hospital setting typically record at least one rhythm strip at the bottom of the printout.

Note that the information contained on the upper left corner of Fig. 2.3 includes measurements of intervals in milliseconds (msec). This information is provided by the computer's interpretive program, which is usually very accurate when calculating heart rates, axes, and intervals.

Consider This

When a simultaneous tracing is obtained, the beats in a vertical column are all the product of the same ventricular depolarization. Likewise, beats in a horizontal row are continuous, even as the leads change.

Fig. **2.3**

Female Caucasian	Vent. rate	77 bpm	Normal sinus rhythm
	PR interval	156 msec	Normal ECG
	QRS duration	80 msec	
Room:	QT/QTc	356/402 msec	
Loc:	P-R-T axes	73 56 60	

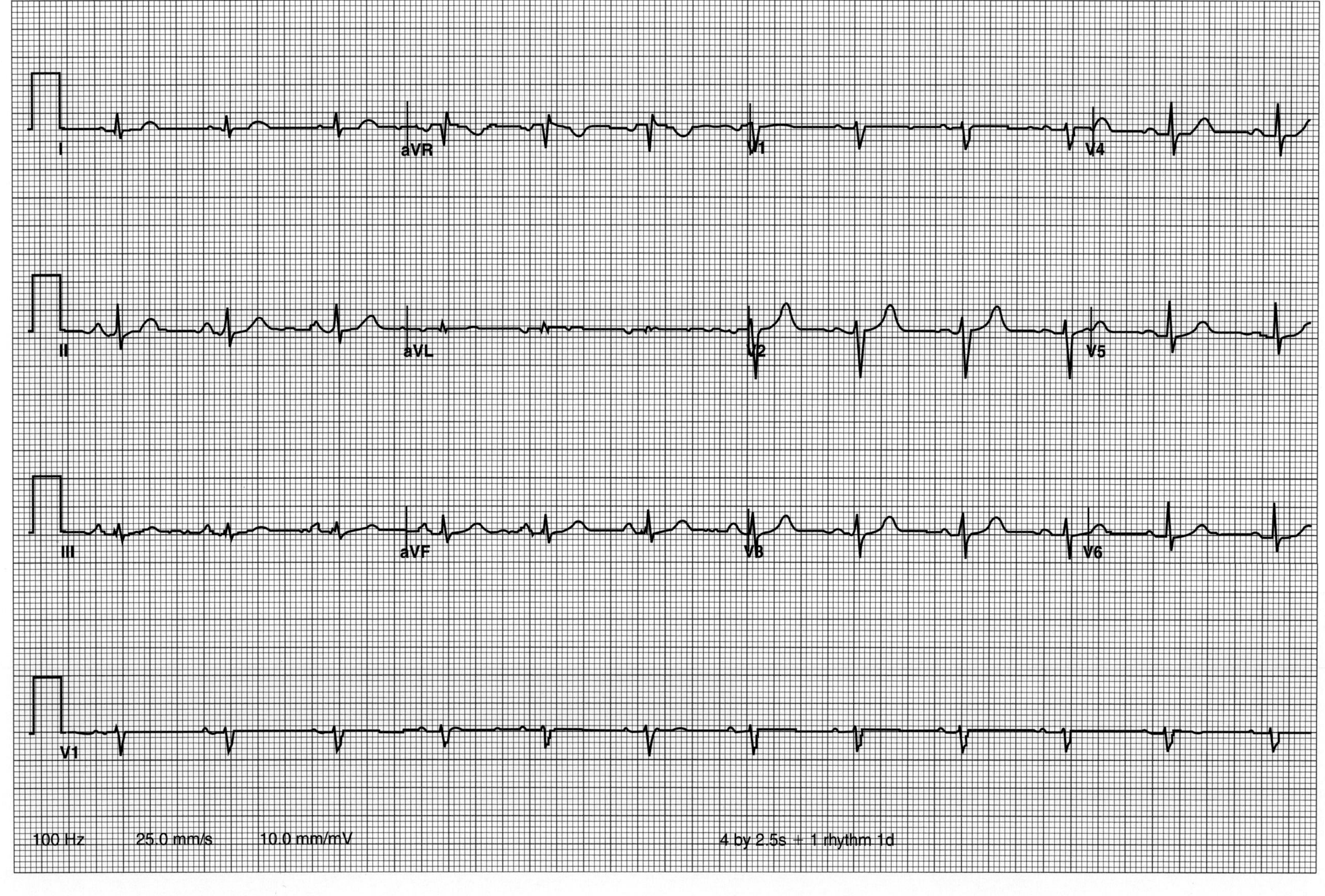

Right Chest Leads

Other chest leads that are not part of a standard 12-lead ECG may be used to view specific surfaces of the heart. Right chest leads are used to evaluate the right ventricle when a right ventricular infarction is suspected (Fig. 2.4). Placement of right chest leads is identical to placement of the standard chest leads except it is done on the right side of the chest. If time does not permit obtaining all of the right chest leads, the lead of choice is V_4R. A summary of the right chest leads can be found in Table 2.2.

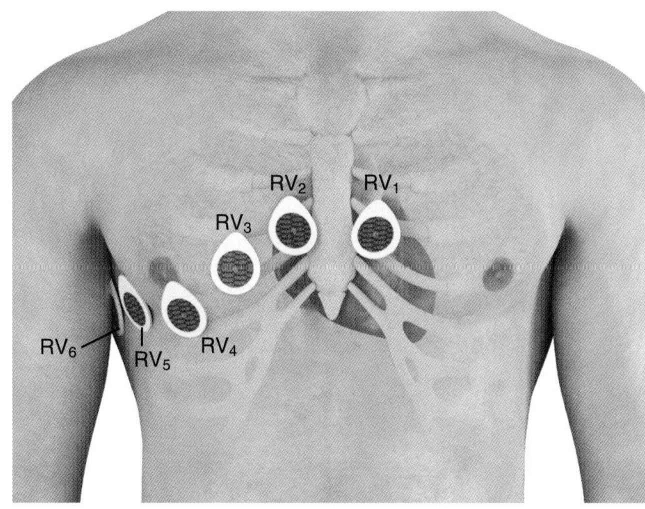

Fig. **2.4** Electrode locations for recording a right chest electrocardiogram (ECG). Right chest leads are not part of a standard 12-lead ECG but are used when a right ventricular infarction is suspected. (From Hedges, J. R. [2014]. *Roberts and Hedges' clinical procedures in emergency medicine* [6th ed.]. Philadelphia, PA: Saunders.)

TABLE 2.2 Right Chest Lead Placement

Lead	Placement
V_1R	Lead V_2
V_2R	Lead V_1
V_3R	Midway between V_2R and V_4R
V_4R	Right midclavicular line, fifth intercostal space
V_5R	Right anterior axillary line, fifth intercostal space
V_6R	Right midaxillary line, fifth intercostal space

Posterior Chest Leads

Posterior chest leads can be used to evaluate the heart's posterior surface when an infarction affecting this area is suspected. These leads are placed further left and toward the back. All of the leads are placed on the same horizontal line as V_4 to V_6. Lead V_7 is placed at the posterior axillary line. Lead V_8 is placed at the angle of the scapula (i.e., the posterior scapular line), and lead V_9 is placed over the left border of the spine (Fig. 2.5).

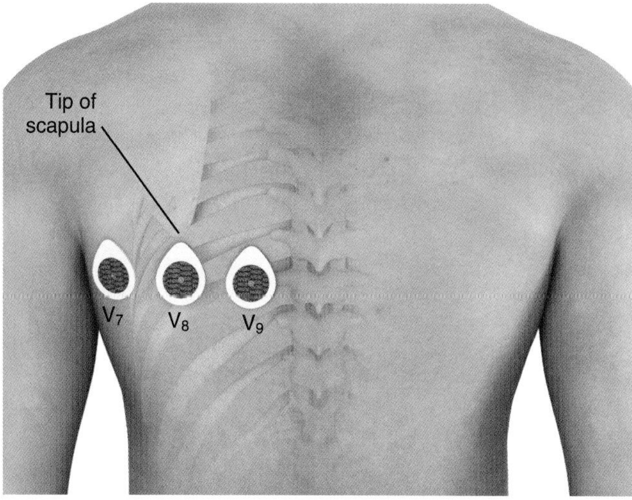

Fig. **2.5** Electrode locations for left posterior chest lead placement. (From Hedges, J. R. [2014]. *Roberts and Hedges' clinical procedures in emergency medicine* [6th ed.]. Philadelphia, PA: Saunders.)

VECTORS AND AXIS

Leads have a negative (−) and positive (+) electrode pole that senses the magnitude and direction of the electrical force caused by the spread of waves of depolarization and repolarization throughout the myocardium. A **vector** (arrow) is a symbol representing this force. A vector's angle of orientation represents the average direction of current flow, and its length represents the voltage (i.e., amplitude). Leads that face the tip or point of a vector record a positive deflection on ECG paper.

An imaginary line joining the positive and negative electrodes of a lead is called the *axis* of the lead. **Electrical axis** refers to the net direction, or angle in degrees, in which the main vector of depolarization is pointed. When *axis* is used by itself, it refers to the QRS axis.

During normal ventricular depolarization, the left side of the interventricular septum is stimulated first. The electrical impulse then crosses the septum to stimulate the right side. The left and right ventricles are then depolarized simultaneously. Because the left ventricle is considerably larger than the right, right ventricular depolarization forces are overshadowed on the ECG.

The axes of leads I, II, and III form an equilateral triangle with the heart at the center (i.e., Einthoven's triangle). Einthoven's law states that the sum of the electrical currents recorded in leads I and III equals the sum of the electrical current recorded in lead II. This can be expressed as lead I + lead III = lead II. If the augmented limb leads are added to the equilateral triangle, and the axes of the six leads moved in a way in which they bisect each other, the result is the *hexaxial reference system* (Fig. 2.6). The hexaxial reference system represents all of the frontal plane (limb) leads with the heart in the center and is the means used to express the location of the frontal plane axis. This system forms a 360-degree circle surrounding the heart. The positive end of lead I is designated at 0 degrees. The six frontal plane leads divide the circle into segments, each representing 30 degrees. All degrees in the upper hemisphere are labeled as negative degrees, and all degrees in the lower hemisphere are labeled as positive degrees.

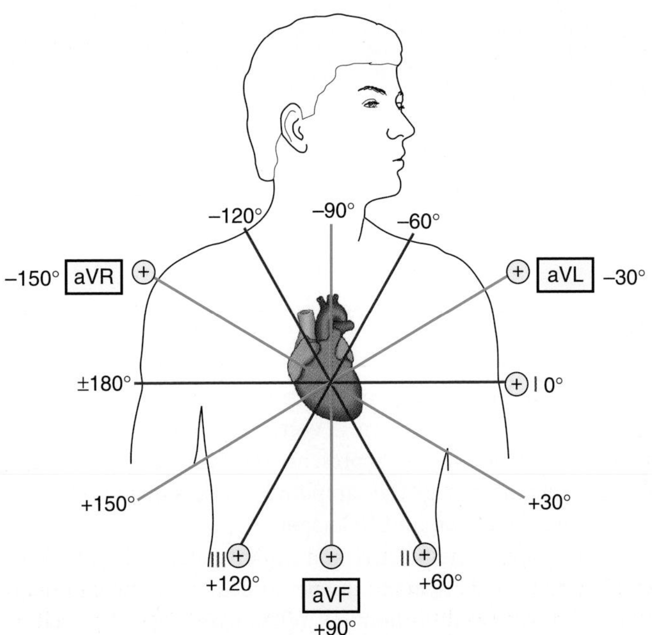

Fig. **2.6** The hexaxial reference system. (From Beachey, W. [2013]. *Respiratory care anatomy and physiology: Foundations for clinical practice* [3rd ed.]. St. Louis, MO: Mosby.)

In the hexaxial reference system, the axes of some leads are perpendicular to each other. Lead I is perpendicular to lead aVF. Lead II is perpendicular to aVL, and lead III is perpendicular to lead aVR. If the electrical force moves toward a positive electrode, a positive (upright) deflection will be recorded. If the electrical force moves away from a positive electrode, a negative (downward) deflection will be recorded. If the electrical force is parallel to a given lead, the largest deflection in that lead will be recorded. If the electrical force is perpendicular to a lead axis, the resulting ECG complex will be isoelectric and/or equiphasic in that lead. Notice that leads III and aVL are positioned on opposite (reciprocal) sides of the hexaxial reference system.

To determine electrical axis, look again at Fig. 2.3. Because the hexaxial reference system is derived from the limb leads, we will be focusing on the leads shown in the two columns on the left side of the figure (lead I, II, III, aVR, aVL, and aVF). Look for the most equiphasic or isoelectric QRS complexes in these leads. Lead aVL shows QRS complexes that most closely reflect our criteria. The patient's QRS axis is perpendicular to the positive electrode in lead aVL. Look at the hexaxial reference system diagram (see Fig. 2.6) to determine which ECG lead is perpendicular to lead aVL. Lead II is perpendicular to lead aVL. Now we know that the patient's QRS axis is moving along the same vector as lead II. Note that the values associated with lead II in the hexaxial reference system diagram are −120 degrees and +60 degrees. To determine whether the QRS axis is moving in a positive or negative direction, look at lead II in Fig. 2.3 and determine whether the QRS complex is primarily positive or negative in this lead. You will see that the QRS is primarily positive in lead II; therefore, this patient's QRS axis is about +60 degrees. At the top of Fig. 2.3 you will see the computer's calculation of the patient's P-QRS-T axes. The computer calculated the patient's QRS axis at +56 degrees. Our estimate of +60 degrees was very close!

In adults, the normal QRS axis is considered to be between −30 and +90 degrees in the frontal plane (Ganz, 2016). Current flow to the right of normal is called *right axis deviation* (between +90 and ±180 degrees). Current flow in the direction opposite of normal is called *indeterminate*, "no man's land," *northwest,* or *extreme right axis deviation* (between −90 and ±180 degrees). Current flow to the left of normal is called *left axis deviation* (between −30 and −90 degrees).

Shortcuts exist to determine axis deviation. Leads I and aVF divide the heart into four quadrants (Fig. 2.7). These two leads can be used to quickly estimate electrical axis. In leads I and aVF, the QRS complex is normally positive. If the QRS complex in either or both of these leads is negative, axis deviation is present (Table 2.3).

Right axis deviation may be a normal variant, particularly in the young and in thin individuals. Other causes of right axis deviation include mechanical shifts associated with inspiration or emphysema, right ventricular hypertrophy, chronic obstructive pulmonary disease, Wolff-Parkinson-White syndrome, and acute or chronic pulmonary thromboembolism.

Left axis deviation may be a normal variant, particularly in older and obese individuals. Other causes of left axis deviation include mechanical shifts associated with expiration; a high diaphragm caused by pregnancy, ascites, or abdominal tumors; hyperkalemia; emphysema; dextrocardia, and left ventricular hypertrophy.

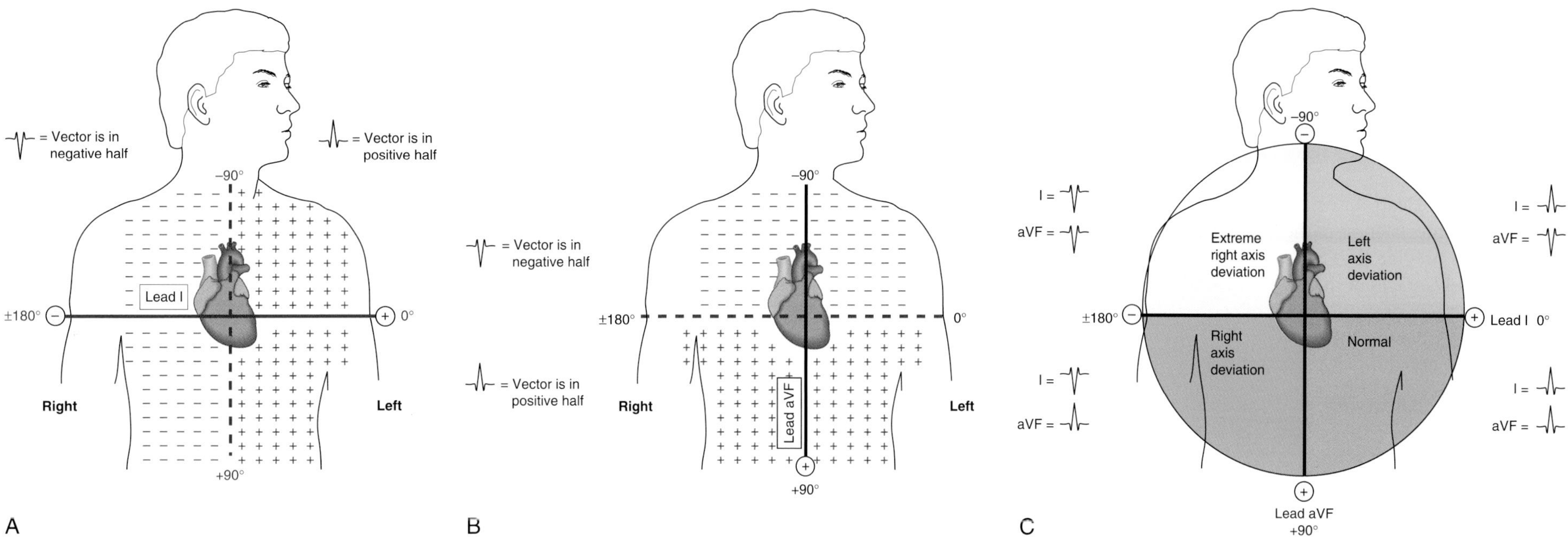

Fig. 2.7 **A,** Lead I divides the chest into positive and negative halves with respect to the QRS it records. **B,** Lead aVF divides the chest into positive and negative lower and upper halves with respect to the QRS it records. **C,** Using leads I and aVF together locates the mean cardiac vector within a 90-degree quadrant. (From Beachey, W. [2013]. *Respiratory care anatomy and physiology: Foundations for clinical practice* [3rd ed.]. St. Louis, MO: Mosby.)

TABLE 2.3 Two-Lead Method of Axis Determination

Axis	Normal	Left	Right	Extreme Right
Lead I QRS direction	Positive	Positive	Negative	Negative
Lead aVF QRS direction	Positive	Negative	Positive	Negative

Cabrera Display Format

The 12-lead ECG layout previously described has been in use for many years worldwide. The national standard in Sweden is the Cabrera format, which has been in use for more than 40 years. With this display format, the frontal plane leads are displayed in the logical sequence of impulse progression through the heart in the frontal plane, and then in the horizontal plane (Fig. 2.8).

To review, a standard 12-lead ECG displays leads in the following sequence: I, II, III, aVR, aVL, aVF (frontal plane leads), V_1, V_2, V_3, V_4, V_5, and V_6 (horizontal plane leads). In contrast, the Cabrera format displays the frontal plane leads in anatomical sequence (i.e., aVL, I, −aVR, II, aVF, III), followed by the horizontal plane leads (i.e., V_1, V_2, V_3, V_4, V_5, and V_6) (Lam, Wagner, & Pahlm, 2015). Note that the inverted form of lead aVR is used with the Cabrera format and is indicated as −aVR. This refers to lead aVR with reversed polarity. In the hexaxial reference system, the inverted form of lead aVR exists at 30 degrees in the frontal plane, filling the gap between lead I, which is at 0 degrees, and lead II, which is at 60 degrees.

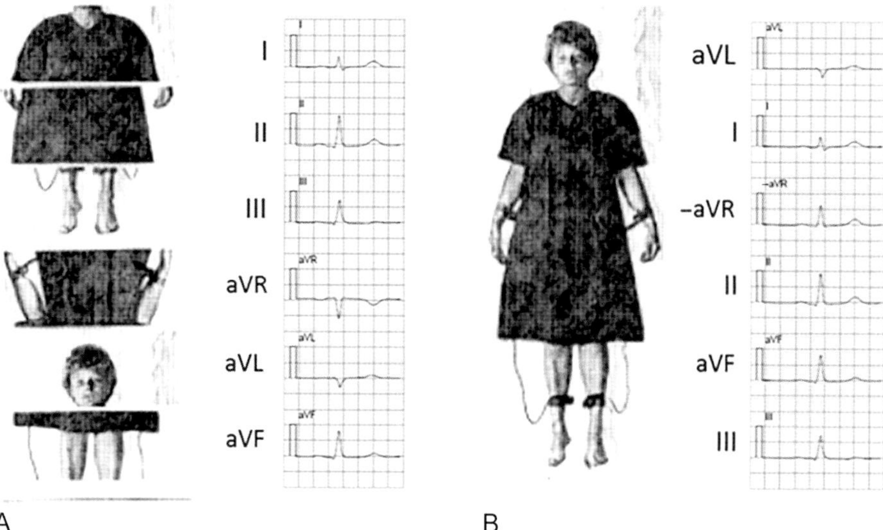

Fig. 2.8 When taking a picture of a person, one does not expect the various parts of the body to be shown in "jumbled" order (**A**) or even one of the subpictures shown upside down. This is akin to displaying the limb leads of the 12-lead ECG in the classical way. The Cabrera display (**B**) shows the limb leads in sequential, "anatomic" order. (From Lam, A., Wagner, G. S., & Pahlm, O. [2015]. The classical versus the Cabrera presentation system for resting electrocardiography: Impact on recognition and understanding of clinically important electrocardiographic changes. *Journal of Electrocardiology, 48*(4), 476–482).

Examples of potential advantages with regard to the use of the Cabrera format include the following: (1) the ECG reader's visualization of the electrical activity of the heart is enhanced with anatomical sequencing of the frontal plane leads, (2) the inverted form of lead aVR can be viewed as a transition lead between the lateral (i.e., lead I) and inferior (i.e., lead II) areas of the heart, improving recognition of lateral and inferior ischemia and infarction, and (3) the ECG reader can calculate electrical axis faster and with greater accuracy.

The American Heart Association and the American Journal of Cardiology have recognized the appropriateness of the Cabrera system and recommended that all vendors of ECG machines provide the Cabrera system as an option (Wagner et al., 2009). Despite the potential advantages of the Cabrera format, experts say it is likely that the more traditional format will prevail because of conservatism within the cardiology community (Lam, Wagner, & Pahlm, 2015).

WHAT EACH LEAD "SEES"

Think of the positive electrode as an eye looking in at the heart. The part of the heart that each lead "sees" is determined by two factors. The first factor is the dominance of the left ventricle on the ECG, and the second is the position of the positive electrode on the body. Because the ECG does not directly measure the heart's electrical activity, it does not "see" all of the current flowing through the heart. What the ECG sees from its vantage point on the body's surface is the net result of countless individual currents competing in a tug-of-war. For example, the QRS complex, which represents ventricular depolarization, is not a display of all the electrical activity occurring in the right and left ventricles. It is the net result of a tug-of-war produced by the many individual currents in both the right and left ventricles. Because the left ventricle is much larger than the right, the left overpowers it. What is seen in the QRS complex is the additional electrical activity of the left ventricle (i.e., the portion that exceeds the right ventricle). Therefore, in a normally conducted beat, the QRS complex primarily represents the electrical activity occurring in the left ventricle.

The second factor, the position of the positive electrode on the body, determines which portion of the left ventricle is seen by each lead. You can commit the view of each lead to memory, or you can easily reason it by remembering where the positive electrode is located. Fig. 2.9 demonstrates the portion of the left ventricle that each lead views.

Contiguous Leads

The sudden blockage of a coronary artery will result in myocardial ischemia, injury, and/or death of the area of the myocardium supplied by the affected artery. Remember that the positive electrode of each ECG lead is like an eye looking in at the heart. Therefore, the ECG changes associated with ischemia, injury, or infarction will not be seen in every

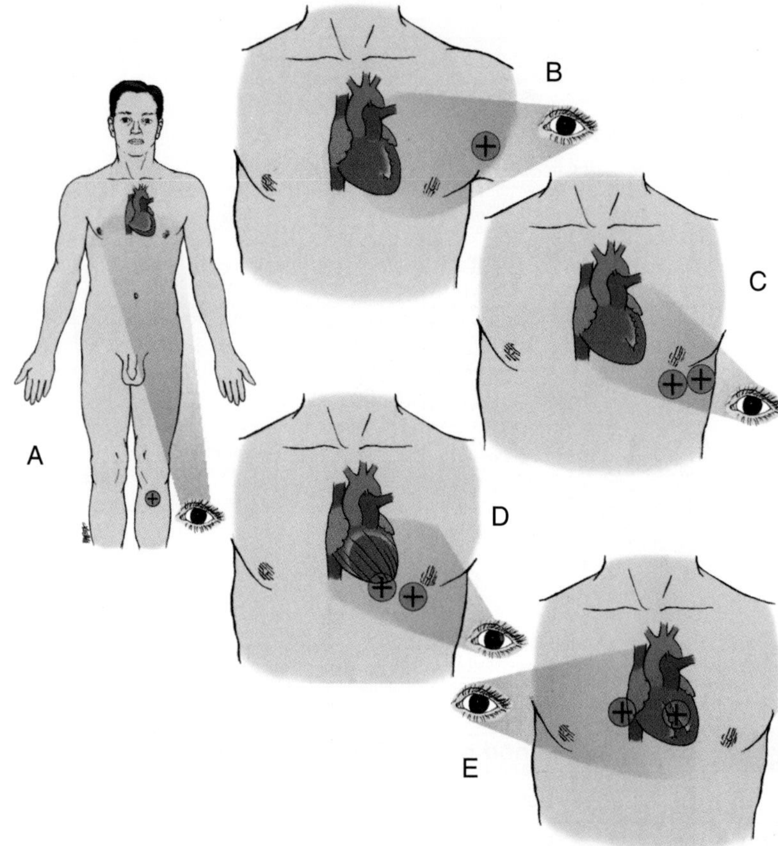

Fig. 2.9 Lead viewpoints. **A,** Leads II, III, and aVF each have their positive electrode positioned on the left leg. From the perspective of the left leg, each of them "sees" the inferior wall of the left ventricle. **B,** From their vantage point on the left arm, leads I and aVL "look" in at the lateral wall of the left ventricle. **C,** Leads V_5 and V_6 also "view" the lateral wall because they are positioned on the axillary area of the left chest. **D,** Leads V_3 and V_4 are positioned in the area of the anterior chest. From this perspective, these leads "see" the anterior wall of the left ventricle. **E,** The septal wall is "seen" by leads V_1 and V_2, which are positioned next to the sternum. Lead aVR, which is not shown, views the heart from the right shoulder. It "sees" the basal ventricular septum and the inferior and lateral apex of the heart.

lead. If ECG findings are seen in leads that look directly at the area fed by the blocked vessel, they are called *indicative changes* (Fig. 2.10). If ECG findings are seen in leads opposite the affected area, they are called *reciprocal changes*, discussed later.

Indicative changes are significant when they are seen in two *anatomically contiguous* leads. Two leads are contiguous if they look at the same or adjacent areas of the heart or they are numerically consecutive chest leads. To better understand this, look at Table 2.4, which shows the area viewed by each lead of a standard 12-lead ECG. The colors in the table were added so that you can quickly see the areas of the heart viewed by the same

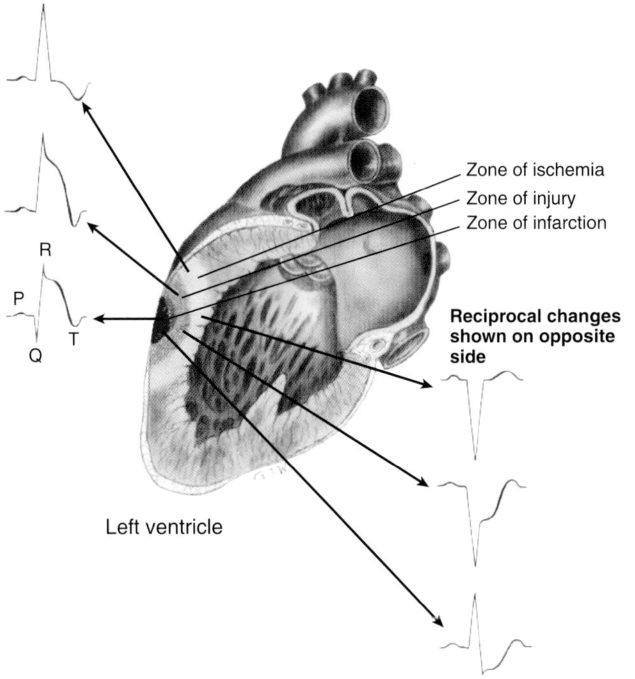

Fig. **2.10** Zones of ischemia, injury, and infarction showing indicative electrocardiogram changes and reciprocal changes corresponding to each zone. (Modified from Urden, L. D., Stacy, K. M., & Lough, M. E. [2014]. *Critical care nursing* [7th ed.]. St. Louis: Mosby.)

TABLE 2.4 Localizing Electrocardiogram Changes

I: Lateral	aVR: —	V_1: Septum	V_4: Anterior
II: Inferior	aVL: Lateral	V_2: Septum	V_5: Lateral
III: Inferior	aVF: Inferior	V_3: Anterior	V_6: Lateral

leads. For example, leads II, III, and aVF appear the same color in the table because they view the inferior wall of the left ventricle. Because these leads "see" the same part of the heart, they are considered contiguous leads.

Leads I, aVL, V_5, and V_6 are contiguous because they all look at adjoining tissue in the lateral wall of the left ventricle. Leads V_1 and V_2 are contiguous because both leads look at the septum. Leads V_3 and V_4 are contiguous because both leads look at the anterior wall of the left ventricle. If right chest leads such as V_4R, V_5R, and V_6R are used, they are contiguous because they view the right ventricle. Leads V_7, V_8, and V_9 are contiguous because they look at the posterior (i.e., inferobasal) surface of the heart.

Reciprocal Leads

ECG changes associated with ischemia, injury, or infarction may be associated with reciprocal ("mirror image") ECG changes in leads opposite (i.e., about 180 degrees away from) the leads that show the indicative change (see Fig. 2.10). For example, STE in lead III, an indicative change, will show ST-segment depression, a reciprocal change, in lead aVL. Reasons why reciprocal changes may be subtle or may not be apparent on a standard 12-lead ECG include the following (Wagner et al., 2009):

- The standard 12-lead ECG may not reflect the leads opposite the indicative change.
- The magnitude of the voltage transmitted to the body surface is inadequate to meet diagnostic criteria. For example, conditions that may cause a low QRS voltage include chronic obstructive pulmonary disease, myocardial infarction, cardiomyopathy, and hypothyroidism.
- The presence of confounding ECG abnormalities, such as intraventricular conduction disturbances.

Experts note that lead aVR does not have any contiguous leads; however, it is reciprocal to limb leads I and II and partly reciprocal to chest leads V_5, V_6, and V_7 (Talebi et al., 2015). For example, infarction of the basal portion of the interventricular septum can produce STE in aVR and ST depression in leads I, II, and V_5 through V_7 (Talebi et al., 2015).

12-LEAD ECG ACQUISITION

The goals of 12-lead acquisition are to obtain an ECG that is free of distortion (clear), with the leads placed correctly (accurate), and done quickly (fast).

Goal 1: Clear

Accurate 12-lead ECG interpretation requires a tracing in which the waveforms and intervals are free of distortion. Distortion of an ECG tracing by electrical activity that is noncardiac in origin is called **artifact**, which may result from external or internal sources. The presence of artifact can interfere with a 12-lead machine's ability to acquire and/or interpret the ECG. Possible causes of external artifact include loose electrodes, broken ECG cables or broken lead wires, external chest compressions, and 60-cycle interference. Internal artifact may result from patient movement, shivering, muscle tremors (e.g., seizures, Parkinson disease), or hiccups (Pelter & Carey, 2017).

A wandering baseline may occur because of patient movement. Subtle patient movements, such as those caused by the patient's breathing (particularly when electrodes have been applied directly over the ribs), talking, shivering, tapping toes, or rolling fingers can be enough to produce artifact. Efforts made to reduce muscle tension and the source of patient movement, such as having the patient relax and take a deep breath before acquisition, can improve the tracing quality. When the tracing quality precludes a good interpretation, the tracing should be repeated.

Evaluation of the monitoring equipment (e.g., electrodes, cables, wires) before use and proper preparation of the patient's skin can minimize the problems associated with artifact. The signal from the patient's heart is conducted through lead wires and a cable to the monitor. If a lead wire is frayed or broken or the cable's insulation is cracked, the signal to the monitor is affected and artifact can result. Inspect the monitoring cable and lead wires and replace them if damaged. If not preconnected, the limb lead and chest lead wires are inserted into a main cable and the cable connector is inserted into the ECG port on the monitor.

Consider This

When the baseline wanders, ST segments may appear elevated when in fact they are not. This ST-segment elevation (STE) may not be the result of infarction but may simply be an expected finding that occurs as the monitor centers the isoelectric line in the screen. Therefore, it is important to be cautious about analyzing STE in leads with a wandering baseline.

When preparing the patient's skin for electrode application, small areas may need to be shaved or clipped to ensure proper adhesion of the electrodes to the skin if excessive hair is present at electrode sites. Ensure that the skin areas where the electrodes will be applied are clean and dry; if these areas are oily, cleanse them with an alcohol pad. Fresh electrodes should be attached to the lead wires before applying the electrodes to the skin to minimize patient discomfort. When removing pregelled electrodes from their packaging, ensure that the conductive jelly in the center of the electrode is moist. If the electrode gel has dried out, it is not able to penetrate the skin. If the gel does not penetrate the skin, the signal to the monitor will be weak and artifact results. To promote impulse transmission, lightly abrade the skin to remove oil and dead skin cells. Many electrode manufacturers include an abrasive area on the disposable backing of the electrode for this purpose, but skin prep tape or a gauze pad also work well.

Some electrical devices may interfere with the 12-lead monitor. If artifact persists after removing hair, prepping the skin, and normal troubleshooting did not turn up any problems, electromagnetic interference (EMI) might be the reason. The problem might be corrected by ensuring that power cords are not touching or lying near the ECG cable. If equipment is causing EMI (such as an electric blanket, radio transmitter, or bed control), it needs to be relocated or unplugged; alternately, the patient could be moved to a different area.

Although artifact is sometimes easy to discern, it can mimic serious dysrhythmias (Fig. 2.11) and lead to unnecessary testing and treatment (Harrigan, Chan, & Brady, 2012).

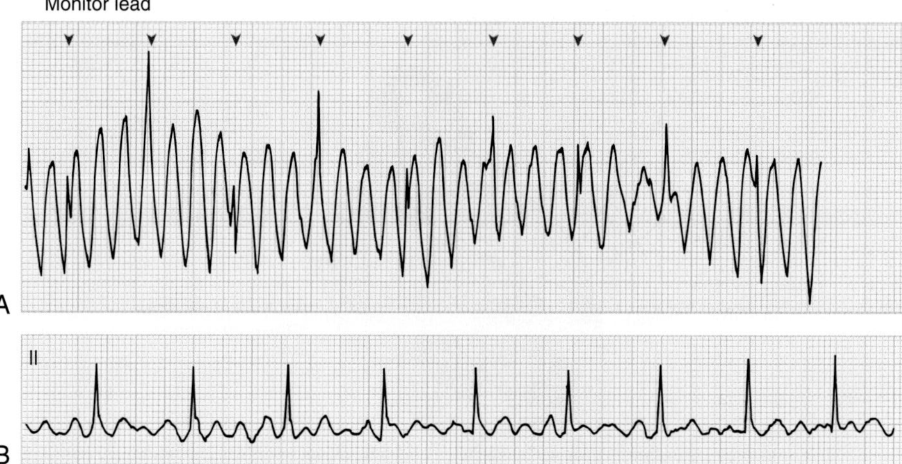

Fig. 2.11 Artifact simulating serious dysrhythmias. **A,** Motion artifact mimicking ventricular tachyarrhythmia. Partly obscured normal QRS complexes (*arrowheads*) can be seen with a heart rate of approximately 100 beats/minute. **B,** Parkinsonian tremor causing baseline oscillations mimicking atrial fibrillation. The regularity of QRS complexes may provide a clue to the source of this artifact. (From Mann, D.L., Zipes, D.P., Libby, P., Bonow, R.O., & Braunwald, E. [2015]. *Braunwald's heart disease: A textbook of cardiovascular medicine* [10th ed.]. Philadelphia, PA: Saunders.)

Consider This

A study surveying physicians presented with rhythm strips containing artifact simulating ventricular tachycardia (VT) found that 94% of the internists, 58% of the cardiologists, and 38% of the electrophysiologists who participated in the study failed to recognize the rhythm as artifact (Knight, Pelosi, Michaud, Strickberger, & Morady, 2001). In this study, 31% of the internists, 53% of the cardiologists, and 88% of the electrophysiologists who misdiagnosed the rhythm as VT recommended an invasive procedure for further evaluation or therapy.

Goal 2: Accurate

An accurate 12-lead ECG requires placing the electrodes correctly, positioning the patient, and selecting the correct settings for a diagnostic quality tracing. Although most 12-lead devices will default to the proper setting for these considerations, it is important to understand the significance of each and be able to verify that they have been properly set.

Electrode Positioning

Although there are several indications for obtaining a 12-lead ECG, one of its most important uses is in the diagnosis and triage of patients with acute coronary syndromes. Accurate positioning of electrodes is essential because ECG changes resulting from electrode misplacement can affect clinical decision-making and treatment.

Proper placement of limb electrodes has been debated for years, and there is considerable variability in clinical practice. A 2007 article pertaining to standardization of the ECG mentions an American Heart Association recommendation for placement of the limb lead electrodes on the arms and legs distal to the shoulders and hips, and thus not necessarily on the wrists and ankles (Kligfield et al., 2007). It is common practice in many hospital and prehospital settings to use an alternative electrode configuration to reduce motion artifact from the extremities. With Mason-Likar electrode placement, the limb electrodes are moved to the torso, but chest electrode placement is unchanged. Although rhythm diagnosis is not adversely affected with Mason-Likar electrode placement, there is concern that Q waves in the inferior leads may be masked, making detection of inferior infarction more difficult (Francis, 2016; Sejersten et al., 2006). Another alternative electrode configuration is the Lund system, in which the limb electrodes are placed on the proximal areas of the limbs and chest electrode placement is unchanged. The Lund system has been found to more closely replicate the ECG recordings obtained with conventional electrode positioning (Pahlm & Wagner, 2008).

Incorrect Electrode Positioning

Studies have shown 17% to 24% of patients were given a different diagnosis when the 12-lead ECG was acquired using an incorrect electrode configuration (Bond et al., 2012). Examples of possible differences in interpretation with correct versus incorrect electrode placement are shown in Fig. 2.12.

Most recording errors are the result of placing electrodes on the wrong extremity. However, transposing the lead wires in the monitoring cable can produce similar results (Greenfield Jr., 2008). Reversal of the right and left arm lead wires is common and results in significant ECG changes (Fig. 2.13). Key findings for detecting right arm/left arm reversal include the following (Harrigan, Chan, & Brady, 2012):

- Negative PQRST waveforms in lead I
- Positive PQRST waveforms in lead aVR

Errors in placement of the chest electrodes is common because their positioning is relative to anatomic landmarks. Obesity and the female anatomy are two variables that make consistent chest electrode positioning difficult (Harrigan, Chan, & Brady, 2012).

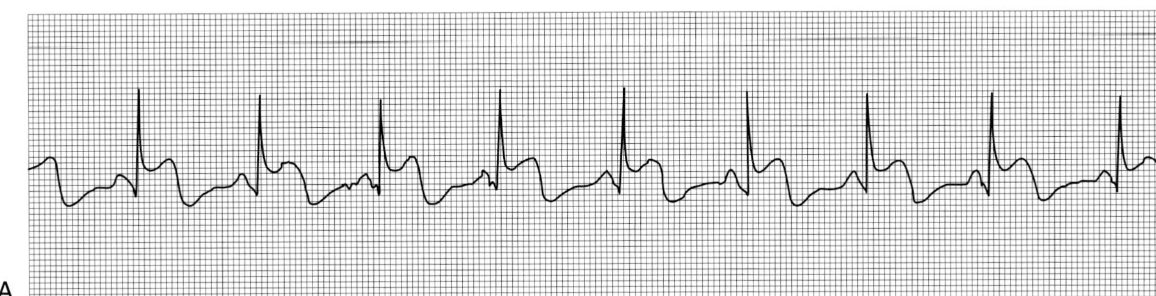

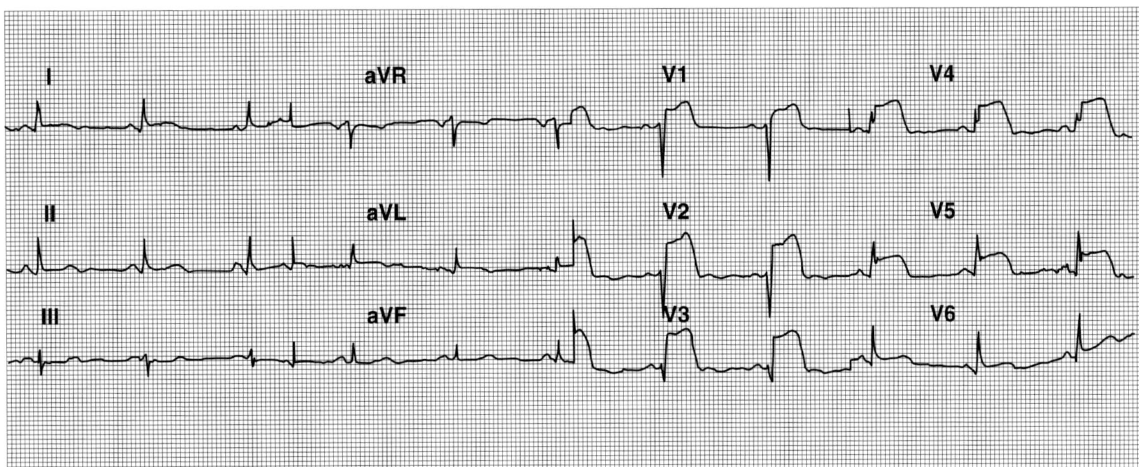

Fig. 2.12 **A,** This tracing demonstrates ST-segment elevation (STE) in what was labeled as lead II. The electrode used to obtain this lead II rhythm strip was not positioned on the left leg. Instead, it was positioned on the trunk, near the V_5 position. **B,** The 12-lead electrocardiogram from the same patient. No STE is seen in lead II. Note how similar the initial lead II tracing is to the V_5 tracing. In this instance, improper limb lead placement resulted in a tracing that more closely resembled a chest lead than a limb lead.

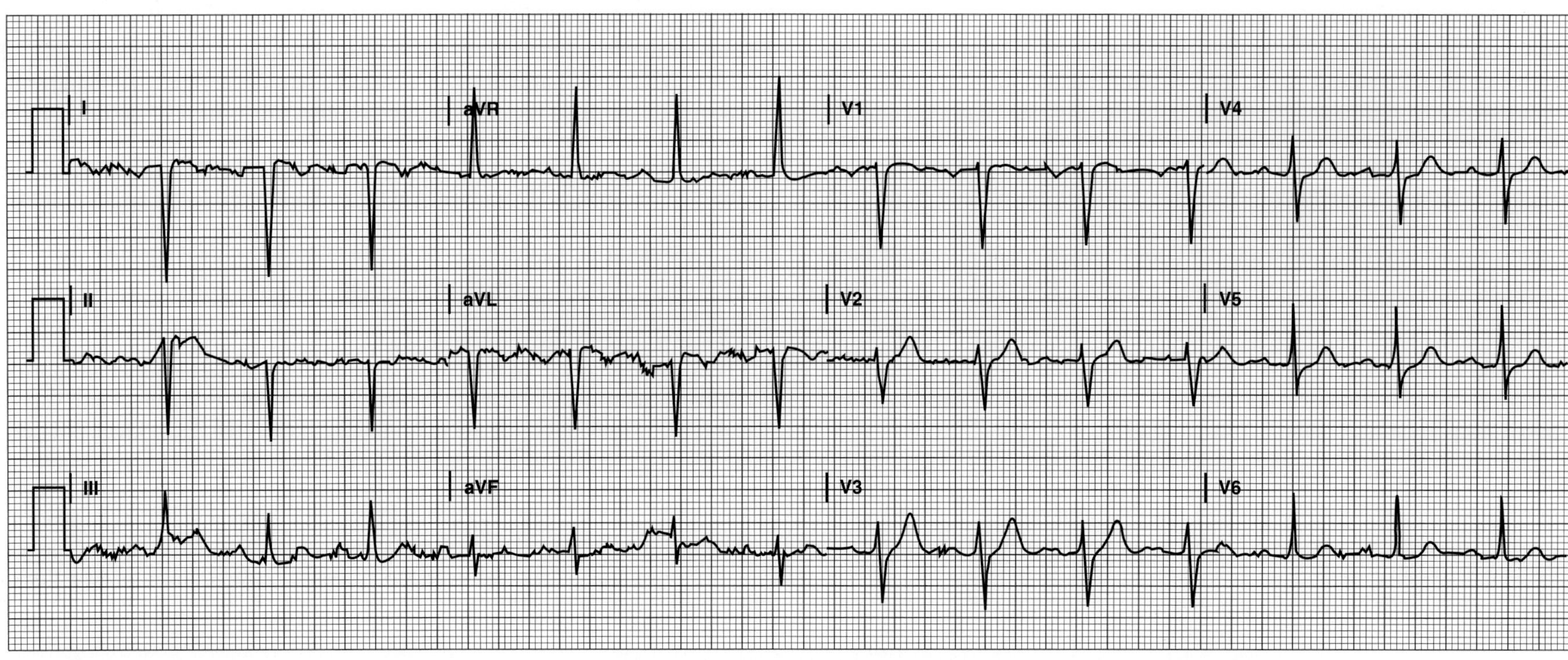

Fig. 2.13 A 12-lead electrocardiogram showing reversed arm leads. Note the negative PQRST waveforms in lead I and the positive PQRST waveforms in lead aVR.

When placing chest electrodes on these patients, place the electrodes for leads V_3 through V_6 *under* the breast rather than *on* the breast.

The most common errors in chest electrode placement are positioning the V_1 and V_2 electrodes in the second or third rather than in the fourth intercostal space and placing the V_4 to V_6 electrodes too high on the lateral chest (Mirvis & Goldberger, 2015). Placing the right chest electrodes too high on the chest can produce patterns that mimic those of anterior myocardial infarction or an intraventricular conduction delay (Mirvis & Goldberger, 2015).

Patient Positioning

Although it may not be immediately obvious, the position of the patient can affect the ECG. One reason for differences between tracings obtained in various positions is that while the electrode does not move when the patient changes position, the position of the heart does move relative to that electrode. As a result, body position changes (e.g., side-lying, elevation of the torso) can cause changes in amplitudes and axes on the ECG recording (Kligfield et al., 2007).

Ideally, a patient should be supine when the ECG is acquired. This position is preferred because it provides adequate support for the limbs so that muscle activity is minimal (Wung, 2017). If the patient is not supine when the tracing is obtained, simply note the patient's position on the 12-lead printout.

Frequency Response

The heart is not the only source of electrical activity that is detected by the ECG. Competing with the heart are such things as muscle tremor, movement artifact, 60-cycle interference, and other types of background "noise." Therefore, engineers work to produce a situation in which the monitor clearly sees the signal produced by the heart but ignores those signals that produce artifact.

To better understand this concept, once again, think of the ECG monitor as a voltmeter. Like any other voltmeter, it functions within a certain range or spectrum. If electrical activity occurs within that spectrum, the monitor senses it; if it occurs outside of the spectrum, the monitor does not sense it. The spectrum in which an ECG can accurately reproduce the signals it is sensing is referred to as the **frequency response**. Frequency response can be considered the window through which the ECG looks. If the window is wide, the ECG sees a lot; if the window is narrow, the ECG sees less. Fig. 2.14 demonstrates how changes in frequency response affect what the monitor can and cannot see.

Which is better? The answer depends on the purpose for which the ECG monitor is being used. A narrow frequency response can be referred to as *monitor quality* and a wide frequency response can be referred to as *diagnostic quality*. Monitor quality aids in rhythm analysis, while diagnostic quality is necessary for accurate ST-segment analysis. The frequency response for *monitor* quality is often 0.05 Hertz (Hz, cycles per second) to 40 Hz. The frequency response for *diagnostic* quality is 0.05 to 150 Hz. The 12-lead machine's interpretive program uses ECG data obtained at this frequency when formulating its analysis.

Some slight variation among manufacturers and ECG models may be found. Newer monitors are designed to allow the user to instantly switch between monitor quality and diagnostic quality. This allows health care professionals to use monitor quality when determining rate and rhythm and to later switch to diagnostic quality for ST-segment analysis. The frequency response is printed on the ECG paper (see Fig. 2.3).

The ECG in Fig. 2.15 was obtained from a healthy 30-year-old emergency care provider. The ST segment is elevated by about 2 mm in V_1 when recorded in monitor quality. While this tracing was being recorded, the monitor was switched from monitor quality into diagnostic quality. The fifth beat was the first to be captured in diagnostic quality. Notice that the ST segment is no longer elevated. ECG tracings obtained in monitor quality frequency response display STE that is not present in diagnostic quality. This could lead to misidentification of acute coronary syndrome patients. Furthermore, the ST segment may appear normal in monitor quality but show STE when obtained in diagnostic quality. Also note that there is more artifact in the later portion of the tracing. This demonstrates the trade-off: increased fidelity often results in greater artifact.

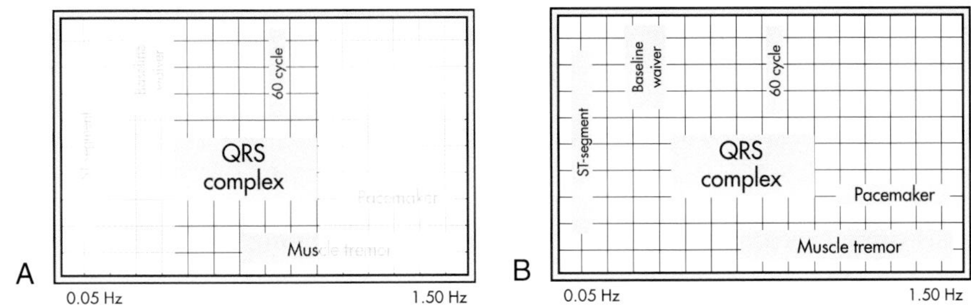

Fig. **2.14** **A,** With a limited frequency response, the monitor can clearly "see" the QRS complex but cannot see the other features as clearly. **B,** With a wider frequency response, the monitor can see the QRS complex and the ST-segment as well.

Consider This

To use STE as an indicator of infarction, the monitor must be set to standard calibration and in diagnostic quality.

Another example of how frequency response can change the ECG is demonstrated in Fig. 2.16. These strips were obtained within seconds of each other, first using monitor quality, and then using diagnostic quality. A monitor quality recording has produced STE beyond the amount present in a diagnostic quality tracing. In addition, the pacemaker spike is not clearly visible in the first tracing (monitor quality) but is prominent in the second tracing (diagnostic quality).

Goal 3: Fast

When treating patients experiencing an ACS, much has to be accomplished in a short time. Fortunately, a 12-lead ECG can be obtained very quickly, even in these circumstances. Speed of acquisition is particularly important to prehospital professionals because the goal is to be able to obtain a 12-lead ECG without an increase in scene time.

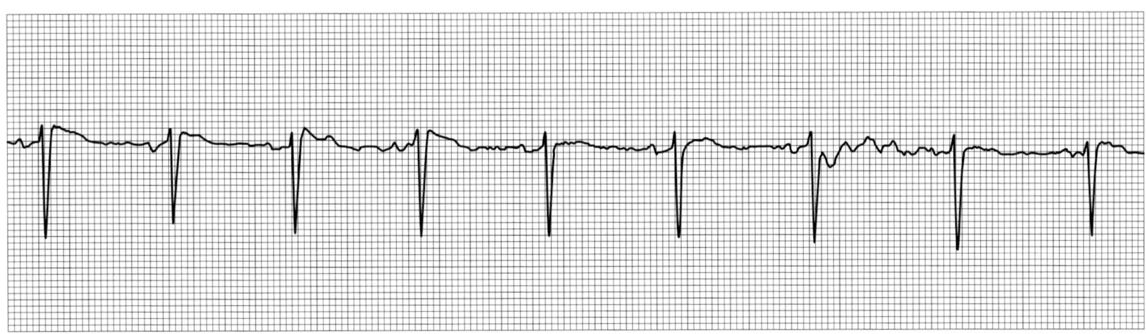

Fig. **2.15** The first four beats were obtained in monitor quality and demonstrate 2 mm of STE. The fifth beat was obtained in diagnostic quality and shows no STE.

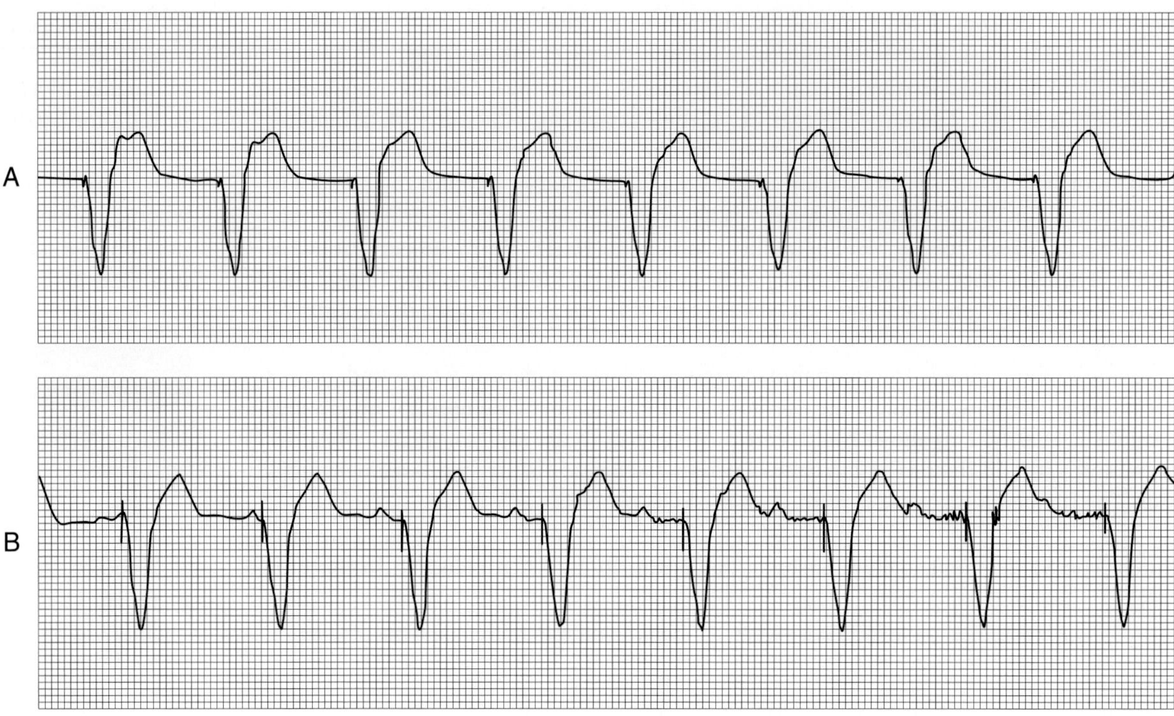

Fig. 2.16 **A,** Tracing obtained in monitor quality. The patient's pacemaker was firing, but no pacemaker spikes are visible. The STE is prominent. **B,** The same patient, with the tracing obtained in diagnostic quality. The pacemaker spikes are now visible, as are some P waves with PR intervals that gradually lengthen.

The solution is to gain proficiency in the skill. Just as with virtually every other skill, 12-lead acquisition can be done more quickly with practice. Ideally, practice would be gained on various body types and genders.

REFERENCES

Bond, R. R., Finlay, D. D., Nugent, C. D., Breen, C., Guldenring, D., & Daly, M. J. (2012). The effects of electrode misplacement on clinicians' interpretation of the standard 12-lead electrocardiogram. *European Journal of Internal Medicine, 23*(7), 610–615.

Ching, S., & Ting, S. M. (2015). The forgotten lead: aVR in left main disease. *American Journal of Medicine, 128*(12), e11–e13.

Francis, J. (2016). ECG monitoring leads and special leads. *Indian Pacing and Electrophysiology Journal, 16*(3), 92–95.

Ganz, L. (2016). Electrocardiography. In L. Goldman & A. I. Schafer (Eds.), *Goldman's Cecil medicine* (25th ed., pp. 267–273). Philadelphia, PA: Saunders.

Greenfield Jr., J. C. (2008). Erroneous electrocardiogram recordings because of switched electrode leads. *Journal of Electrocardiology, 41*(5), 376–377.

Harrigan, R. A., Chan, T. C., & Brady, W. J. (2012). Electrocardiographic electrode misplacement, misconnection, and artifact. *Journal of Emergency Medicine, 43*(6), 1038–1044.

Kligfield, P., Gettes, L. S., Bailey, J. J., Childers, R., Deal, B. J., Hancock, E. W., et al. (2007). Recommendations for the standardization and interpretation of the electrocardiogram part I: The electrocardiogram and its technology. *Journal of the American College of Cardiology, 49*(10), 1109–1127.

Knight, B. P., Pelosi, F., Michaud, G. F., Strickberger, S. A., & Morady, F. (2001). Physician interpretation of electrocardiographic artifact that mimics ventricular tachycardia. *American Journal of Medicine, 110*(5), 335–338.

Lam, A., Wagner, G. S., & Pahlm, O. (2015). The classical versus the Cabrera presentation system for resting electrocardiography: Impact on recognition and understanding of clinically important electrocardiographic changes. *Journal of Electrocardiology, 48*(4), 476–482.

Lederer, W. J. (2017). Cardiac electrophysiology and the electrocardiogram. In W. F. Boron & E. L. Boulpaep (Eds.), *Medical physiology* (3rd ed., pp. 483–506). Philadelphia, PA: Elsevier.

Mirvis, D. M., & Goldberger, A. L. (2015). Electrocardiography. In D. L. Mann, D. P. Zipes, P. Libby, R. O. Bonow, & E. Braunwald (Eds.), *Braunwald's heart disease: A textbook of cardiovascular medicine* (10th ed., pp. 114–154). Philadelphia, PA: Saunders.

Omar, H. R., & Camporesi, E. M. (2014). The importance of lead aVR interpretation by emergency physicians. *American Journal of Emergency Medicine, 32*(10), 1289–1290.

Pahlm, O., & Wagner, G. S. (2008). Proximal placement of limb electrodes: a potential solution for acquiring standard electrocardiogram waveforms from monitoring electrode positions. *Journal of Electrocardiology, 41*(6), 454–457.

Pelter, M. M., & Carey, M. G. (2017). Cardiac monitoring and electrocardiographic leads. In D. J. Lynn-McHale Wiegand (Ed.), *AACN procedure manual for high acuity, progressive, and critical care* (7th ed., pp. 467–476). St. Louis, MO: Elsevier.

Sejersten, M., Pahlm, O., Pettersson, J., Zhou, S., Maynard, C., Feldman, C. L., et al. (2006). Comparison of EASI-derived 12-lead electrocardiograms versus paramedic-acquired 12-lead electrocardiograms using Mason-Likar limb lead configuration in patients with chest pain. *Journal of Electrocardiology*, 39(1), 13–31.

Surawicz, B., Childers, R., Deal, B. J., & Gettes, L. S. (2009). AHA/ACCF/HRS Recommendations for the standardization and interpretation of the electrocardiogram: Part III: Intraventricular conduction disturbances: A scientific statement from the American Heart Association Electrocardiography and Arrhythmias Committee. *Journal of the American College of Cardiology, 53*(11), 976–981.

Talebi, S., Visco, F., Pekler, G., Savi, M., Fernaine, G., Chaudhari, S., et al. (2015). Diagnostic value of lead aVR in acute coronary syndrome. *American Journal of Emergency Medicine, 33*(10), 1527–1530.

Vorobiof, G., & Ellestad, M. H. (2011). Lead aVR: Dead or simply forgotten? *JACC. Cardiovascular Imaging, 4*(2), 187–190.

Wagner, G. S., Macfarlane, P., Wellens, H., Josephson, M., Gorgels, A., Mirvis, D. M., et al. (2009). AHA/ACCF/HRS recommendations for the standardization and interpretation of the electrocardiogram: Part VI: Acute ischemia/infarction; a scientific statement from the American Heart Association Electrocardiography and Arrhythmias Committee. *Journal of the American College of Cardiology, 53*(11), 1003–1011.

Wung, S. F. (2017). Twelve-lead electrocardiogram. In D. J. Lynn-McHale Wiegand (Ed.), *AACN procedure manual for high acuity, progressive, and critical care* (7th ed., pp. 494–500). St. Louis: Elsevier.

QUICK REVIEW

1. Which of the following view the lateral surface of the left ventricle?
   a. Leads V_1 and V_2
   b. Leads V_3 and V_4
   c. Leads II, III, and aVF
   d. Leads I, aVL, V_5, and V_6

2. Which of the following are chest (i.e., precordial) leads?
   a. Leads I and aVL
   b. Leads I, II, and III
   c. Leads V_1, V_2, V_3, V_4, V_5, and V_6
   d. Leads I, II, III, aVR, aVL, and aVF

3. Where should the positive electrode for lead V_5 be positioned?
   a. Left midaxillary line at same level as V_4
   b. Left anterior axillary line at same level as V_4
   c. Left side of sternum, fourth intercostal space
   d. Right side of sternum, fourth intercostal space

4. In the hexaxial reference system, lead I is perpendicular to lead
   a. II.
   b. III.
   c. aVF.
   d. aVL.

5. Which leads look at adjoining tissue in the anterior region of the left ventricle?
   a. V_2, V_3, V_4
   b. II, III, aVF
   c. I, aVL, V_5
   d. aVR, aVL, aVF

6. When leads I and aVF are used to determine electrical axis, left axis deviation is present if the QRS is
   a. positive in lead I and positive in lead aVF.
   b. positive in lead I and negative in lead aVF.
   c. negative in lead I and negative in lead aVF.
   d. negative in lead I and positive in lead aVF.

ANSWERS

1. **D**. Leads I, aVL, V_5, and V_6 view the lateral surface of the left ventricle.

2. **C**. Six chest (i.e., precordial or "V") leads view the heart in the horizontal plane. The chest leads are identified as V_1, V_2, V_3, V_4, V_5, and V_6.

3. **B**. Lead V_4 is recorded with the positive electrode in the left midclavicular line in the fifth intercostal space. Lead V_5 is recorded with the positive electrode in the left anterior axillary line at the same level as V_4.

4. **C**. In the hexaxial reference system, the axes of some leads are perpendicular to each other. Lead I is perpendicular to lead aVF. Lead II is perpendicular to aVL, and lead III is perpendicular to lead aVR.

5. **A**. Leads V_2, V_3, and V_4 are next to each other on the patient's chest. Leads V_1 and V_2 view the septum. Leads V_3 and V_4 look at the anterior wall of the left ventricle. Therefore, leads V_2, V_3, and V_4 look at adjoining tissue in the anterior region of the left ventricle.

6. **B**. Leads I and aVF divide the heart into four quadrants. These two leads can be used to quickly estimate electrical axis. If the QRS is positive in lead I and negative in lead aVF, left axis deviation is present.

Acute Coronary Syndromes

3

CHAPTER

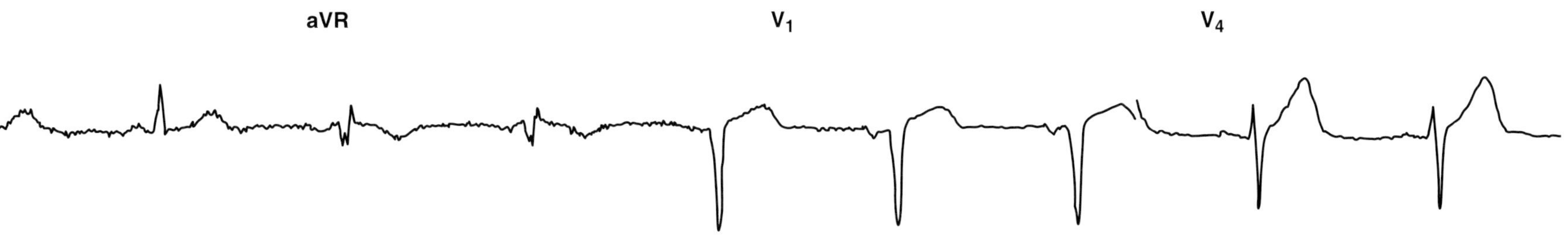

LEARNING OBJECTIVES

After reading this chapter, you should be able to:

1. Describe the pathophysiology of coronary heart disease.
2. Differentiate the characteristics of stable (classic) angina, unstable angina (UA), and acute myocardial infarction (MI).
3. Recognize the electrocardiographic (ECG) changes produced by myocardial ischemia, injury, and infarction.
4. Localize the area of MI and predict which coronary artery is occluded.
5. Explain the importance of the 12-lead ECG in acute coronary syndromes (ACSs).
6. Discuss the three groups used when categorizing the ECG findings of the patient experiencing an ACS.

KEY TERMS

angina pectoris: Chest discomfort of sudden onset that occurs when the increased oxygen demand of the heart temporarily exceeds the blood supply
anginal equivalents: Symptoms of myocardial ischemia other than chest pain or discomfort
coronary heart disease: Atherosclerosis of the coronary arteries
transmural MI: An MI extending from the endocardium to the epicardium

CORONARY HEART DISEASE

Recall from Chapter 1 that acute coronary syndrome (ACS) refers to distinct conditions caused by a similar sequence of pathologic events involving abruptly reduced coronary artery blood flow (Amsterdam et al., 2014). The usual cause of an ACS is the rupture of an atherosclerotic plaque.

Atherosclerosis is a systemic disease in which the innermost layer of large- and middle-sized muscular arteries undergoes changes in response to endothelial injury. This layer is vulnerable to damage arising from conditions including hypertension, high cholesterol, and smoking (Fig. 3.1). The arteries that are the most heavily affected by atherosclerosis include the abdominal aorta, coronary arteries, ilio-femoral arteries, and carotid bifurcations (Falk & Bentzon, 2017). In coronary heart disease, atherosclerosis builds up in the coronary arteries. The major risk factors that promote the development of atherosclerosis appear in Box 3.1.

Atherosclerotic lesions include the fatty streak, fibrous plaque, and the complicated lesion. Fatty streaks are thin lesions composed of lipids (mostly cholesterol) or smooth muscle cells that protrude slightly into the arterial opening. They appear in all populations, even those with a low incidence of coronary artery disease (CAD). Once formed, fatty streaks produce more toxic oxygen radicals and cause immunologic and inflammatory changes, resulting in progressive damage to the vessel wall (Brashers, 2014). Progression from a fatty streak to a complicated lesion is associated with injured endothelium that activates the inflammatory response. As the inflammatory response continues, the fatty streak becomes a fatty plaque, then a fibrous plaque, and finally, a complicated lesion where hemorrhage occurs within the plaque and a thrombus forms.

Atherosclerotic plaques differ with regard to their makeup, their vulnerability to rupture, and their tendency to form a blood clot. A "stable" or "nonvulnerable" atherosclerotic plaque has a relatively thick fibrous cap that separates it from contact with the blood and covers a core that contains a large amount of collagen and smooth muscle cells but a relatively small lipid pool (Fig. 3.2). As these plaques increase in size, the artery can become severely narrowed (i.e., stenosed). Narrowing of the coronary artery may cause different clinical symptoms depending on the extent of occlusion and the speed at which it develops (Fig. 3.3) (Damjanov, 2017).

The walls of an artery outwardly expand (i.e., remodel) as plaque builds up inside it. This occurs so that the size of the vessel stays relatively constant, despite the increased size of the plaque. When the plaque fills about 40% of the vessel lumen, remodeling stops because the artery can no longer expand to make room for the increase in plaque size. Because the plaque usually increases in size over months and years, other vascular pathways may enlarge as portions of a coronary artery become blocked. These vascular pathways (i.e., collateral circulation) serve as an alternative route for blood flow around the blocked artery to the heart muscle. Thus, the presence of collateral arteries may prevent infarction despite complete blockage of the artery.

Factors that contribute to the transformation of a stable atherosclerotic plaque to a so-called vulnerable plaque include local and systemic inflammation, mechanical features, and anatomic changes (Lange & Hillis, 2016). If the fibrous cap tears or ruptures, the contents of the plaque (i.e., collagen, smooth muscle cells, tissue factor, inflammatory cells, and lipid material) are exposed to flowing blood. Platelets stick to the damaged lining of the vessel and to each other and form a plug. "Sticky platelets" secrete several chemicals, including thromboxane A_2. These substances stimulate vasoconstriction, reducing blood flow at the site. Once platelets are activated, thrombin is generated and fibrin is formed, ultimately producing a fibrin-rich thrombus (i.e., clot) (Anderson, 2016).

Consider This

Aspirin (an antiplatelet agent) blocks the production of thromboxane A_2, slowing down the clumping of platelets and lowering the risk of complete blockage of the vessel. Glycoprotein IIb/IIIa receptor inhibitors are medications that prevent fibrinogen binding and platelet clumping. Fibrinolytics are medications that stimulate the conversion of plasminogen to plasmin, which dissolves clots.

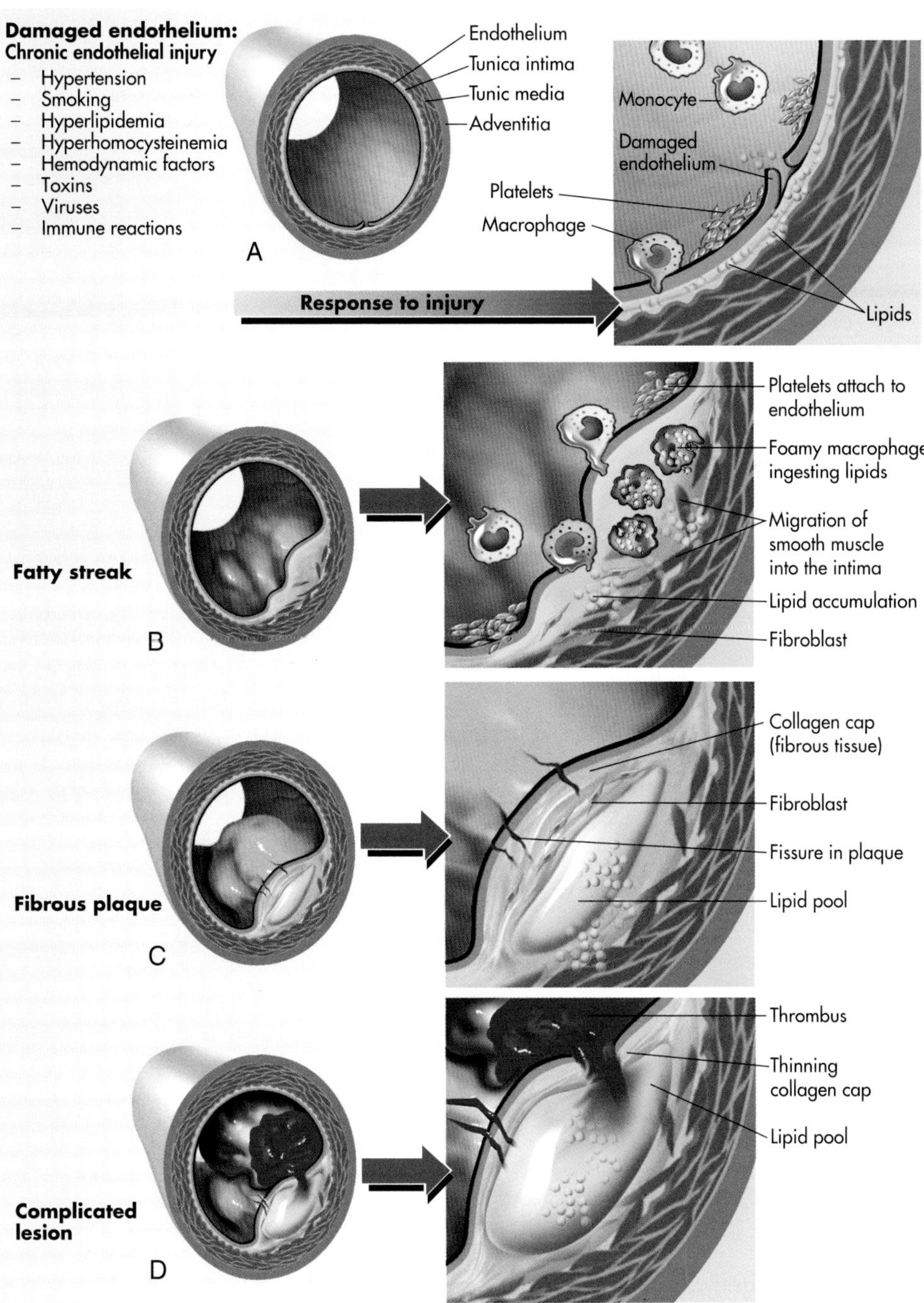

Fig. 3.1 Pathogenesis of atherosclerosis. **A,** Damaged endothelium. **B,** Diagram of fatty streak and lipid core formation. **C,** Diagram of fibrous plaque. Raised plaques are visible: Some are yellow; others are white. **D,** Diagram of complicated lesion: Thrombus is red; collagen is blue. Plaque is complicated by red thrombus deposition. (From McCance, K. L., Huether, S. E., Brashers, V. L., & Rote, N. S. [2014]. *Pathophysiology, the pathological basis for disease in adults and children* [7th ed.]. St. Louis, MO: Mosby.)

Box 3.1 Cardiovascular Disease Risk Factors

NONMODIFIABLE (FIXED) FACTORS
- Advancing age
- Family history of coronary heart disease, ischemic stroke, or peripheral arterial disease
- Gender
- Race

MODIFIABLE FACTORS
- Abdominal obesity
- Cigarette smoking
- Elevated low-density lipoprotein cholesterol level
- Elevated triglyceride level
- Hypertension
- Low high-density lipoprotein level
- Physical inactivity
- Type 2 diabetes

CONTRIBUTING FACTORS
- Elevated inflammatory markers
- Psychosocial factors (e.g., job stress, life events, reactions to stress)

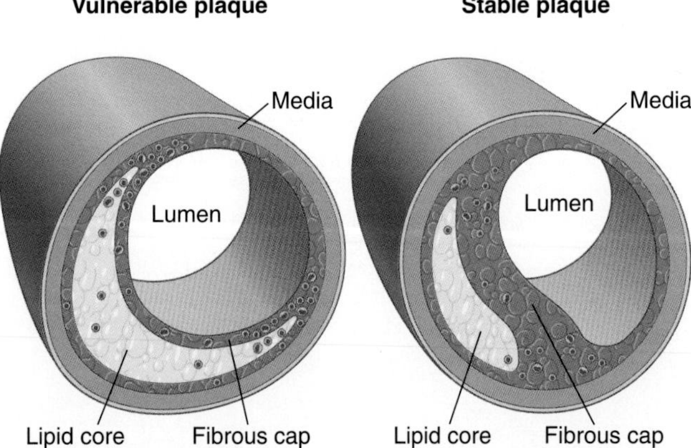

Fig. 3.2 Vulnerable and stable atherosclerotic plaque. (From Kumar, V., Abbas, A. K., & Aster, J. C. [2013]. *Robbins basic pathology* [9th ed.]. Philadelphia, PA: Saunders.)

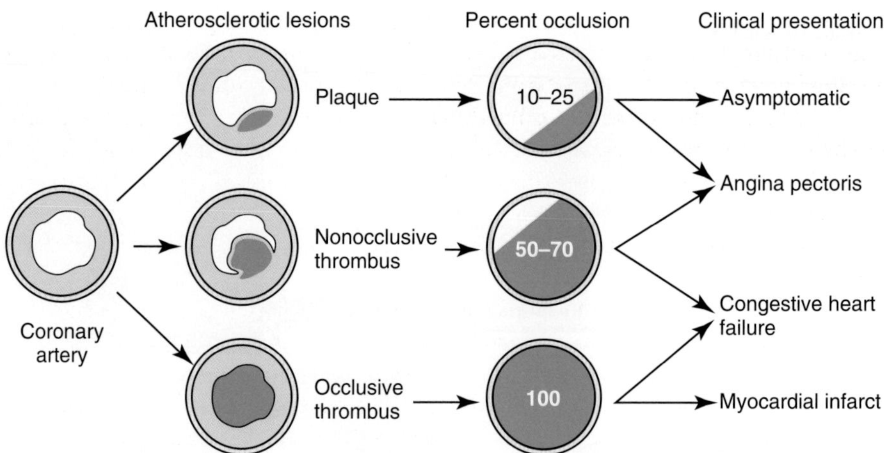

Fig. 3.3 Narrowing of the coronary artery may cause different clinical symptoms depending on the extent of occlusion and the speed at which it develops. (From Damjanov, I. [2017]. *Pathology for the health professions* [5th ed.]. St. Louis, MO: Elsevier.)

ISCHEMIC HEART DISEASE

Myocardial ischemia is usually the result of the blockage or gradual narrowing of one or more of the epicardial coronary arteries by atheromatous plaque (Morrow & Boden, 2015). Factors such as endothelial dysfunction, microvascular disease, and vasospasm may also exist alone or in combination with coronary atherosclerosis and may be the major cause of myocardial ischemia in some patients (Morrow & Boden, 2015) (Fig. 3.4).

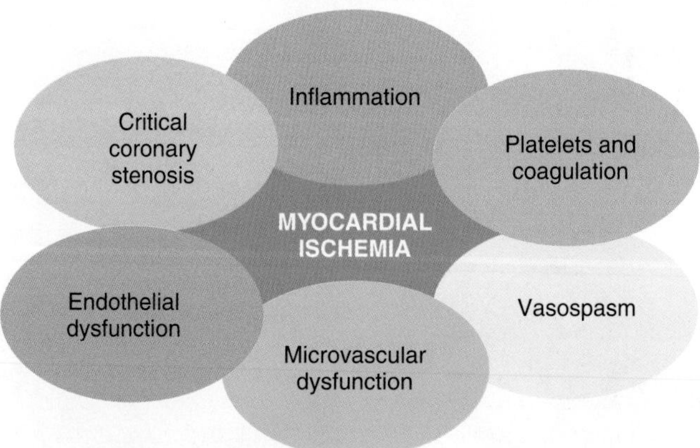

Fig. 3.4 Pathophysiology of ischemic heart disease. (From Mann, D. L., Zipes, D. P., Libby, P., Bonow, R. O., & Braunwald, E. [2015]. *Braunwald's heart disease: A textbook of cardiovascular medicine* [10th ed.]. Philadelphia, PA: Saunders.)

Narrowing or blockage of a coronary artery can disrupt the oxygen supply to the area of the heart supplied by the affected vessel(s). If the cause of the ischemia is not reversed and blood flow is not restored to the affected area of the heart muscle, ischemia may lead to cellular injury and, ultimately, cellular death (i.e., infarction). Clinical presentations of ischemic heart disease may include angina pectoris, silent myocardial ischemia, acute myocardial infarction (MI), or sudden cardiac death. Early assessment and emergency care are essential to prevent worsening ischemia.

Angina pectoris is the most common clinical expression of myocardial ischemia (Boden, 2016). It most often occurs in patients with CAD involving at least one coronary artery. However, it can be present in patients with normal coronary arteries. Angina also occurs in persons with uncontrolled hypertension or valvular heart disease. Angina typically occurs because of an imbalance between myocardial oxygen demand (i.e., increased myocardial oxygen requirements) and myocardial oxygen supply (i.e., decreased coronary blood flow). Ischemia can quickly resolve by reducing the heart's oxygen demand (by resting or slowing the heart rate with medications such as beta-blockers) or increasing blood flow by dilating the coronary arteries with medications such as nitroglycerin (NTG).

Clinical Features

The discomfort associated with angina is thought to be caused by substances such as lactate, histamine, adenosine, bradykinin, and serotonin that build up during periods of lactic acidosis and then irritate nerve endings when they are released into the circulation (Tobin & Eagle, 2017). Although ischemic chest discomfort can occur anywhere in the chest, neck, arms, or back, it usually begins in the central or left chest and then radiates to the arm (especially the little finger [ulnar] side of the left arm), the wrist, the jaw, the epigastrium, the left shoulder, or between the shoulder blades (Fig. 3.5). Common words used by patients experiencing angina to describe the sensation they are feeling are shown in Box 3.2.

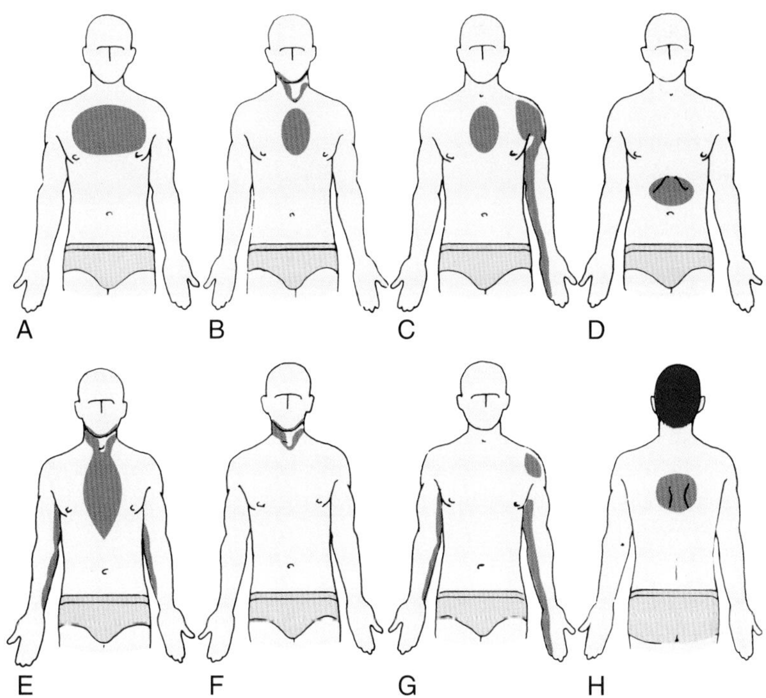

Fig. 3.5 Common sites for anginal discomfort. **A,** Upper part of chest. **B,** Beneath the sternum radiating to neck and jaw. **C,** Beneath the sternum radiating down left arm. **D,** Epigastric. **E,** Epigastric radiating to the neck, jaw, and arms. **F,** Neck and jaw. **G,** Left shoulder. **H,** Interscapular. (From Urden, L. D., Stacy, K. M., & Lough, M. E. [2018]. *Critical care nursing: Diagnosis and management* [8th ed.]. St. Louis, MO; Mosby.)

Consider This

Not all chest discomfort is cardiac related. Obtaining an accurate history is important to help determine if a patient's signs and symptoms are most likely related to ischemia secondary to coronary artery disease.

Box 3.2 Words Patients Often Use to Describe Angina

"Heaviness"
"Pressing"
"Suffocating"
"Squeezing"
"Strangling"
"Constricting"
"Bursting"
"Burning"
"Grip-like"
"A band across my chest"
"A weight in the center of my chest"
"A vise tightening around my chest"

Although chest discomfort is the classic symptom associated with ischemic heart disease, anginal equivalents (i.e., symptoms of myocardial ischemia other than chest pain or discomfort) may be present. Box 3.3 lists examples of anginal equivalents.

Anginal equivalents are common, particularly in older adults, individuals with diabetes, women, patients with prior cardiac surgery, and patients in the immediate postoperative period of noncardiac surgery (Karve, Bossone, & Mehta, 2007). Older adults may have atypical symptoms such as dyspnea, syncope, upper extremity pain, weakness, a

Box 3.3 Examples of Anginal Equivalents

- Abdominal or epigastric discomfort
- Acute change in mental status
- Difficulty breathing
- Dizziness
- Dysrhythmias
- Excessive sweating
- Generalized weakness
- Isolated arm or jaw pain
- Lightheadedness
- Palpitations
- Shoulder or back pain
- Sudden fatigue
- Syncope or near-syncope
- Unexplained nausea or vomiting

change in mental status, unexplained nausea, and abdominal or epigastric discomfort (Glickman et al., 2012). They are also more likely to present with more severe preexisting conditions, such as hypertension, heart failure, or a previous acute MI, than a younger patient. Diabetic individuals may present atypically because of autonomic dysfunction. Common signs and symptoms include generalized weakness, syncope, lightheadedness, or a change in mental status.

Women with ischemic heart disease often have anginal equivalent symptoms (Table 3.1). Failing to recognize the significance of their symptoms, some patients ignore them, whereas others seek medical assistance but find that their symptoms are minimized,

TABLE 3.1 Cardiovascular Symptoms Experienced by Women

Symptom 1 month before acute MI	Percentage	Symptom during acute MI	Percentage
Unusual fatigue	71%	Shortness of breath	58%
Sleep disturbance	48%	Weakness	55%
Shortness of breath	42%	Unusual fatigue	43%
Indigestion	39%	Cold sweat	39%
Anxiety	36%	Dizziness	39%
Heart racing	27%	Nausea	36%
Arm heaviness or weakness	25%	Arm heaviness or weakness	35%
Changes in thinking or memory	24%	Ache in arms	32%
Vision change	23%	Heat or flushing	32%
Loss of appetite	22%	Indigestion	31%
Hands or arm tingling	22%	Pain centered high in the chest	31%
Difficulty breathing at night	19%	Heart racing	23%

MI, Myocardial infarction.
Source: McSweeney et al. (2003)

misdiagnosed, or ignored by clinicians (McSweeney, Cody, O'Sullivan, Elberson, Moser, & Garvin, 2003). Several interesting findings were reported in a 2003 study of 515 women with a diagnosis of acute MI (McSweeney et al., 2003):

- About 78% of women reported at least one prodromal symptom for more than 1 month either daily or several times a week before the acute MI. Only about 30% reported chest discomfort, which they described as aching (33%), tightness (33%), pressure (32%), sharpness (23%), burning (21%), fullness (18%), and tingling (18%). Descriptors were not mutually exclusive.
- The most frequent acute symptoms were shortness of breath (58%), weakness (55%), unusual fatigue (43%), cold sweat (39%), and dizziness (39%). Descriptors were not mutually exclusive. Forty-three percent did not experience any type of chest discomfort with acute MI. When chest discomfort/pain was present, the main locations were in the back (37%) and high chest (28%), and the pain was most commonly described as pressure (22%), an ache (15%), or tightness (15%) and was frequently rated as severe in intensity (59%). Selections were not mutually exclusive.

Diagnosis

Possible diagnostic studies that may be obtained in a patient with a complaint of chest discomfort include laboratory tests (including cardiac biomarkers), a 12-lead electrocardiogram (ECG), a chest radiograph, and echocardiography. Noninvasive stress testing or coronary angiography, or both, may be performed to define the amount of ischemic myocardium and determine an overall treatment plan (Tobin & Eagle, 2017).

Consider This

Injured myocardial cells release enzymes and proteins that pass through broken cell membranes and leak into the bloodstream. Examples include myoglobin, cardiac troponins T (TnT) and I (TnI), creatine kinase (CK) and its myocardial band (MB) isoform, and lactate dehydrogenase, among others (Halim, Newby, & Ohman, 2010). The presence of these substances in the blood, which are called *cardiac biomarkers, serum cardiac markers, or serum biomarkers,* can subsequently be measured by means of blood tests to verify the presence of an infarction.

The 12-lead ECG is an important diagnostic tool for patients presenting with ischemic chest discomfort or anginal equivalent symptoms. The first 12-lead ECG should be obtained within 10 minutes of patient contact. Although ECG findings may be normal at rest, they become abnormal during an episode of angina in 50% or more of patients with ischemic heart disease (Morrow & Boden, 2015). The most common finding is transient ST-segment depression, reflecting subendocardial ischemia (Cinquegrani, 2016). Because ischemia affects repolarization, its effects can be viewed on the ECG as changes in ST segments and T waves (Fig. 3.6). When measured at the J point, an ST-segment depression of 0.5 mm or more is suggestive of myocardial ischemia when viewed in two or more anatomically contiguous

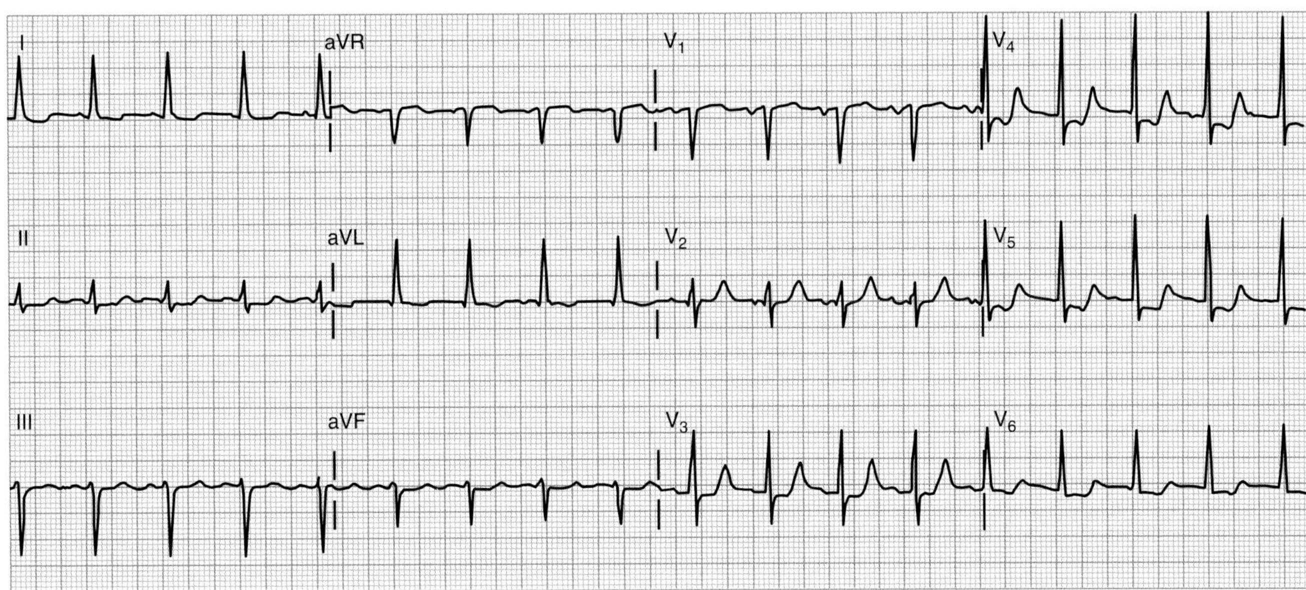

A

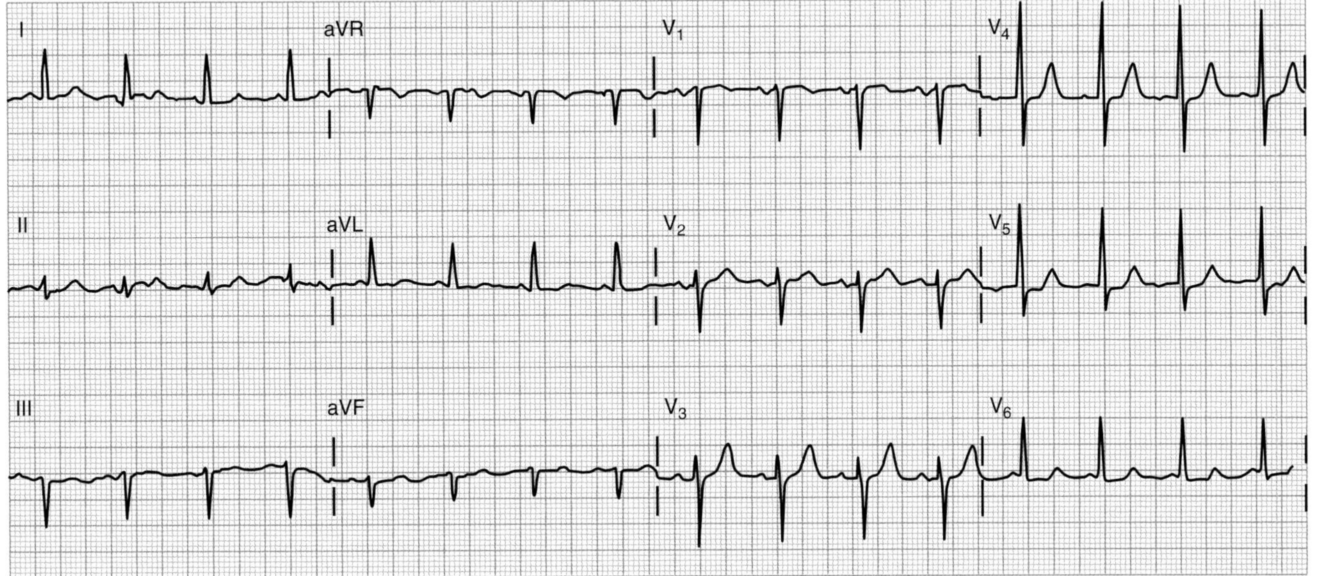

B

Fig. 3.6 Electrocardiogram obtained **(A)** during angina and **(B)** after the administration of sublingual nitroglycerin and subsequent resolution of angina. During angina, transient ST-segment depression and T-wave abnormalities are present. (From Benjamin, I. J., Griggs, R. C., Wing, E. J., & Fitz, J. G. [2016]. *Andreoli and Carpenter's Cecil essentials of medicine* [9th ed.]. Philadelphia, PA: Saunders.)

leads (Thygesen et al., 2012). Negative (i.e., inverted) T waves may also be present. After the episode of chest discomfort is resolved, ST segments usually return to the baseline.

Stable Angina

Stable (i.e., classic) angina remains relatively constant and predictable in terms of severity, signs and symptoms, precipitating events, and response to treatment. It is characterized by brief episodes of chest discomfort related to activities that increase the heart's need for oxygen. Common precipitating events and possible related signs and symptoms are shown in Box 3.4. Symptoms typically last less than 5 minutes and are usually relieved within 5 minutes with rest, short-acting NTG, or both (Amsterdam et al., 2014). A delay of more than 5 to 10 minutes before relief is obtained with rest and NTG suggests that the symptoms are either not caused by ischemia or are caused by severe ischemia, as with unstable angina (UA) or acute MI (Morrow & Boden, 2015).

Variant Angina

Variant angina, also called *Prinzmetal angina* or *Prinzmetal variant angina*, is an uncommon form of angina. It is the result of intense spasm of a segment of a coronary artery. This variant angina may occur in otherwise healthy individuals with no demonstrable coronary heart disease or in patients with a nonobstructive atheromatous plaque. It can be difficult to suspect variant angina from the patient's clinical presentation. Patients with variant angina are generally younger and have fewer coronary risk factors (except for smoking) compared with patients with chronic stable angina. In some patients, variant angina has been associated with migraine headache and Raynaud phenomenon, suggesting a possible association with a more generalized vasospastic disorder (Boden, 2016).

Variant angina usually occurs at rest, often occurs between midnight and 8 a.m., and may awaken the patient from sleep (Kawano et al., 2002). Episodes may occur in clusters of two or three within 30 to 60 minutes. Contributing factors include cigarette smoking, cocaine use, exposure to cold, hyperventilation, hypomagnesemia, insulin resistance, medications (e.g., antimigraine agents, chemotherapy, anesthetics, antibiotics), and vitamin E deficiency (Kaski & Arroyo-Espliguero, 2010).

Although episodes usually last only a few minutes, they are often described as severe and may be accompanied by syncope related to atrioventricular (AV) block or ventricular dysrhythmias (Kaski & Arroyo-Espliguero, 2010). If the spasm is prolonged, it may lead to subendocardial or transmural MI (i.e., extending from the endocardium to the epicardium) and sudden cardiac death (Kaski & Arroyo-Espliguero, 2010).

Recall that ECG changes observed with classic angina include ST-segment *depression*. By contrast, variant angina usually produces ST-segment *elevation* (STE) during anginal episodes. Chest discomfort and ECG changes may resolve spontaneously or they can be relieved by NTG. After the episode is resolved, ST segments usually return to the baseline. Because NTG is effective at relieving coronary spasm, the ECG evidence of variant angina may be lost if no pretreatment ECG is obtained.

A multilead ECG showing STE in leads supplied by the left coronary artery (LCA) is shown in Fig. 3.7. This tracing was obtained a few moments before the administration of NTG. The patient reported that the NTG had relieved the chest pain, and a second tracing was then obtained. The obvious STE noted in the first example is no longer present, suggesting the possibility of variant angina (Fig. 3.8).

It is important to recognize that patients with near-complete coronary artery occlusion in the presence of exertional or physiologic stress can also demonstrate STE that resolves with NTG administration. The importance of considering the patient's clinical picture, history, etc., and not just his or her ECG changes, cannot be overemphasized when managing these patients.

Box 3.4 Stable Angina Pectoris

COMMON PRECIPITATING EVENTS
- Emotional upset
- Exercise/exertion
- Exposure to cold weather

RELATED SIGNS AND SYMPTOMS
- Shortness of breath
- Palpitations
- Sweating
- Nausea or vomiting

Microvascular Angina

Angina sometimes occurs in the absence of significant atherosclerosis or vasospasm of the epicardial coronary arteries. With microvascular angina, angina is related to disease of the small, distal branches of the coronary arteries (i.e., coronary microvascular disease [CMD]). Ischemia and angina occur because functional and structural changes in the coronary microvasculature disrupt the ability of the vessels to dilate and increase

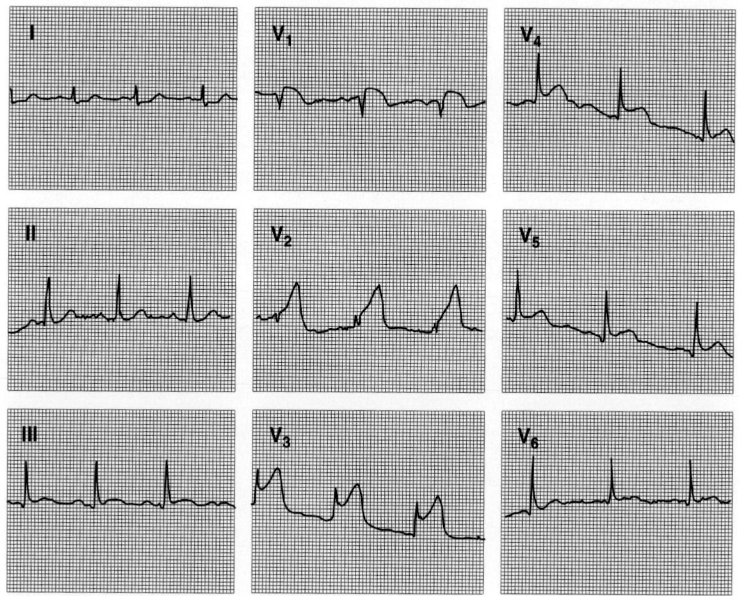

Fig. 3.7 A multilead electrocardiogram showing ST-elevation in leads supplied by the left coronary artery. This tracing was obtained a few moments before the administration of nitroglycerin.

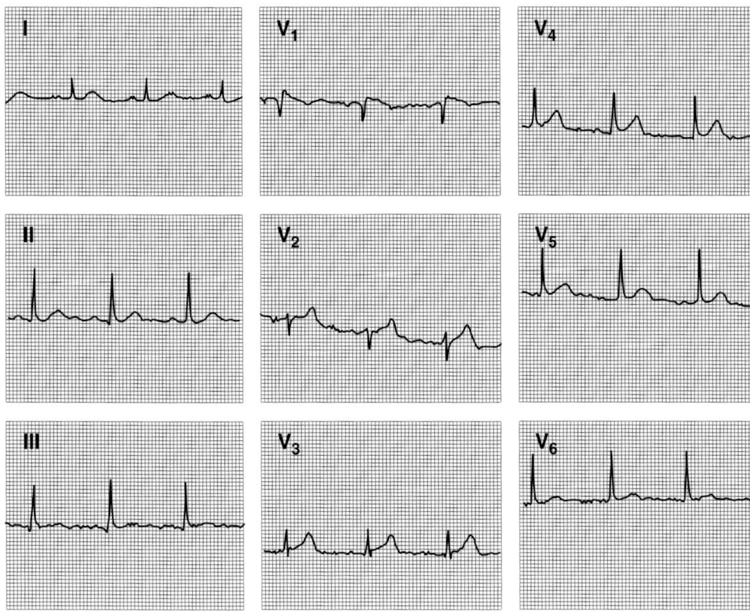

Fig. 3.8 Electrocardiogram obtained after nitroglycerin administration.

coronary blood flow in response to increased myocardial oxygen demand (Chen, Wei, AlBadri, Zarrini, & Bairey Merz, 2016). Patients with CMD have significantly higher rates of cardiovascular events, including hospitalization for heart failure, sudden cardiac death, and MI (Chen et al., 2016).

Consider This

Microvascular angina can be present in patients with and without obstructive epicardial CAD (Löffler & Bourque, 2016).

The pathophysiology of this type of angina is complex. Possible mechanisms include endothelial dysfunction, microvascular spasm, generalized vascular disorder, and abnormal subendocardial perfusion. Possible contributing factors include increased systemic inflammation, insulin resistance, abnormal vasoconstriction and impaired vasodilation of the microvascular bed, estrogen deficiency, and increased cardiac pain sensitivity, among others. Patients with microvascular angina have risk factors similar to those of epicardial CAD (Löffler & Bourque, 2016).

Microvascular angina is most often seen in perimenopausal and postmenopausal women (Naderi & Cho, 2016). Anginal episodes are often characterized by dull chest pain after exertion (Naderi & Cho, 2016) that typically persists for several minutes after interrupting efforts and/or shows a poor or slow response to NTG (Crea, Camici, & Bairey Merz, 2014). There is conflicting evidence with regard to current treatment strategies.

The types of angina are compared in Table 3.2.

TABLE 3.2 Angina Pectoris

Type	Pathology	Characteristics	Therapy
Stable	70% or greater luminal narrowing of one or more coronary arteries from atherosclerosis	• Predictable pattern provoked by emotional upset, exercise or exertion, exposure to cold • Symptoms usually last less than 5 minutes • ST-segment depression during anginal episodes • Relieved with rest or NTG	• Aspirin • Sublingual NTG • Attention given to reduction of modifiable risk factors (e.g., smoking cessation, exercise, weight control, BP control, statins)
Variant	Coronary vasospasm	• Typically occurs at rest • Transient STE during episodes	• Calcium channel blockers • Nitrates
Microvascular	Disease affecting the distal branches of coronary arteries	• More common in women • Episodes often associated with lingering discomfort after exertion • ST-segment depression during anginal episodes	• Nitrates (inconsistent beneficial effects) • ACE inhibitors • Estrogen • Transcutaneous electrical nerve stimulation • Lifestyle modification
Unstable	Plaque rupture with platelet and fibrin thrombus, causing worsening coronary obstruction	• Increase in frequency, duration, or severity of anginal episodes • New-onset angina or now occurring at rest or with low level of activity • Discomfort that may be described as painful • Symptoms last for 10 minutes or more • ST-segment depression during anginal episodes	• Aspirin and clopidogrel • Anti-ischemic medications • Heparin or LMWH • Glycoprotein IIb/IIIa inhibitors

ACE, Angiotensin-converting enzyme; *BP,* blood pressure; *ECG,* electrocardiogram; *LMWH,* low-molecular-weight heparin; *MI,* myocardial infarction; *NTG,* nitroglycerin; *STE,* ST-segment elevation.
Source: Modified from Cinquegrani (2016)

ACUTE CORONARY SYNDROMES

In most patients, UA, infarction, and sudden cardiac death occur because of abrupt plaque change followed by thrombosis (Kumar, Abbas, & Aster, 2018) (Fig. 3.9). If the coronary artery obstruction is partial or intermittent, the result may be no signs and symptoms (i.e., silent ischemia), UA, non–ST-elevation MI (NSTEMI), or, possibly, sudden death. Complete blockage of a coronary artery may result in ST-elevation MI (STEMI) or sudden death. Although both NSTEMI and STEMI are life-threatening, they are discussed separately because their management strategies differ.

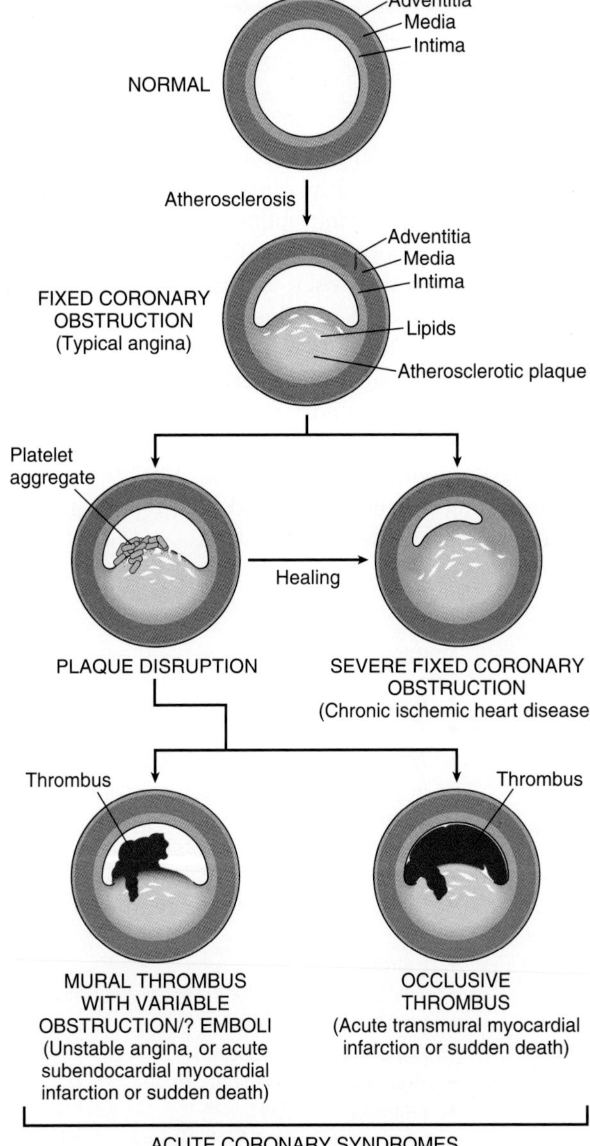

Fig. 3.9 Diagram of sequential progression of coronary artery lesions leading to various acute coronary syndromes. (From Kumar, V., Abbas, A. K., & Aster, J. C. [2018]. *Robbins basic pathology* [10th ed.]. Philadelphia, PA: Elsevier. Modified and redrawn from Schoen F. J. [1989]. *Interventional and surgical cardiovascular pathology: Clinical correlations and basic principles.* Philadelphia, PA: Saunders, p 63.)

UA and NSTEMI are often grouped together as *non-ST-elevation acute coronary syndromes* (NSTE-ACS) because ECG changes associated with these conditions usually include ST-segment depression and T-wave inversion in the leads that face the affected area. UA and NSTEMI differ primarily by whether myocardial ischemia is severe enough to cause cellular damage leading to detectable quantities of cardiac biomarkers (Amsterdam et al., 2014).

Consider This

Cardiac biomarkers are elevated when an infarction is present; they are not elevated in patients with UA because there is no tissue death.

The subendocardial area is the innermost half of the myocardium, and the subepicardial area is the outermost half (Fig. 3.10). The endocardial and subendocardial areas of the myocardial wall are the least perfused areas of the heart and the most vulnerable to ischemia because these areas have a high demand for oxygen and are fed by the most distal

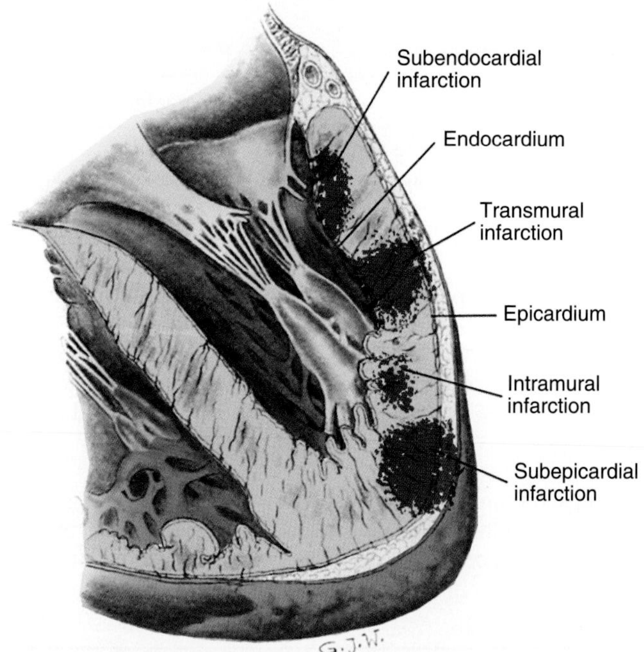

Fig. 3.10 Possible locations of infarctions in the ventricular wall. (From Urden, L. D., Stacy, K. M., & Lough, M. E. [2018]. *Critical care nursing: Diagnosis and management* [8th ed.]. St. Louis, MO: Mosby.)

branches of the coronary arteries. *Transmural* is a term used to describe ischemia, injury, or infarction that extends from the endocardium to the epicardium. For example, a transmural MI describes an infarction involving the entire thickness of the left ventricular wall.

When a coronary artery is blocked, the region of the heart supplied by the affected artery is called the *area at risk* (Fig. 3.11). Ischemia occurs immediately in the area supplied by the affected artery. Anaerobic metabolism ensues and lactic acid accumulates in the cardiac cells, which quickly results in a loss of myocardial contractility (Schoen & Mitchell, 2015). Diastolic and systolic dysfunctions appear within 30 to 45 seconds of blood flow deprivation (Blanc-Brude, 2011). Ischemia also contributes to dysrhythmias, probably by causing electrical instability of ischemic areas of the heart (Schoen & Mitchell, 2015).

If blood flow is not restored to the affected artery, myocardial cells within the subendocardial area begin to reveal signs of injury within 20 to 40 minutes. If blood flow is quickly restored, the area at risk can potentially be salvaged; aerobic metabolism resumes, cellular repair begins, and myocardial contractility is restored.

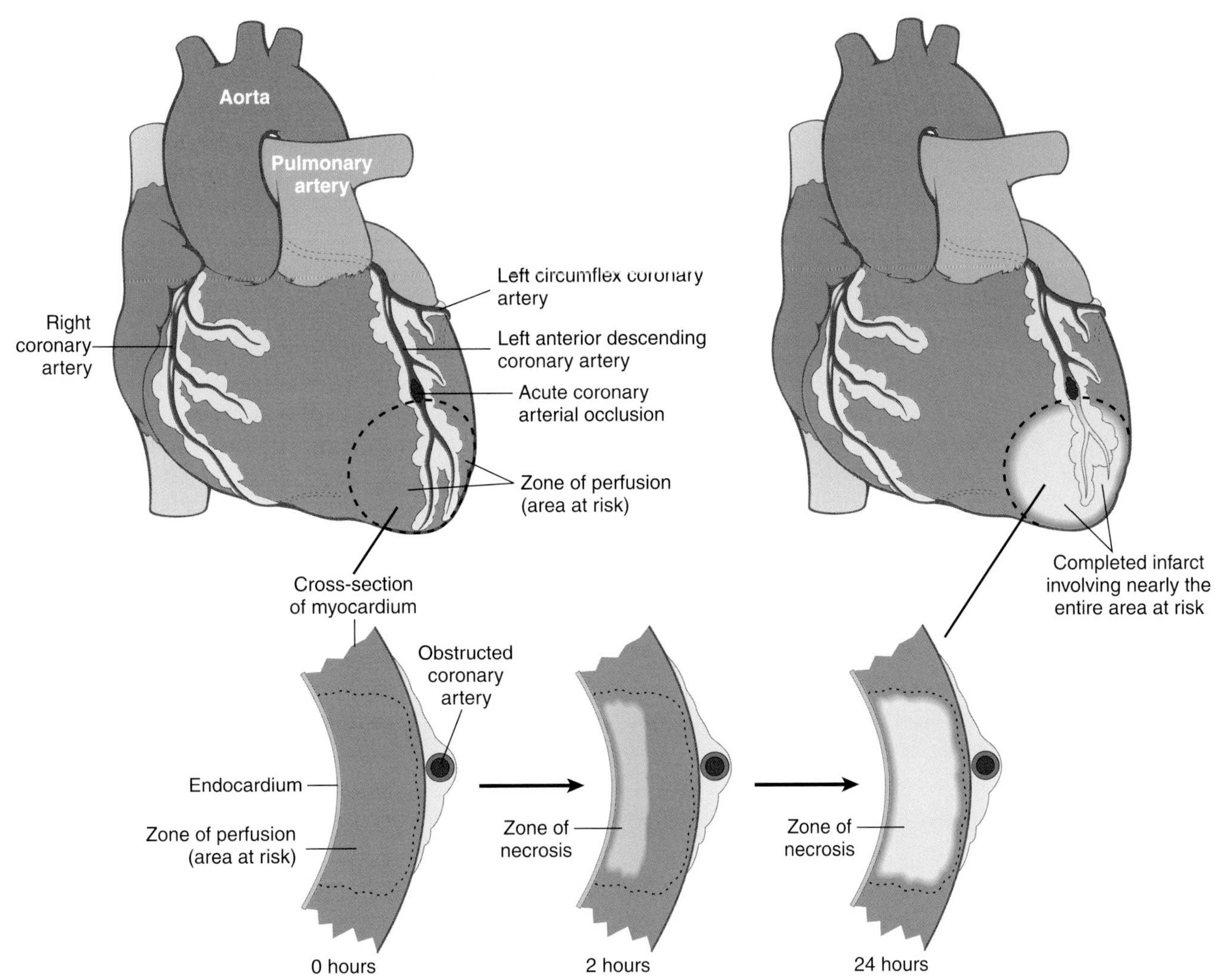

Fig. **3.11** Progression of myocardial necrosis after coronary artery occlusion. A transmural segment of the myocardium dependent on the occluded vessel for perfusion constitutes the area at risk (outlined). Necrosis begins in the subendocardial region in the center of the ischemic zone and, with time, expands to involve the entire wall thickness. Note that a very narrow zone of myocardium immediately beneath the endocardium is spared from necrosis because it can be oxygenated by diffusion from the ventricle. (From Kumar, V., Abbas, A. K., & Aster, J. C. [2018]. *Robbins basic pathology* [10th ed.]. Philadelphia, PA: Elsevier.)

Death of myocardial cells occurs when the area at risk has been deprived of blood flow for an extended interval, usually 2 to 4 hours or longer, depending on factors such as the presence of collateral circulation to the ischemic area, persistent or intermittent coronary vessel blockage, the metabolic/oxygen needs of the myocardium at risk, and the sensitivity of the myocardial cells to ischemia (Schoen & Mitchell, 2015; Thygesen et al., 2012). Without clinical intervention (i.e., reperfusion therapy), the infarction can expand to involve the entire thickness of the myocardial wall. Because time is muscle when caring for patients with an ACS, the benefits of reperfusion therapy are greatest when it is performed early.

The diagnosis of an ACS is made on the basis of the following: (1) the patient's ECG findings, (2) cardiac biomarker results, and (3) the patient's history and clinical presentation (Fig. 3.12). The patient's clinical presentation and outcome depend on factors that include the following:

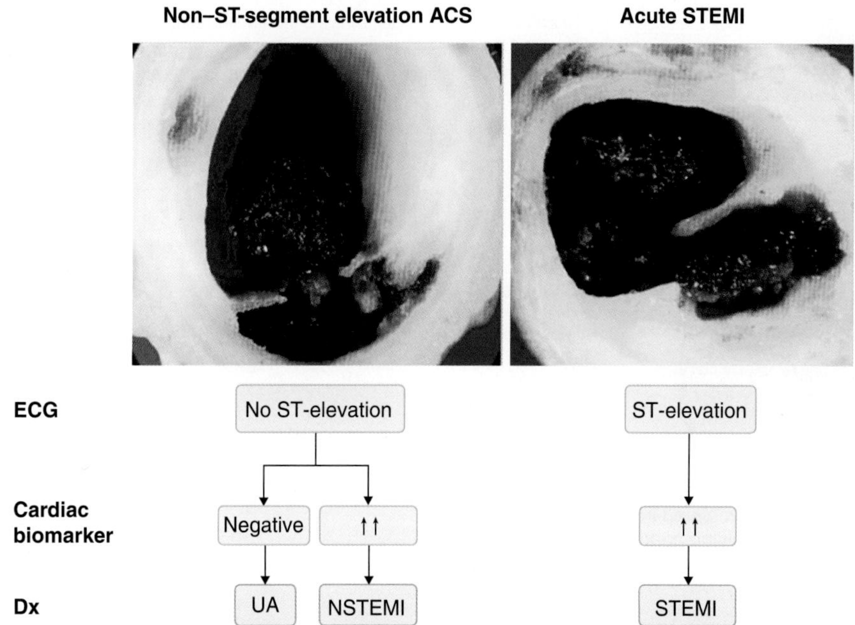

Fig. 3.12 Acute coronary syndrome (ACS). Symptomatic, morphologic, electrocardiographic, and serologic findings in patients with various kinds of ACS. Individuals with an ACS usually complain of chest pain or discomfort. If the involved coronary artery is totally occluded by fresh thrombus (shown on the right), the patient's electrocardiogram (ECG) reveals ST-segment elevation, cardiac biomarkers subsequently are elevated, and the patient is diagnosed with an ST-segment elevation myocardial infarction (STEMI). If the involved coronary artery is partially occluded by fresh thrombus (shown on the left), the patient's ECG does not show ST-segment elevation. If cardiac biomarkers are not elevated, the patient is diagnosed with unstable angina (UA). If cardiac biomarkers are elevated, the patient is diagnosed with a non-STEMI (NSTEMI). *Dx,* Diagnosis. (From Goldman, L., & Schafer, A. I. [2016]. *Goldman-Cecil medicine* [25th ed.]. Philadelphia, PA: Saunders.)

- Amount of myocardium supplied by the affected artery
- Severity and duration of myocardial ischemia
- Electrical instability of the ischemic myocardium
- Rate of development, degree, and duration of coronary obstruction
- Presence (and extent) or absence of collateral coronary circulation

Clinical Features

The patient experiencing an ACS typically complains of retrosternal pain, pressure, heaviness, or squeezing lasting 10 minutes or longer that usually occurs at rest or with minimal exertion (Amsterdam et al., 2014). Chest discomfort may be accompanied by anginal equivalents such as unexplained new-onset or increased exertional dyspnea (most common equivalent), unexplained fatigue, diaphoresis, nausea and vomiting, or syncope (Amsterdam et al., 2014). Atypical presentations are common and may include pleuritic pain, epigastric pain, acute-onset indigestion, or increasing dyspnea in the absence of chest pain. Atypical complaints are most often observed in younger (25 to 40 years of age) and older (75 years of age and older) patients, women, and patients with diabetes mellitus, chronic renal insufficiency, or dementia (Amsterdam et al., 2014; Lange & Hillis, 2016).

Features that help differentiate ACSs from stable angina include the following: (1) onset of symptoms at rest (or with minimal exertion) and lasting longer than 10 minutes unless treated promptly; (2) severe, oppressive pressure or chest discomfort; and (3) an accelerating pattern of symptoms that develop more frequently, occur with greater severity, or awaken the patient from sleep (Giugliano, Cannon, & Braunwald, 2015).

When obtaining the patient's history, ask targeted questions to determine the patient's probability of an ACS. Patients often have a history of stable angina or MI. Physical examination findings may be normal. Sinus tachycardia, hypotension, and pale, cool skin are findings that are more common with STEMI than with NSTE-ACS (Giugliano et al., 2015). During the examination, consider the possibility of other conditions that mimic acute MI such as aortic dissection, acute pericarditis, acute myocarditis, and pulmonary embolism.

Diagnosis

Recall that the diagnosis of an ACS is made on the basis of the patient's history and clinical presentation, cardiac biomarker results, and ECG findings. Clinical presentation and ECG findings are discussed later in this chapter.

Cardiac Biomarkers

Cardiac biomarkers are useful for confirming the diagnosis of MI for patients with STEMI (Table 3.3). They are also useful for confirming the diagnosis of MI when patients present without STE on their ECG, when the diagnosis may be unclear, and to distinguish patients with UA from those with NSTEMI.

TABLE 3.3 Cardiac Biomarkers

Biomarker	Initial Rise	Peak	Comments
Troponin (cTnI, cTnT)	2 to 4 hours	10 to 24 hours	Elevation may persist for 14 days (and occasionally longer) with a large infarction
CK-MB	4 to 6 hours	12 to 24 hours	Returns to normal in 48 to 72 hours
Myoglobin	1 to 3 hours	6 to 12 hours	Returns to normal within 24 to 36 hours

cTnI, Cardiac-derived troponin I; *cTnT,* cardiac-derived troponin T; *CK-MB,* creatine kinase isoenzyme.

Cardiac troponins (i.e., TnI and TnT) are the biomarkers of choice for diagnosing MI. Troponins are proteins found in skeletal and cardiac muscle that attach to tropomyosin. After ischemia, muscle injury, or destruction of muscle, these substances are released into the blood. Because the ranges of normal biomarker levels vary among laboratories, current clinical practice guidelines define an increased cardiac troponin concentration as a value that exceeds the 99th percentile as compared with a normal reference population (Amsterdam et al., 2014).

For patients presenting with symptoms suggestive of an ACS, cardiac biomarkers (i.e., troponin levels) should be obtained on initial presentation and again between 3 and 6 hours later after symptom onset to determine a rising or falling pattern (Amsterdam et al., 2014). If cardiac biomarkers are not present in the patient's circulation based on two or more samples collected at least 6 hours apart, the diagnosis is UA. If elevated biomarker levels are present (and STE is absent), the diagnosis is NSTEMI. If elevated biomarker levels are present and the ECG shows STE in two or more contiguous leads, the diagnosis is STEMI.

Creatine kinase isoenzyme (CK-MB) may be used to estimate the size of an MI (Amsterdam et al., 2014) and is the preferred alternative when cardiac troponin markers are unavailable (Thygesen et al., 2012).

Consider This

Elevated cardiac troponin levels may be present with a number of conditions other than MI. For example, abnormal elevations have been observed with heart failure, chronic kidney disease, pulmonary embolism, myocarditis, pericarditis, sepsis, transplant rejection, chemotherapy, and direct or indirect cardiac trauma (Giugliano et al., 2015).

TABLE 3.4 Localization of a Myocardial Infarction

Anatomic Region	Indicative Changes	Reciprocal Changes	Affected (Culprit) Coronary Artery
Anterior LV	V_3, V_4	V_7, V_8, V_9	LCA (LAD)
Septum	V_1, V_2	V_7, V_8, V_9	LCA (LAD)
Inferior LV	II, III, aVF	I, aVL	RCA (most common) or LCA (Cx branch)
Right ventricle	V_1R–V_6R	I, aVL	RCA
Lateral LV	I, aVL, V_5, V_6	II, III, aVF (if a high-lateral infarction)	LCA (LAD and/or Cx branch) or RCA
Posterior LV	V_7, V_8, V_9	V_1 through V_4	Cx or RCA
Diffuse subendocardial ischemia	aVR, V_1	I, II, aVL, V_4, V_5, V_6 (may involve additional leads)	LMCA, proximal LAD, or three-vessel disease

Cx, Circumflex; *LAD,* left anterior descending; *LCA,* left coronary artery; *LMCA,* left main coronary artery, *LV,* left ventricle; *RCA,* right coronary artery.

12-Lead ECG

To recognize ECG signs of ischemia, injury, and infarction, you need to be able to spot changes in the shape of the QRS complex, ST segment, and T wave. To localize the area at risk, note which leads are displaying that evidence and consider which part of the heart that those leads "see." Once the area at risk has been recognized, an understanding of coronary artery anatomy makes it possible to predict which coronary artery is affected. Table 3.4 summarizes the pattern in which coronary arteries most commonly supply the myocardium.

One way to gauge the relative extent or size of an infarction is to evaluate how many leads are showing indicative changes. An ECG showing changes in only a few leads suggests a smaller infarction than one that produces changes in many leads. In general, the more proximal the blockage in the vessel, the larger the infarction and the greater the number of leads showing indicative changes.

The left ventricle is divided into regions where an MI may occur—septal, anterior, lateral, inferior, and inferobasal (posterior) (Fig. 3.13). If an ECG shows changes in leads II, III, and aVF, the inferior wall is affected. Because the inferior wall of the left ventricle is supplied by the right coronary artery (RCA) in most people, it is reasonable to suppose that these ECG changes are the result of partial or complete blockage of the RCA. When indicative changes are seen in the leads viewing the septal, anterior, and/or lateral walls of the left ventricle (V_1–V_6, I, and aVL), it is reasonable to suspect that these ECG changes are the result of partial or complete blockage of the LCA. Locating an MI on the basis of ECG changes is discussed in more detail later in this chapter.

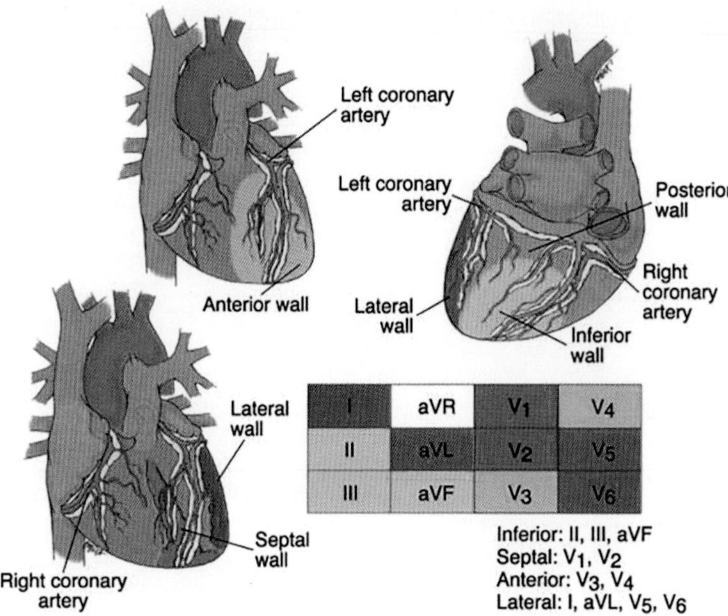

Fig. **3.13** The surfaces of the heart and facing leads.

Unstable Angina and Non-ST-Elevation Myocardial Infarction

UA, which is also known as *preinfarction angina, accelerating or crescendo angina, intermediate coronary syndrome*, and *preocclusive syndrome*, is a condition of intermediate severity between stable angina and acute MI. With UA and NSTEMI, partial occlusion of a coronary artery occurs that limits coronary blood flow, leading to subendocardial ischemia (UA) and possible subendocardial necrosis (NSTEMI) in the distribution of the affected coronary artery (Cinquegrani, 2016).

12-Lead ECG

ECG changes that are most often seen in NSTE-ACS include ST-segment depression and T-wave inversion in the leads facing the affected area (Figs. 3.14 and 3.15). These ECG changes occur in up to 50% of NSTE-ACS patients (Lange & Hillis, 2016). Transient STE (i.e., STE lasting less than 20 minutes) occurs in up to 10% of patients (Giugliano et al., 2015).

Consider This

Up to 50% of patients experiencing an acute MI do not have significant findings on their initial ECG (Cinquegrani, 2016). A normal ECG does not rule out an acute MI, particularly in the early hours of a coronary artery occlusion.

Consider This

If a patient presents with a possible ACS and the only ST-segment change seen on a standard 12-lead ECG is depression (particularly in leads V_1 through V_4), strongly consider obtaining posterior chest leads V_7 through V_9 to assess for a possible inferobasal (i.e., posterior) infarction.

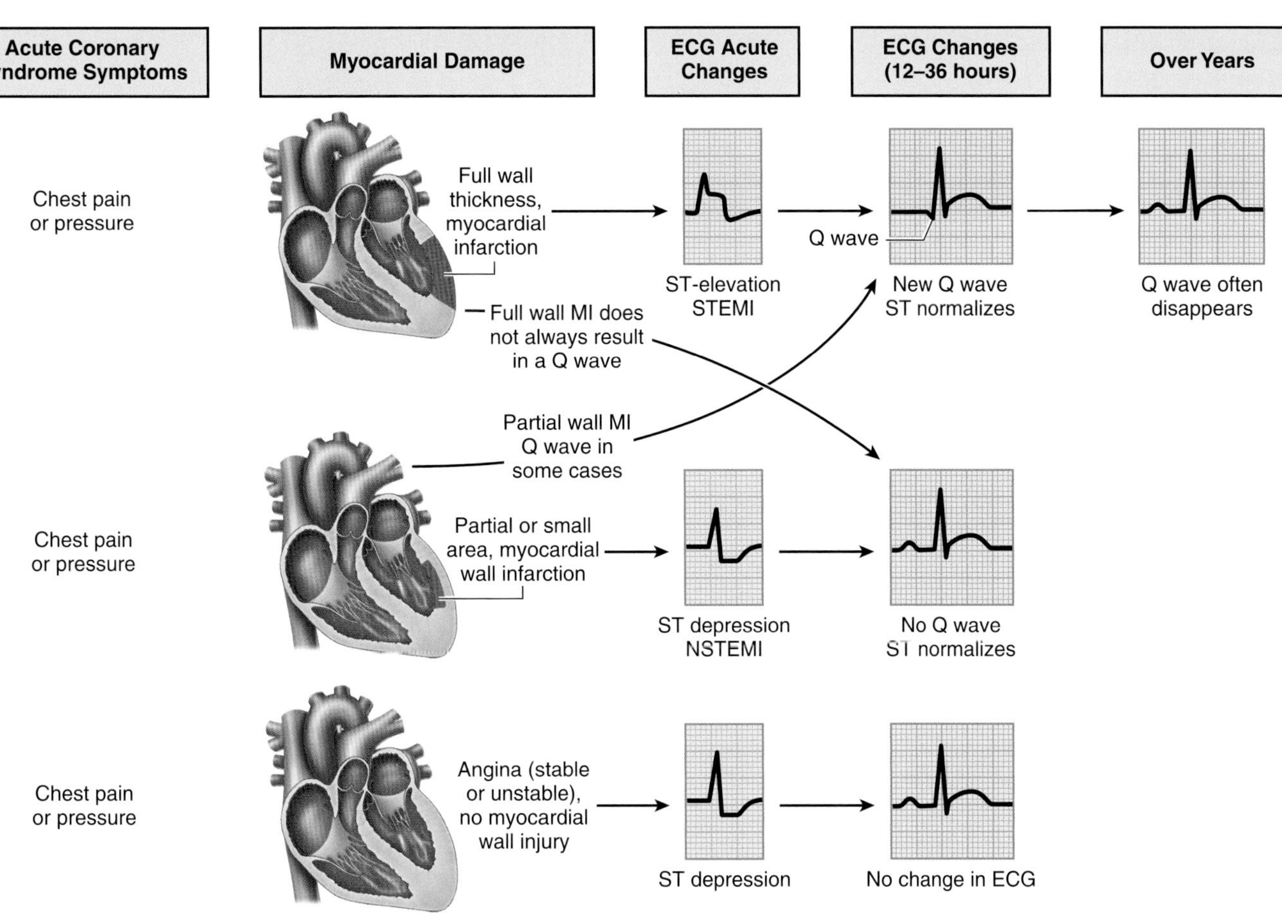

Fig. **3.14** Acute coronary syndromes: ST-elevation myocardial infarction (STEMI), non–ST-elevation myocardial infarction (NSTEMI), unstable angina. Electrocardiography changes over time. (From Urden, L. D., Stacy, K. M., & Lough, M. E. [2018]. *Critical care nursing: Diagnosis and management* [8th ed.]. St. Louis, MO: Mosby.)

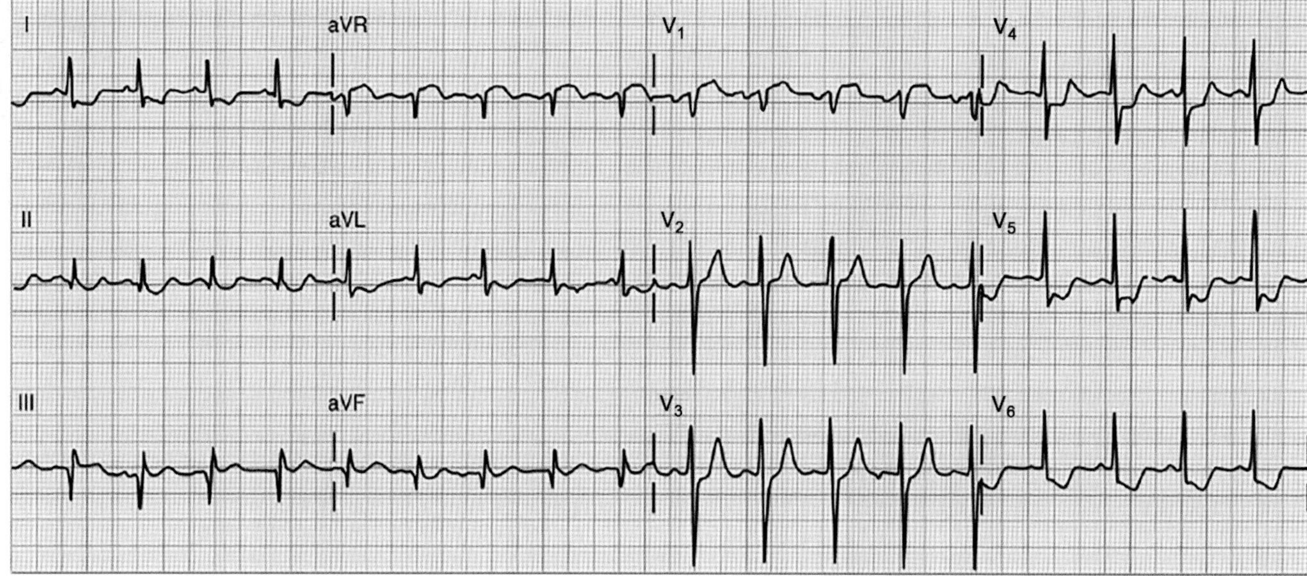

Fig. 3.15 Marked ST-segment depression in a patient with prolonged chest pain is the result of an acute non–ST-segment elevation myocardial infarction. Between 1 and 3 mm of ST-segment depression is seen in leads I, aVL, and V_4 to V_6. The patient is known to have had a previous inferior myocardial infarction. (From Andreoli, T. E., Benjamin, I. J., Griggs, R. C., & Wing, E. J. [2010]. *Andreoli and Carpenter's Cecil essentials of medicine.* Philadelphia, PA: Saunders.)

ST-Elevation Myocardial Infarction

Recall that, with NSTEMI, a coronary artery is *partially* occluded, which can lead to subendocardial ischemia in the distribution of the affected coronary artery. With STEMI, an epicardial coronary artery is *completely* blocked. This occlusion can result in myocardial ischemia that affects the entire thickness (i.e., transmural) of the ventricular wall (see Fig. 3.10).

12-lead ECG

ECG changes associated with STEMI often occur in a predictable pattern. The ECG changes described here appear in leads looking at the area fed by the blocked (culprit) vessel.

- *Hyperacute T waves.* Within minutes of an interruption of coronary blood flow, hyperacute T waves may be observed on the ECG in the leads facing the affected area. Hyperacute T waves are tall, positive, peaked, and broad based (Fig. 3.16). Clinically, hyperacute T waves are often not observed because these ECG changes have typically resolved by the time the patient seeks medical assistance. In addition to acute myocardial ischemia and infarction, possible causes of tall T waves include hyperkalemia, left ventricular hypertrophy, left bundle branch block (BBB), acute pericarditis, acute central nervous system events (e.g., intracranial hemorrhage), and benign early repolarization, among others.

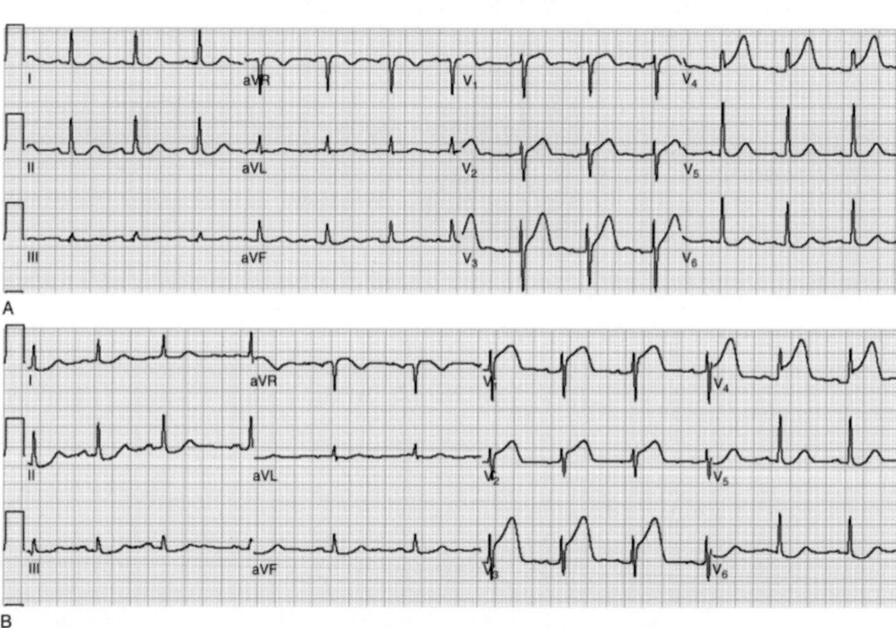

Fig. 3.16 Hyperacute T wave of acute myocardial infarction. **A,** Note the broad, tall T waves in leads V_3 and V_4 in this patient with chest pain and diaphoresis. These are the hyperacute T waves of early ST-segment elevation myocardial infarction. The ST segment is just beginning to rise in leads V_3 and V_4; leads V_1 and V_2 are also suspicious. **B,** This tracing is from the same patient, roughly 30 minutes after the electrocardiogram in A. Note the prominent ST-segment elevation in leads V_1 to V_4. (From Walls, R.M., Hockberger, R.S., & Gausche-Hill, M. [2018]. *Rosen's emergency medicine.* [9th ed.]. Philadelphia, PA: Elsevier.)

Consider This

The presence of hyperacute T waves has been reported as early as 30 minutes after the onset of chest pain and usually appears before elevation in cardiac biomarkers or ST changes on the ECG (Sovari, Assadi, Lakshminarayanan, & Kocheril, 2007).

- *ST-segment changes.* Evidence of myocardial injury can be seen on the ECG as STE (Fig. 3.17). New or presumed new STE of 1 mm or more at the J point in all leads other than V_2 and V_3 in a patient who is experiencing an ACS is suggestive of myocardial injury when observed in two or more anatomically contiguous leads (O'Gara et al., 2013). For leads V_2 and V_3, STE is considered significant if it is elevated by 2 mm or more in men older than 40 years or elevated by 1.5 mm or more in women (O'Gara et al., 2013). Continuous ST-segment monitoring can be helpful for detecting ST-segment changes that confirm the diagnosis of an ACS as well as for detecting silent or unrecognized myocardial ischemia.

Consider This

Conditions other than STEMI can cause STE. Examples of these conditions include benign early repolarization, pericarditis, bundle branch block, and ventricular paced rhythms, among others. These conditions are discussed in Chapter 4.

- *QRS changes.* An MI was once classified according to its location (e.g., anterior, inferior) and whether or not it produced Q waves on the ECG over several days. A *Q-wave infarction* was generally considered to be synonymous with *transmural infarction*, and a *non–Q-wave infarction* was referred to as a *subendocardial infarction* (Morrow & Boden, 2015). This terminology has been replaced because a pathologic Q wave may take hours to develop (and, in some cases, never develop) and because cardiac magnetic resonance studies indicate that the development of a Q wave on the ECG is determined more by the size of the infarction than by the depth of mural involvement (Scirica & Morrow, 2015).

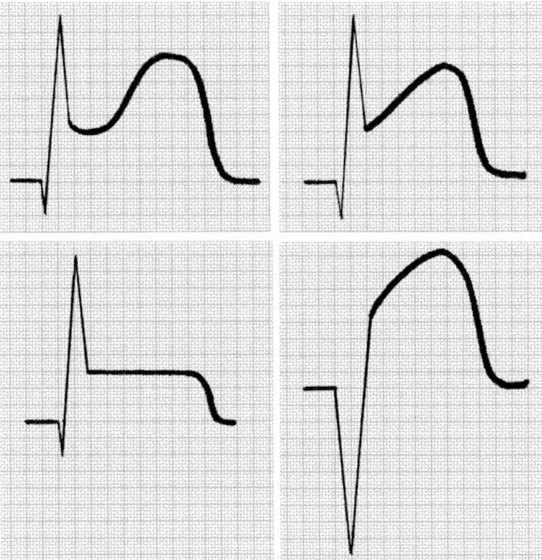

Fig. 3.17 Various shapes of ST-segment elevation seen with acute myocardial infarctions. (From Goldberger, A. L., Goldberger, Z. D., & Shvilkin, A. [2018]. *Goldberger's clinical electrocardiography: A simplified approach* [9th ed.]. Philadelphia, PA: Elsevier.)

Consider This

The 12-lead ECG is used to differentiate between patients with STE and those without STE and to guide treatment decisions with regard to reperfusion therapy. Most patients with STEMI will develop ECG evidence of pathologic Q waves (O'Gara et al., 2013).

- *T-wave inversion.* In a patient experiencing an ACS, inverted T waves suggest ischemia. T-wave inversion may precede the development of ST-segment changes or they may occur at the same time. Inverted T waves associated with ischemia and infarction are usually narrow and symmetrically inverted (Kurz, Mattu, & Brady, 2014). They may remain inverted for varying periods ranging from days, weeks, or months, or they may remain permanently (Wagner et al., 2009).

Localizing a Myocardial Infarction

Leads that view the same surfaces of the heart can be grouped together and analyzed for ECG evidence of myocardial ischemia, injury, or infarction. Because ECG evidence must be found in at least two contiguous leads, assessing lead groupings for indicative changes is helpful in determining the location of the area at risk and predicting which coronary artery is affected. In general, the more proximal the blockage in the vessel, the larger the infarction and the greater the number of leads showing indicative changes (Morris & Brady, 2002).

Localization of an infarction works reasonably well for STEMI. However, ST-segment depression and T-wave changes that suggest the presence of myocardial ischemia, as in NSTE-ACS, are less reliable in localizing the culprit vessel because these ECG changes reflect subendocardial rather than transmural ischemia (Halim et al., 2010).

Consider This

Factors including the anatomic position and size of the heart, the patient's unique pattern of coronary artery distribution, the location of the occlusion along the length of the coronary artery, the presence of collateral circulation, previous infarctions, and concomitant medication- and electrolyte-related ECG changes may also affect the perceived location of an infarction versus its actual location.

When viewing the 12-lead ECG of a patient experiencing an ACS, look at each lead for the presence of ST-segment displacement (i.e., elevation or depression). If ST-segment displacement is present, note its displacement in millimeters. Inspect the T waves for any changes in orientation, shape, and size. Examine each lead for the presence of a Q wave. If a Q wave is present, measure its duration.

Anterior Infarction

An anterior infarction occurs when the blood supply to the left anterior descending (LAD) artery is disrupted (Fig. 3.18). Evidence can be seen in leads V_3 and V_4, which face the anterior wall of the left ventricle. Septal involvement is evidenced by changes in leads V_1 and V_2 (Fig. 3.19). Proximal occlusion of the LAD may become an anteroseptal infarction if the septal branch is involved (Table 3.5). ECG changes of an anteroseptal infarction should be visible in leads V_1 through V_4 (Fig. 3.20). An anterolateral infarction may result if the marginal branch is involved.

If the chest leads indicate ECG changes in leads V_3 and V_4 (suggestive of an anterior MI) and indicative changes are also present in V_5 and V_6, the infarction would be called an *anterolateral infarction* or an *anterior infarction with lateral extension.* ECG changes with this type of infarction are also possible in leads I and aVL. If the blockage occurs proximal to both the septal and diagonal branches, an extensive anterior infarction (anteroseptal-lateral MI) will result. ECG changes should be visible in leads V_1 through V_6, as well as leads I and aVL. Reciprocal changes in an anterior or anteroseptal MI appear in leads V_7, V_8, and V_9. Reciprocal changes with an anterior or anteroseptal MI do not appear in the limb leads because they are in a different plane.

Poor R-wave progression is a phrase used to describe R waves that decrease in size from V_1 to V_4. Possible causes include right or left ventricular hypertrophy and left BBB, among other causes. Poor R-wave progression may also be a nonspecific indicator of anterior wall infarction.

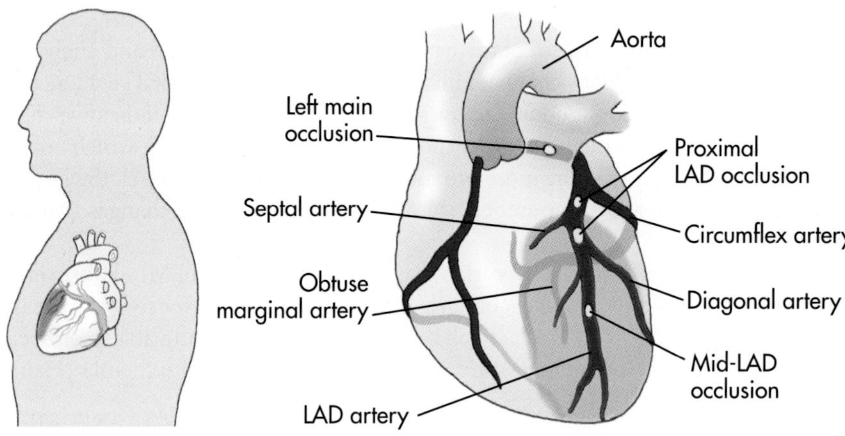

I Lateral	aVR	V_1 Septum	V_4 Anterior
II Inferior	aVL Lateral	V_2 Septum	V_5 Lateral
III Inferior	aVF Inferior	V_3 Anterior	V_6 Lateral

Fig. **3.18** Anterior infarction. Occlusion of the midportion of the left anterior descending (LAD) artery results in an anterior infarction. Proximal occlusion of the LAD may become an anteroseptal infarction if the septal branch is involved or an anterolateral infarction if the marginal branch is involved. If the occlusion occurs proximal to both the septal and diagonal branches, an extensive anterior infarction will result.

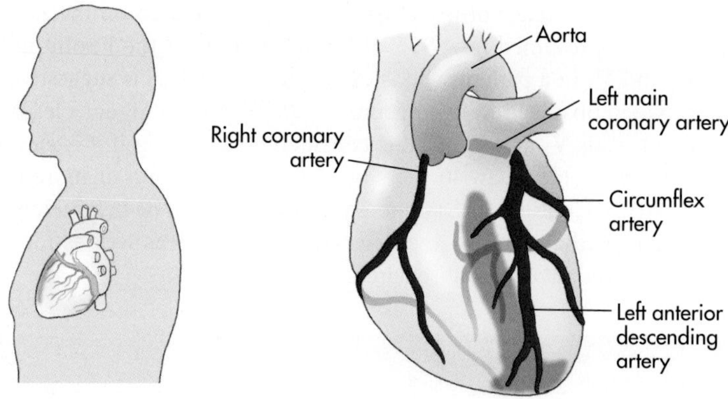

I Lateral	aVR	V_1 Septum	V_4 Anterior
II Inferior	aVL Lateral	V_2 Septum	V_5 Lateral
III Inferior	aVF Inferior	V_3 Anterior	V_6 Lateral

Fig. **3.19** Septal infarction.

TABLE 3.5 Anterior and Septal Infarctions

Anatomic Region	Indicative Changes	Reciprocal Changes	Possible Complications
Anterior LV	V_3, V_4	V_7, V_8, V_9	Left ventricular dysfunction, including heart failure and cardiogenic shock; AV blocks, BBBs, PVCs, atrial flutter, AFib
Septum	V_1, V_2	V_7, V_8, V_9	
Anteroseptal LV	V_1, V_2, V_3, V_4	V_7, V_8, V_9	
Anterolateral LV	I, aVL, V_3, V_4, V_5, V_6	II, III, aVF (if high lateral infarction), V_7, V_8, V_9	

AFib, Atrial fibrillation; *AV,* atrioventricular; *BBB,* bundle branch block; *LV,* left ventricle; *PVC,* premature ventricular complex.

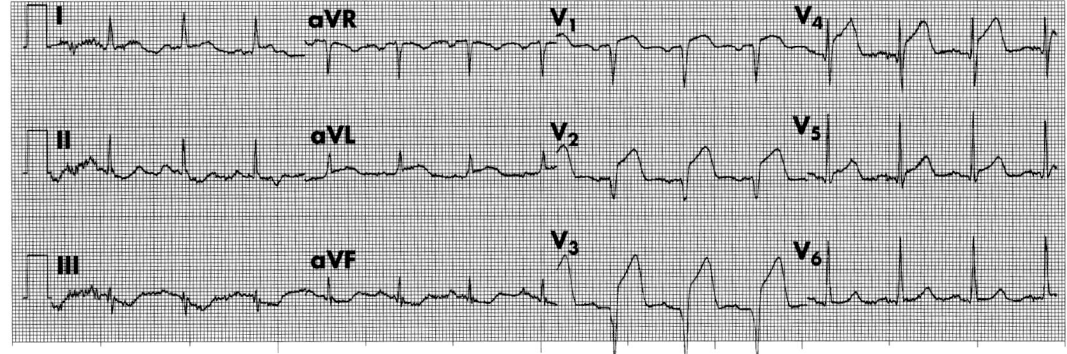

Fig. 3.20 Extensive anteroseptal infarction.

Consider This

Wellens' syndrome, also called *LAD coronary T-wave syndrome*, is an ECG pattern associated with severe proximal LAD stenosis. Patients with Wellens' syndrome typically have a history of chest pain or discomfort. The ECG pattern, which can be transient, is characterized by inverted or biphasic T waves in leads V_2 through V_4 during a pain-free period. There is little or no cardiac enzyme elevation and little or no ST-segment elevation (Mao et al., 2013).

de Winter syndrome, considered an anterior STEMI-equivalent, is associated with acute occlusion of the LAD artery (Martínez-Losas & Fernández-Jiménez, 2016). Patients present with chest pain or discomfort but lack the ECG changes that are typical of an anterior STEMI. The de Winter ECG pattern includes upsloping ST-segment depression greater than 1 mm at the J point in the chest leads; tall, prominent, and symmetrically peaked T waves with no classic STE in the chest leads; and slight (0.5 to 1 mm) STE in lead aVR (Goktas, Sogut, Yigit, & Kaplan, 2017). With both syndromes, rapid recognition and emergent reperfusion therapy can help avert the development of an anterior infarction.

Inferior Infarction

Leads II, III, and aVF view the inferior surface of the left ventricle. In most individuals, the inferior wall of the left ventricle is supplied by the posterior descending branch of the RCA ("right dominant system"). Blockage of the RCA proximal to the marginal branch will result in an inferior MI and right ventricular infarction (RVI). Blockage of the RCA distal to the marginal branch will result in an inferior infarction, sparing the right ventricle (Fig. 3.21, Table 3.6). Reciprocal changes are observed in leads I and aVL.

In some individuals, the circumflex (Cx) artery supplies the inferior wall through the posterior descending artery ("left dominant system"). Blockage of the posterior descending artery will result in an inferior infarction; however, a proximal occlusion of the Cx artery may result in infarction in the lateral and posterior walls. STE in lead V_1 in the presence of an inferior STEMI (with elevation greater in lead III than in lead II) suggests associated RVI (Kurz et al., 2014). Fig. 3.22 is an example of an acute inferior infarction.

Right Ventricular Infarction

RVI should be suspected when ECG changes suggesting an inferior infarction (STE in leads II, III, and/or aVF) are observed. The right ventricle is supplied by the right ventricular marginal branch of the RCA (Fig. 3.23). Blockage of the right ventricular marginal branch results in an isolated RVI. Blockage of the RCA proximal to the right ventricular marginal branch results in an inferior and RVI.

To view the right ventricle, right chest leads are used (Table 3.7). These leads then "look" directly at the right ventricle and can show the STE created by the infarction. If time does not permit the acquisition of all six right-sided chest leads, the leads of choice are V_3R and V_4R (Wagner et al., 2009). The most sensitive ECG signs of right ventricular injury include 1-mm STE in lead V_1 and in lead V_4R (O'Gara et al., 2013). Some researchers have found that the sensitivity of V_4R in detecting RVI is greater when measured 0.06 second after the J point than when measured at the J point (Seo et al., 2011). Be sure to record the right chest leads as quickly as possible after the onset of ACS symptoms because the STE associated with RVI persists for a much shorter period than the STE associated with inferior infarction observed in the limb leads (Wagner et al., 2009). Fig. 3.24 shows an example of RVI.

It has been estimated that 25% of patients with RVI develop clinically evident hemodynamic manifestations (Goldstein, 2012). Patients may present with, or subsequently develop, hypotension caused by bradydysrhythmias or caused by a reduction in preload after the administration of vasodilators such as NTG (Goldstein, 2012).

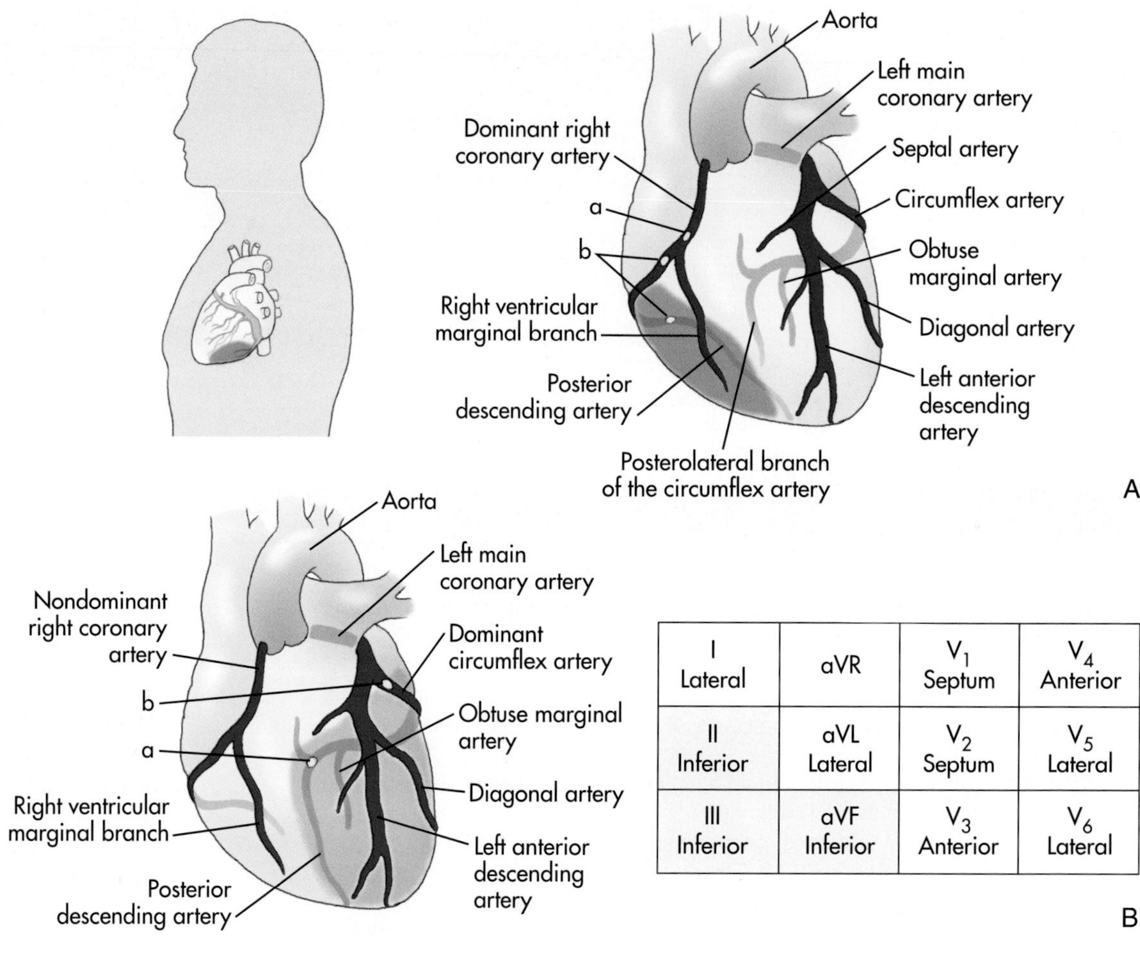

Fig. 3.21 **A,** Inferior wall infarction. Coronary anatomy shows a dominant right coronary artery (RCA). A blockage at point "a" results in an inferior infarction and right ventricular infarction. A blockage at point "b" involves only the inferior wall, sparing the right ventricle. **B,** Inferior wall infarction. Coronary anatomy shows a dominant circumflex artery. A blockage at point "a" results in an inferior infarction. A blockage at "b" may result in a lateral and inferobasal infarction.

Consider This

It is sometimes possible to detect the presence of RVI by close examination of lead V_1. Occasionally, V_1 and V_2 may show STE from an RVI because V_1 is located in the same position as V_2R, and V_2 is also V_1R. When an inferior infarction exists and the ST segment is elevated in V_1 and/or V_2, an RVI is presumed to exist when the amount of STE is greater in V_1 than in V_2. Conversely, when V_1 and V_2 show STE because of a septal infarction, the amount of STE is typically greater in V_2 than in V_1. The use of V_1 as an indicator for RVI is fairly specific but not very sensitive.

TABLE 3.6 Inferior Infarction

Anatomic Region	Indicative Changes	Reciprocal Changes	Possible Complications
Inferior LV	II, III, aVF	I, aVL	Bradydysrhythmias; AV blocks

AV, Atrioventricular; *LV,* left ventricle.

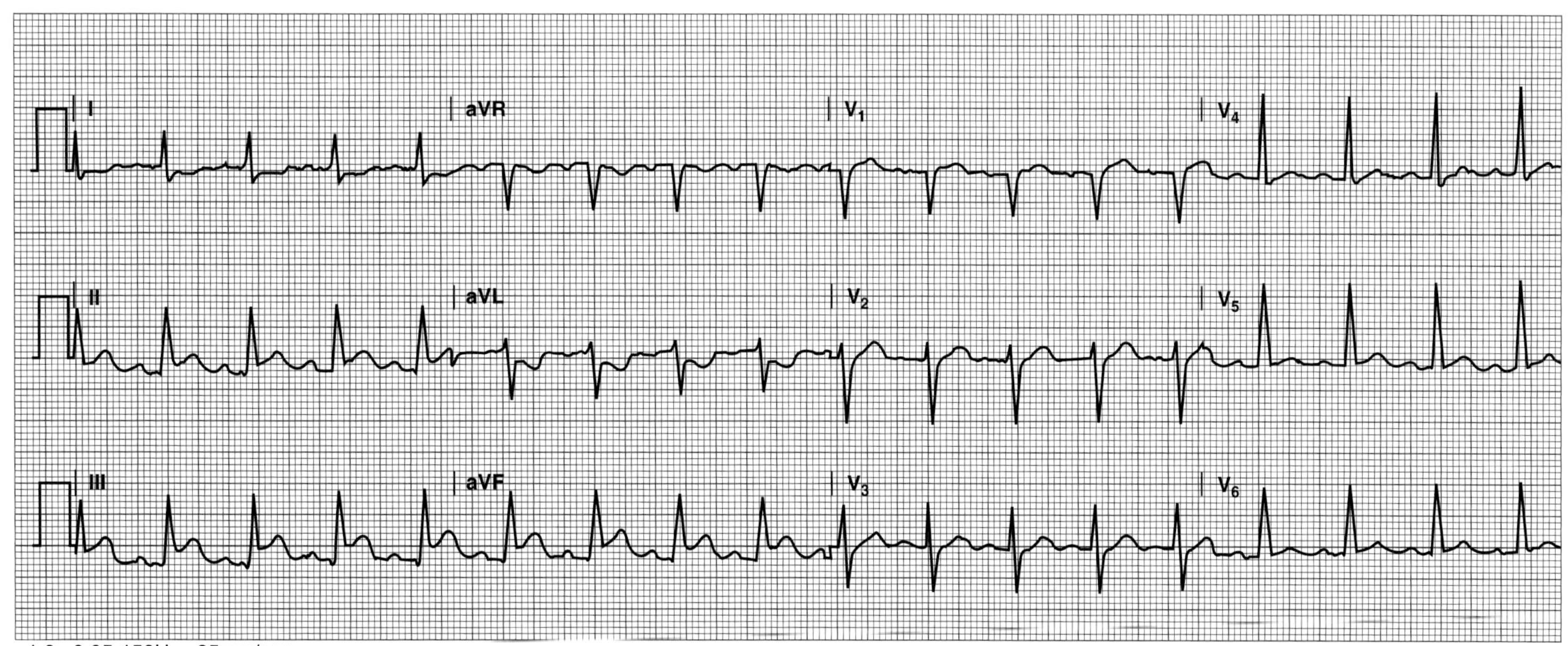

Fig. **3.22** Acute inferior infarction. Note the ST-segment elevation in leads II, III, and aVF and the reciprocal ST depression in leads I and aVL. Abnormal Q waves are also present in leads II, III, and aVF.

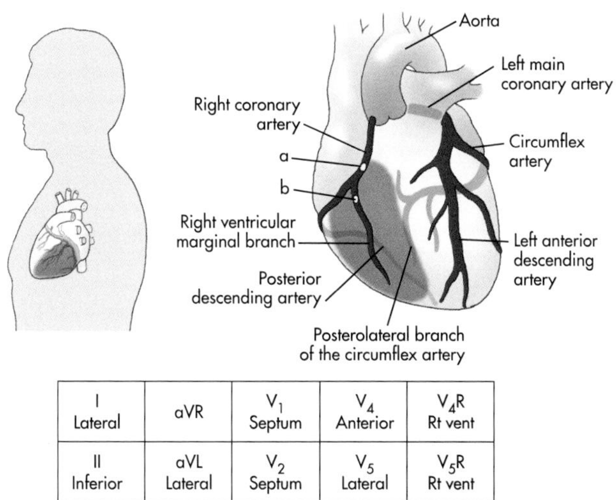

I Lateral	aVR	V_1 Septum	V_4 Anterior	V_4R Rt vent
II Inferior	aVL Lateral	V_2 Septum	V_5 Lateral	V_5R Rt vent
III Inferior	aVF Inferior	V_3 Anterior	V_6 Lateral	V_6R Rt vent

Fig. **3.23** Right ventricular infarction (RVI). At "a," blockage of the right coronary artery proximal to the right ventricular marginal branch results in an inferior and RVI. At "b," blockage of the right ventricular marginal branch results in an isolated RVI.

TABLE 3.7 Right Ventricular Infarction

Anatomic Region	Indicative Changes	Reciprocal Changes	Possible Complications
Right ventricle	V_1R to V_6R	I, aVL	Bradydysrhythmias, AV blocks, ventricular dysrhythmias, hypotension, right-sided heart failure, preload dependent
Inferior and RVI	II, III, aVF, V_1R to V_6R	I, aVL	

AV, Atrioventricular; *RVI,* right ventricular infarction.

Lateral Infarction

Lateral wall infarctions often occur as extensions of anterior or inferior infarctions because the lateral wall of the left ventricle may be supplied by the Cx artery, the LAD artery, or a branch of the RCA. Because the lateral wall of the left ventricle is viewed by a combination of chest (V_5 and V_6) and limb (I and aVL) leads, evidence of a lateral wall infarction may be seen in some or all of the following leads: I, aVL, V_5, and V_6 (Fig. 3.25, Table 3.8). The term *high lateral infarction* is used to describe ST changes viewed in leads I and aVL.

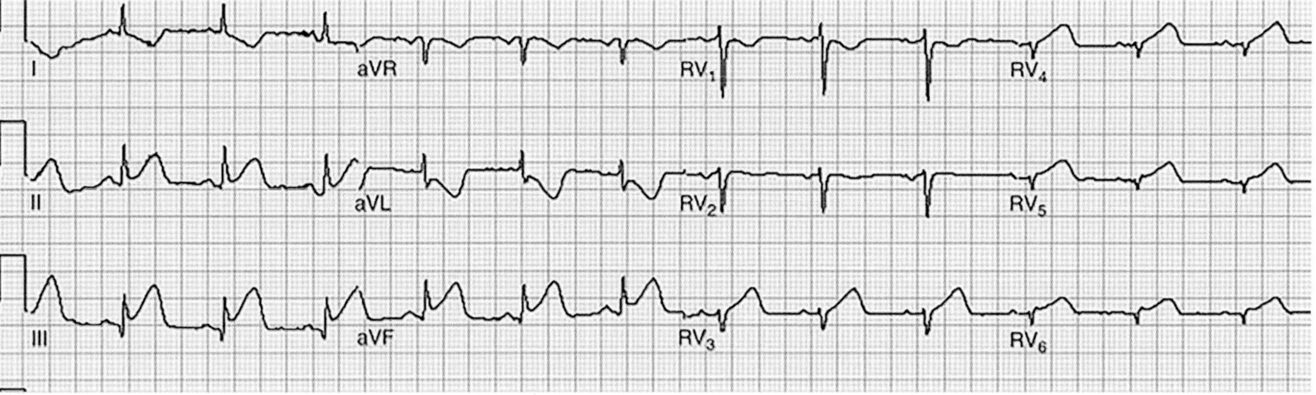

Fig. 3.24 Inferior infarction with right ventricular infarction (RVI). ST-segment elevation (STE) of inferior acute myocardial infarction is present, as is reciprocal ST-segment depression in leads I and aVL. STE is noted in leads RV_3 to RV_6 (V_3R to V_6R), consistent with RVI. (From Walls, R. M., Hockberger, R. S., & Gausche-Hill, M. [2018]. *Rosen's emergency medicine: Concepts and clinical practice* [9th ed]. Philadelphia, PA: Elsevier.)

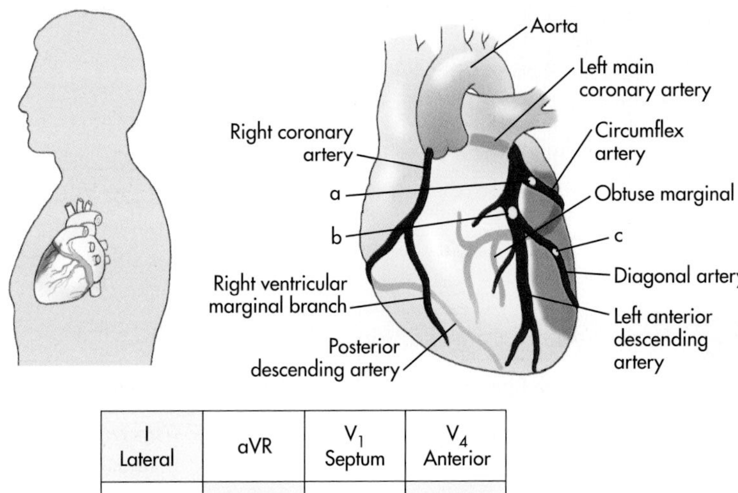

I Lateral	aVR	V_1 Septum	V_4 Anterior
II Inferior	aVL Lateral	V_2 Septum	V_5 Lateral
III Inferior	aVF Inferior	V_3 Anterior	V_6 Lateral

Fig. 3.25 Lateral infarction. Coronary artery anatomy shows (a) blockage of the circumflex artery, (b) blockage of the proximal left anterior descending artery, and (c) blockage of the diagonal artery.

TABLE 3.8 Lateral Infarction

Anatomic Region	Indicative Changes	Reciprocal Changes	Possible Complications
Lateral LV	I, aVL, V_5, V_6	II, III, aVF (if high lateral infarction); aVR	Dysrhythmias

LV, Left ventricle.

The term *low lateral infarction* is used to describe ST changes viewed in leads V_5 and V_6. Reciprocal changes of a high lateral infarction can usually be seen in leads II, III, and aVF.

Isolated lateral wall infarctions usually involve occlusion of the Cx artery and are often missed. More commonly, the lateral wall is involved with proximal occlusion of the LAD (anterolateral MI) or a branch of the RCA (inferolateral MI). An example of a lateral infarction is shown in Fig. 3.26.

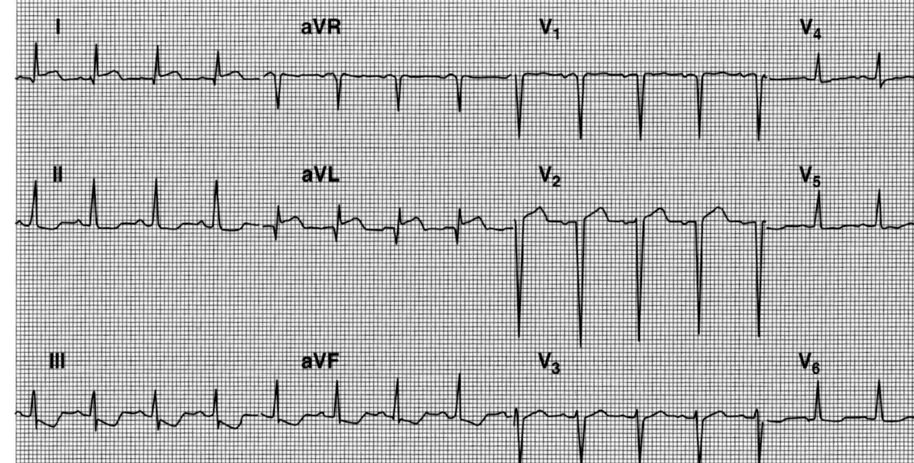

Fig. 3.26 Lateral wall infarction. Lead I shows a small Q wave with ST-segment elevation (STE). A larger Q wave with STE can be seen in lead aVL. This patient had an anterior non–ST-elevation infarction 4 days earlier with STE and T-wave inversion in leads V_2 through V_6. A coronary arteriogram at that time showed a blocked left anterior descending artery distal to its first large septal perforator. The STE evolved and the T waves in all of the chest leads had become upright the day before this tracing was recorded. The patient then had another episode of chest pain associated with the appearance of signs of acute lateral infarction, as shown in this tracing. A repeat coronary arteriogram showed new blockage of the obtuse marginal branch of the circumflex artery. (From Surawicz, B., & Knilans, T. K. [2001]. *Chou's electrocardiography in clinical practice: Adult and pediatric* [5th ed.]. Philadelphia, PA: Saunders.)

Inferobasal Infarction

Posterior MIs usually occur in conjunction with an inferior or lateral infarction. Experts recommend that the term *inferobasal wall* be used instead of *posterior wall* (Thygesen et al., 2012). The inferobasal wall of the left ventricle is supplied by the Cx coronary artery in most patients; however, in some patients, it is supplied by the RCA.

Because no leads of a standard 12-lead ECG directly view the inferobasal wall of the left ventricle, additional chest leads (e.g., V_7, V_8, V_9) should be used to view the heart's posterior surface. Indicative changes of an inferobasal infarction include STE in these leads (Fig. 3.27, Table 3.9). Reciprocal changes, such as tall R waves and ST-segment depression, may be seen in leads V_1 through V_4 (Anderson, 2016). An example of an inferobasal infarction is shown in Fig. 3.28.

Exceptions

The indicative changes described in this chapter are by no means absolute, and not every infarction follows this pattern. However, once these indicative changes are understood, they can be applied to individual patient settings and used as a reference point. There are several notable exceptions to the "classic" pattern of indicative changes.

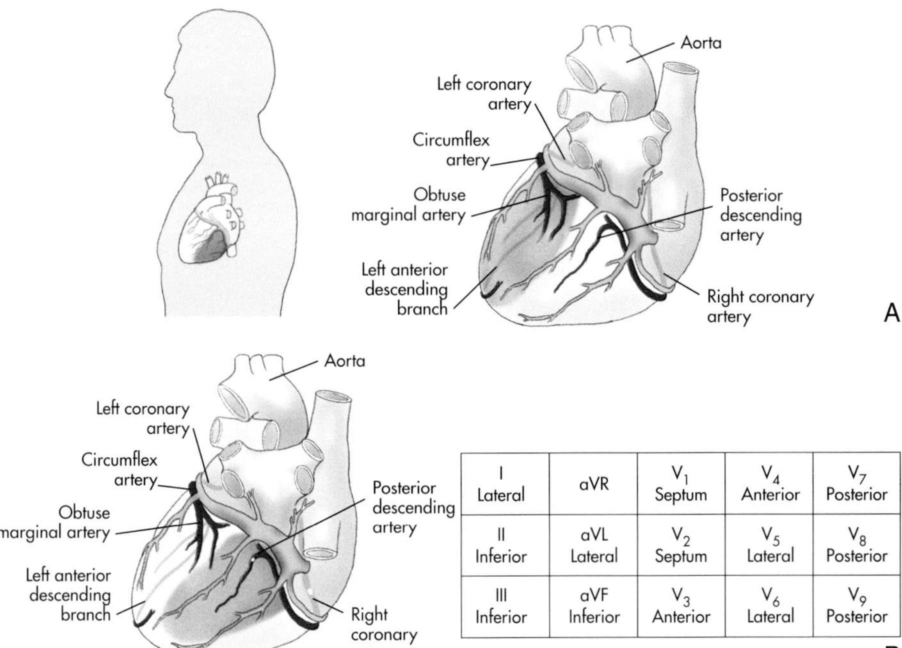

Fig. **3.27** Location of an inferobasal (posterior) infarction. **A,** Coronary anatomy shows a dominant right coronary artery (RCA). Occlusion of the RCA commonly results in an inferior and posterior infarction. **B,** Coronary anatomy shows a dominant circumflex artery. Occlusion of a marginal branch is the cause of most isolated posterior infarctions.

TABLE 3.9 Inferobasal (Posterior) Infarction

Anatomic Region	Indicative Changes	Reciprocal Changes	Possible Complications
Inferobasal	V_7, V_8, V_9	Tall R waves, ST depression in V_1 through V_4	SA and AV node dysfunction
	V_8	aVL, aVF, V_3 (Chien, Gregg, & Wen, 2016)	

AV, Atrioventricular; *SA,* sinoatrial.

Indicative changes may occur in a different order or different time frame than described. Some infarctions do not develop a Q wave, whereas others may lose their Q wave sometime after the infarction. Some patients' ECGs continue to show persistent STE indefinitely after the infarction.

Other exceptions relate to the localization of the infarction. While ECG localization of the site of infarction is possible, it is not perfect. For example, what appears to be a lateral wall infarction on the ECG may in fact be an anterior wall infarct. This can occur with any infarct location and is due to the fact that the ECG is simply a measurement of current flow on the patient's skin. As previously mentioned, factors including anatomic variations, patient position, and other underlying conditions may affect the perceived infarct location versus the actual location. The patient's unique pattern of coronary artery distribution can also affect the infarct location and so can the presence of collateral circulation. For these reasons, emergency care professionals occasionally encounter infarctions that are difficult to localize into the previously mentioned regions. Two common variations are apical infarctions and inferolateral infarctions.

The apex of the heart is the ventricular area most distal to the atria or the bottom "tip" of the heart. This region consists of anterior wall tissue (supplied by the LCA) and inferior wall tissue (supplied by the RCA). Therefore, depending upon the individual's coronary artery distribution, an RCA occlusion may not only produce an inferior infarction, but it may also affect a portion of the anterior wall. Likewise, an LCA occlusion in some individuals will not only affect the anterior wall but also extend into the inferior wall. These situations produce what is known as an apical infarction (Fig. 3.29).

Another common variation in coronary anatomy distribution may produce an inferolateral infarction. In the portion of the population in which the LCA supplies the inferior wall, an occlusion of that artery may produce an infarction that involves not only the inferior wall but the lateral wall as well. This is one explanation for the inferolateral infarction seen in Fig. 3.30.

Another possible explanation for both apical and inferolateral infarctions is the presence of extensive collateral circulation. In this situation, each coronary artery, to some extent, provides blood to tissues generally supplied by the other coronary artery. Therefore, an occlusion in either artery can produce injury in unexpected areas and may produce indicative changes in leads typically supplied by the other coronary artery.

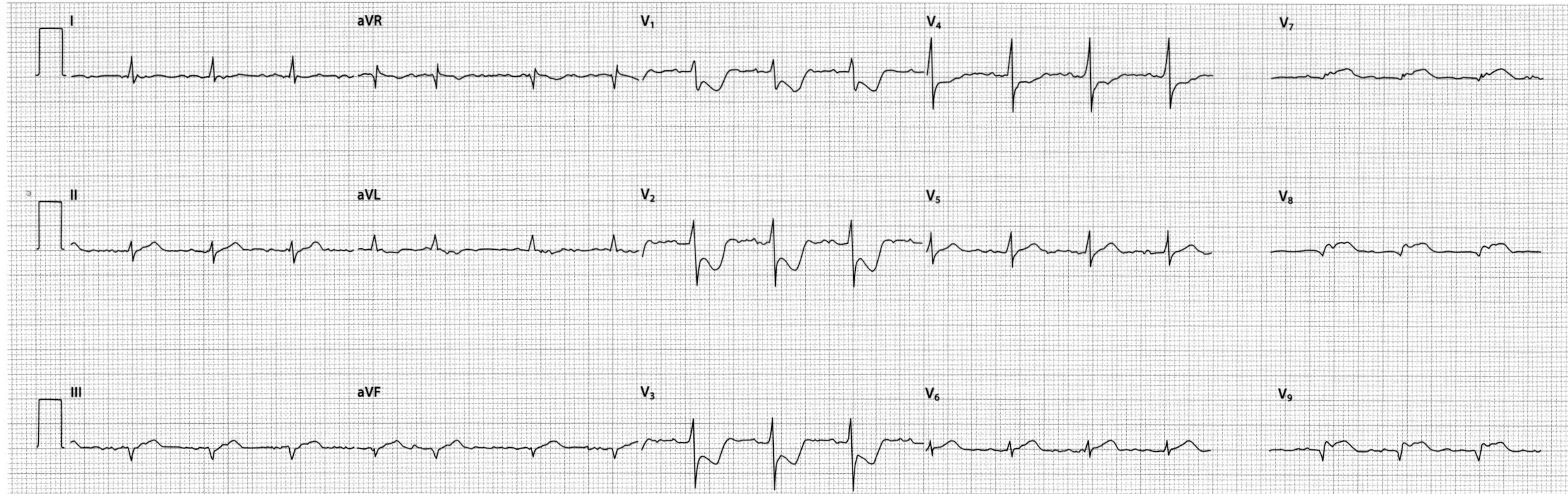

Fig. 3.28 An electrocardiogram recorded in a 76-year-old patient with diabetes during occlusion of the circumflex artery. ST-segment depression is observed in leads V_1 to V_4, which suggests a posterior myocardial infarction (MI) (left panel). Left posterior leads V_7 to V_9 are helpful in recording ST-segment elevation (STE) that confirms posterior myocardial ischemia (right panel). Observing STE in the contiguous posterior leads allows patients with an acute MI to benefit from reperfusion therapy, which would typically be denied based on analysis of the standard 12-lead electrocardiogram alone. (From Wiegand, D. L. [2017]. *AACN procedure manual for high acuity, progressive, and critical care* [7th ed.]. St. Louis, MO: Elsevier.)

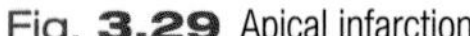

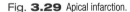

Fig. 3.29 Apical infarction.

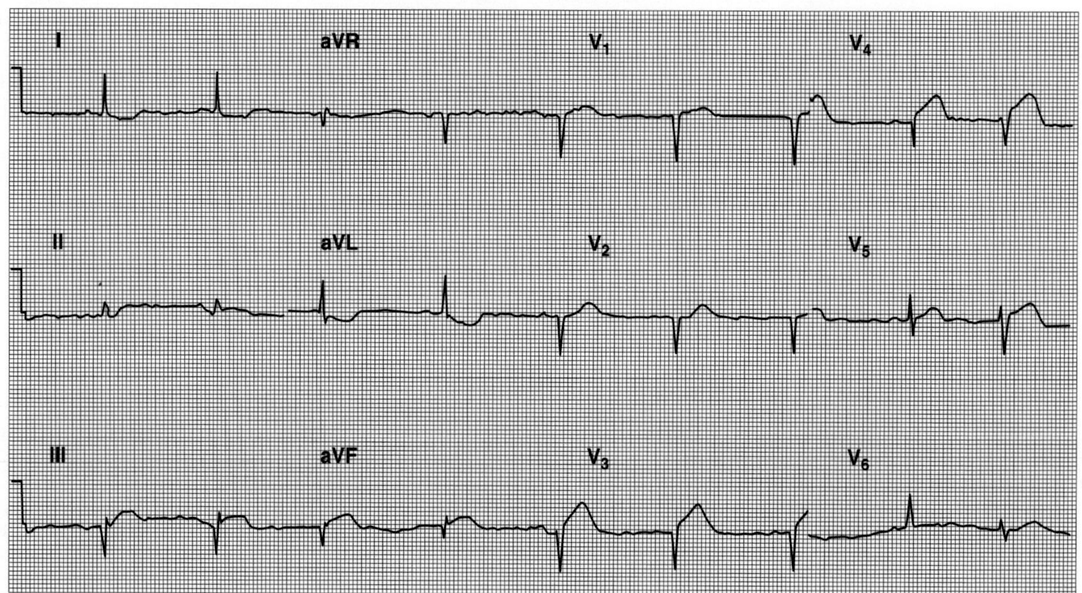

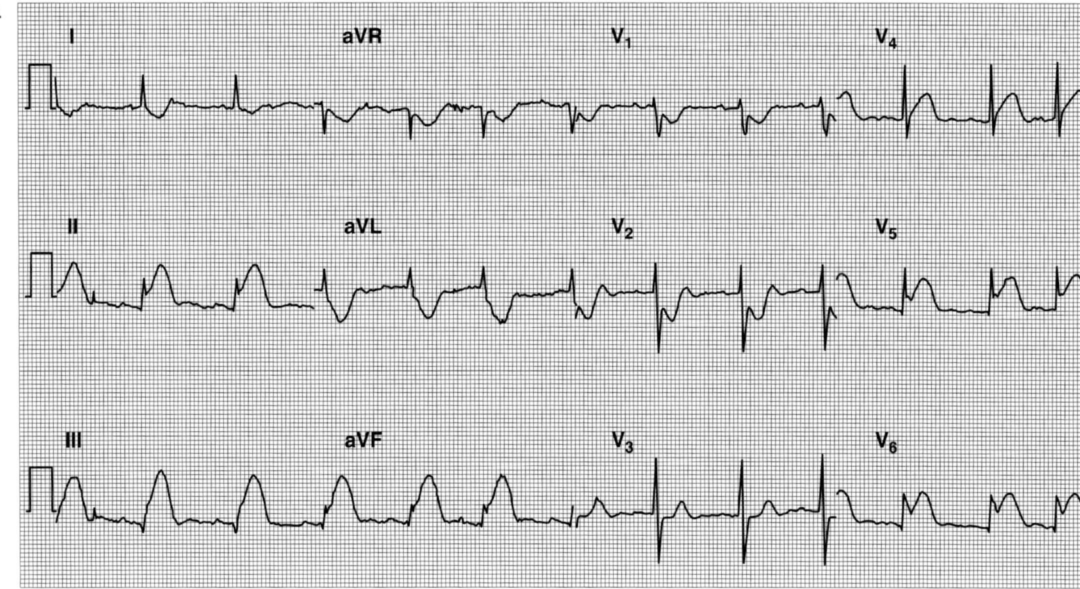

Fig. **3.30** Inferolateral infarction.

INITIAL MANAGEMENT OF ACUTE CORONARY SYNDROMES

Therapeutic interventions for ACSs are aimed at improving myocardial tissue oxygen supply, reducing myocardial oxygen demand, protecting ischemic myocardium, restoring coronary blood flow, and preventing reocclusion of the artery (Brown, 2013). As a health care professional, you must take responsibility for recognizing an ACS, developing a "working diagnosis" of infarction, and taking steps to speed the process of data collection, patient evaluation, and, when appropriate, reperfusion therapy. Early recognition of infarction can greatly reduce *total ischemic time*, which is the time from onset of symptoms of STEMI to successful reperfusion of the blocked coronary artery (O'Gara et al., 2013).

Current guidelines recommend acquiring a 12-lead ECG as soon as possible (i.e., in less than 10 minutes) for all patients exhibiting signs and symptoms of ACS. Recognizing that one-third of all patients with MI do not have chest pain, researchers developed a practical approach to identify patients, particularly those without chest pain, who require an immediate 12-lead ECG in the prehospital setting or at triage in the emergency department (ED) (Glickman et al., 2012). These researchers found that, across all age groups for STEMI, women were less likely than men to present with chest pain. They observed that chest pain decreased in frequency with age; however, a chief complaint of dyspnea, generalized weakness, syncope, or altered mental status all increased in frequency with age. They concluded that those requiring an immediate ECG include patients 30 years or older with chest pain; patients 50 years or older with shortness of breath, altered mental status, upper extremity pain, syncope, or generalized weakness; and those 80 years or older with abdominal pain or nausea/vomiting (Glickman et al., 2012).

Prehospital Management

When arriving on the scene of a patient complaining of chest discomfort or an anginal equivalent, quickly perform a primary survey and stabilize the patient's airway, breathing, and circulation (ABCs) as necessary. Allow the patient to assume a position of comfort. Make sure that the patient does not walk up or down stairs or to the stretcher. Assess vital signs and oxygen saturation. Administer supplemental oxygen if indicated. Titrate oxygen therapy to maintain an oxygen saturation of 94% or greater (O'Connor et al., 2015a).

Consider This

Current consensus documents differ with regard to supplemental oxygen administration. The 2013 American College of Cardiology Foundation/American Heart Association (AHA) guideline for the management of patients with STEMI state that oxygen therapy is appropriate for patients who are hypoxemic (i.e., oxygen saturation less than 90%) (O'Gara et al., 2013). The 2014 AHA/American College of Cardiology guideline for the management of patients with NSTE-ACS recommends supplemental oxygen administration to patients with NSTE-ACS who have an arterial oxygen saturation less than 90%, respiratory distress, or other high-risk features of hypoxemia (Amsterdam et al., 2014). The NSTE-ACS guideline also notes that "the routine use of supplemental oxygen in cardiac patients may have untoward effects, including increased coronary vascular resistance, reduced coronary blood flow, and increased risk of mortality" (Amsterdam et al., 2014). The 2015 AHA resuscitation guidelines state the following: "The provision of supplementary oxygen to patients with suspected ACS who are normoxic has not been shown to reduce mortality or hasten the resolution of chest pain. Withholding supplementary oxygen in these patients has been shown to minimally reduce infarct size. The usefulness of supplementary oxygen therapy has not been established in normoxic patients. In the prehospital, emergency department (ED), and hospital settings, the withholding of supplementary oxygen therapy in normoxic patients with suspected or confirmed ACSs may be considered" (O'Connor et al., 2015b).

Results of the Air Versus Oxygen in ST-Elevation Myocardial Infarction (AVOID) trial, which were published after the systematic review by the International Liaison Committee on Resuscitation, found that supplemental oxygen therapy in patients with STEMI but without hypoxia may increase early myocardial injury and was associated with larger myocardial infarct size assessed at 6 months (Stub et al., 2015).

Obtain a focused history, including the time of symptom onset. Assess and document the degree of the patient's pain or discomfort using a 0-to-10 scale. Antiplatelet and anticoagulant therapies are important components of ACS patient management because exposure of a ruptured plaque's contents triggers activation of the coagulation cascade. Give aspirin as soon as possible if no contraindications are present and establish cardiac monitoring. A diagnostic-quality 12-lead ECG should be obtained as soon as possible during the initial evaluation of any patient with acute nontraumatic chest pain. Perform a secondary assessment during transport as dictated by the patient's condition.

Consider This

In addition to identifying ST-segment changes earlier, prehospital ECGs can detect important transient abnormalities, information not otherwise available from the first ED department ECG (Boothroyd et al., 2013). This information can expedite diagnosis and clinical management decisions among patients suspected of having an acute cardiac event.

STEMI alert programs have been implemented in many emergency medical services systems and hospitals across the country in an attempt to minimize total ischemic time. Although the accuracy of paramedic interpretation of STEMI is high, transmission of the ECG to the ED provider for interpretation can improve the positive predictive value of the prehospital 12-lead ECG for triage and therapeutic decision-making (Davis et al., 2007). If the 12-lead ECG clearly shows evidence of STEMI, alert the receiving hospital and begin completing a fibrinolytic checklist.

Consider This

A 2017 study attempted to determine the causes of software misinterpretation of STEMI compared with clinically identified STEMI. Of 44,611 cases reviewed, the leading causes of false-positives were ECG artifact, early repolarization, probable pericarditis/myocarditis, indeterminate cause, left ventricular hypertrophy, and right bundle branch block. The leading causes of false-negatives were borderline ST-segment elevations less than the software algorithm threshold and tall T waves reducing the ST/T ratio below the algorithm threshold (Bosson et al., 2017).

Establish intravenous (IV) lines in transit and give medications for pain control per local or system protocol. For the hemodynamically stable patient who is experiencing ischemic chest discomfort, up to three doses of sublingual or aerosol NTG can be given at 3- to 5-minute intervals until pain is relieved or low blood pressure limits its use (O'Connor et al., 2015a). Although NTG has several beneficial effects, including dilation of the coronary arteries, the peripheral arterial bed, and venous capacitance vessels, no conclusive evidence has been shown to support the routine use of IV, oral, or topical nitrate therapy in patients with acute MI (O'Connor et al., 2015a). NTG should be avoided in inferior wall MI with a possible associated RVI. Because NTG is a vasodilator, it reduces preload. This reduction in preload can be undesirable in the setting of RVI and may cause profound hypotension. In addition to reassessing and documenting the patient's vital signs and level of discomfort after each dose, it is prudent to obtain a 12-lead ECG before and after interventions, such as NTG administration.

Morphine sulfate is a potent narcotic analgesic and anxiolytic. It causes venodilation, and it can lower heart rate and systolic blood pressure, thereby reducing myocardial oxygen demand. Some studies have demonstrated increased adverse events associated with the use of morphine sulfate in patients with ACS and acute decompensated heart failure (Amsterdam et al., 2014). Many health care professionals use fentanyl (i.e., Sublimaze) for pain relief in place of morphine in patients experiencing an ACS. Fentanyl is a lipid-soluble synthetic opioid that has minimal cardiovascular effects and a more rapid onset and shorter duration of action than morphine. Depending on the patient's hemodynamic stability, the administration of antiarrhythmics, vasopressors, fluid challenges, and/or inotropic agents may be necessary.

Consider This

Caution must be exercised when giving nitroglycerin and morphine to patients experiencing RVI. If hypotension does occur, it can bring with it the serious consequence of a decrease in coronary artery perfusion. Because the coronary arteries are supplied from the aorta, a decrease in blood pressure will reduce blood flow through the coronary arteries. When this occurs in an already infarcting heart, it can reduce collateral circulation to the infarcting areas or create ischemia in previously unaffected areas of the heart. Therefore, hypotension is more than just an inconvenience; it can reduce coronary artery perfusion and worsen the area of injury.

Experts encourage the development of local protocols that allow preregistration and direct transport to the catheterization laboratory of a percutaneous coronary intervention (PCI)–capable hospital (bypassing the ED) for patients who do not require emergent stabilization upon arrival (O'Gara et al., 2013).

In communities where prehospital fibrinolysis is part of a STEMI system of care, prehospital fibrinolysis is reasonable when transport time is more than 30 minutes and in-hospital fibrinolysis is the alternative treatment strategy (O'Connor et al., 2015a). In communities where prehospital fibrinolysis is available and transport directly to a PCI-capable hospital is available, transport directly to the PCI facility may be preferred because the incidence of intracranial hemorrhage, although relatively rare, is greater with fibrinolysis (O'Connor et al., 2015a) (Fig. 3.31).

Emergency Department Management

Although patients experiencing ischemic chest pain symptoms may arrive in the ED by ambulance, many arrive by means of private vehicle. Patients who arrive by private vehicle should be triaged immediately.

Quickly assess and stabilize the patient's ABCs. Frequent assessment of the patient's mental status, vital signs, and oxygen saturation level is important, and continuous ECG monitoring is essential. Administer supplemental oxygen if indicated. If not already done, give aspirin if no contraindications are present and establish IV access. While completing a fibrinolytic checklist, obtain a portable chest radiograph within 30 minutes, and draw initial laboratory tests including cardiac biomarkers, electrolytes, and coagulation studies.

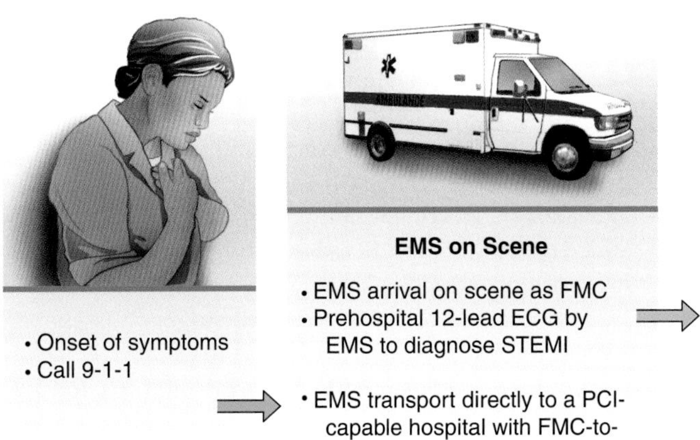

• Onset of symptoms
• Call 9-1-1
EMS on Scene
• EMS arrival on scene as FMC
• Prehospital 12-lead ECG by EMS to diagnose STEMI
• EMS transport directly to a PCI-capable hospital with FMC-to-PCI device goal of ≤90 minutes
• Activate hospital PCI team when en route to hospital
Non-PCI-Capable Hospital
• Immediate interhospital transport to a PCI-capable hospital for patients with STEMI
• Goal is FMC-to-PCI device time of ≤120 minutes.
• When unavoidable time delays will make the FMC-to-PCI device time longer than 120 minutes, fibrinolysis should be selected as the method of reperfusion for patients without contraindications.
• IV fibrinolysis should start within 30 minutes of arrival.
PCI-Capable Hospital
• When a patient is initially seen at a PCI-capable hospital, the goal is a door-to-PCI device time of under 90 minutes.
Goal is Total Ischemic Time ≤ 120 Minutes

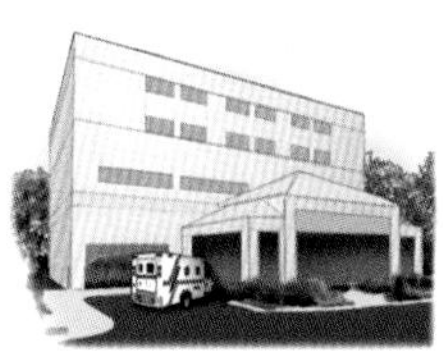

Fig. 3.31 Evaluation of prehospital chest pain and acute coronary syndrome and treatment options. The first step is to call 9-1-1 (green arrow). Transport to a PCI-capable hospital is always the optimal first choice when available (red arrows). Transport to a non-PCI-capable hospital is considered when other options are unavailable (yellow arrow and yellow box). *ECG,* Electrocardiogram; *EMS,* emergency medical services; *FMC,* first medical contact; *PCI,* percutaneous coronary intervention; *STEMI,* ST-segment elevation myocardial infarction. (From Urden, L. D., Stacy, K. M., & Lough, M. E. [2018]. *Critical care nursing: Diagnosis and management* [8th ed.]. St. Louis, MO: Mosby.)

Obtain a targeted history and physical examination. This can be done at the same time as other procedures. Assess and document the character of the patient's chest discomfort, the presence of risk factors for CAD, and the presence of associated signs and symptoms. Consider the possibility of other conditions that mimic ACS such as aortic dissection, acute pericarditis, acute myocarditis, and pulmonary embolism. Continually reassess the degree of the patient's pain or discomfort using a 0-to-10 scale and reassess the patient's response to medications given.

Because of the increased risk of major adverse cardiac events (e.g., reinfarction, hypertension, heart failure, myocardial rupture) associated with the use of nonsteroidal antiinflammatory drugs (NSAIDs), these medications (except for aspirin) should not be initiated in the acute phase of care and should be discontinued in patients using them before hospitalization (Amsterdam et al., 2014; O'Connor et al., 2015a; O'Gara et al., 2013).

Obtain and review a 12-lead ECG. After the 12-lead ECG has been obtained, it should be reviewed carefully for ECG evidence of an ACS. Patients experiencing a STEMI are considered the most emergent, followed by those with NSTE-ACS, and then persons experiencing chest pain of probable cardiac origin. Assess the areas of ischemia or injury by assessing lead groupings. Remember: ECG evidence must be found in at least two contiguous leads.

Consider This

Obtaining and reviewing a 12-lead ECG is an important component of the assessment and management of the patient presenting with ischemic chest discomfort. Obtain the first 12-lead ECG within 10 minutes of patient arrival. Repeat the 12-lead ECG when clinically indicated by a change in patient condition.

On the basis of the 12-lead ECG findings, categorize the patient into one of three groups: (1) STE, (2) ST-segment depression, or (3) normal/nondiagnostic ECG.

1. ***STE***. Patients with STE in two or more contiguous leads are classified as having a STEMI. If STE is seen in leads II, III, and/or aVF, the patient should also be evaluated for a possible RVI.

   The first ED provider who encounters a patient with STEMI should determine the need for reperfusion therapy by means of pharmacologic reperfusion (i.e., fibrinolytics) or mechanical reperfusion (i.e., PCI) (O'Connor et al., 2015b). Because consultation delays therapy, routine consultation with a cardiologist or other physician is not recommended except in equivocal or uncertain cases (O'Connor et al., 2015b). Several factors must be considered when deciding to use fibrinolytic therapy versus PCI, including the time from onset of symptoms, the patient's clinical presentation and hemodynamic status, the patient's age, the location of the infarction, the duration of STEMI at the time of initial ED presentation, patient comorbidities, the risk of bleeding, the presence of contraindications, the time delay to PCI, and the abilities of the PCI cardiologist and hospital (O'Connor et al., 2015a; O'Gara et al., 2013). Although mechanical catheter-based intervention has been proven to produce better outcomes when performed in a timely manner, fibrinolytic therapy continues to play a major role in the treatment of STEMI because only a minority of U.S. hospitals has PCI capabilities (O'Gara et al., 2013). Additional medical therapies for STEMI include antianginal, antiplatelet, and anticoagulant therapy; beta-blockers; angiotensin-converting enzyme inhibitors; and statins.

Consider This

In the event of a cardiac arrest in the patient experiencing an ACS, obtain a 12-lead ECG after the return of spontaneous circulation. Current resuscitation guidelines recommend that coronary angiography be performed emergently for out-of-hospital cardiac arrest (OHCA) patients with suspected cardiac etiology of arrest and STE on the ECG. Further, emergency coronary angiography is reasonable for select (e.g., electrically or hemodynamically unstable) adult patients who are comatose after OHCA of suspected cardiac origin but without STE on the ECG.

2. ***ST-segment depression***. ST depression or transient ST-segment/T-wave changes that occur with pain or discomfort suggest myocardial ischemia. Patients with obvious ST depression in leads V_1 and V_2 should be evaluated for possible inferobasal MI. Patients presenting with NSTE-ACS, including those with recurrent symptoms, ischemic ECG changes, or positive cardiac troponins, should be admitted to a monitored bed for further evaluation (Amsterdam et al., 2014). Stabilized patients with NSTE-ACS should be admitted to an intermediate (or step-down) care unit (Amsterdam et al., 2014). Patients with continuing angina, hemodynamic instability, uncontrolled dysrhythmias, or a large MI should be admitted to a coronary care unit (Amsterdam et al., 2014). Treatment options for NSTE-ACS include antianginal, antiplatelet, and anticoagulant therapy. Because the presence of depressed left ventricular function can influence pharmacologic therapies and can influence revascularization choices (i.e., PCI vs. coronary artery bypass graft surgery), assessment of left ventricular function is recommended (Amsterdam et al., 2014).
3. ***Normal/nondiagnostic ECG***. A normal ECG or nonspecific ST- and T-wave changes are nondiagnostic and should prompt consideration for further evaluation. Consider admission of the patient with signs and symptoms suggesting an ACS and a nondiagnostic ECG to the ED chest pain unit or to an appropriate bed (O'Connor et al., 2015b). Obtaining serial ECGs or continuous monitoring of the ST segment should be performed to detect the potential development of STE if the initial ECG is not diagnostic of STEMI but the patient remains symptomatic and there is a high clinical suspicion of STEMI. Noninvasive tests (e.g., computed tomography angiography, cardiac magnetic resonance, myocardial scintigraphy, stress echocardiography) can be useful in identifying patients suitable for discharge from the ED (O'Connor et al., 2015b). The ACS algorithm appears in Fig. 3.32.

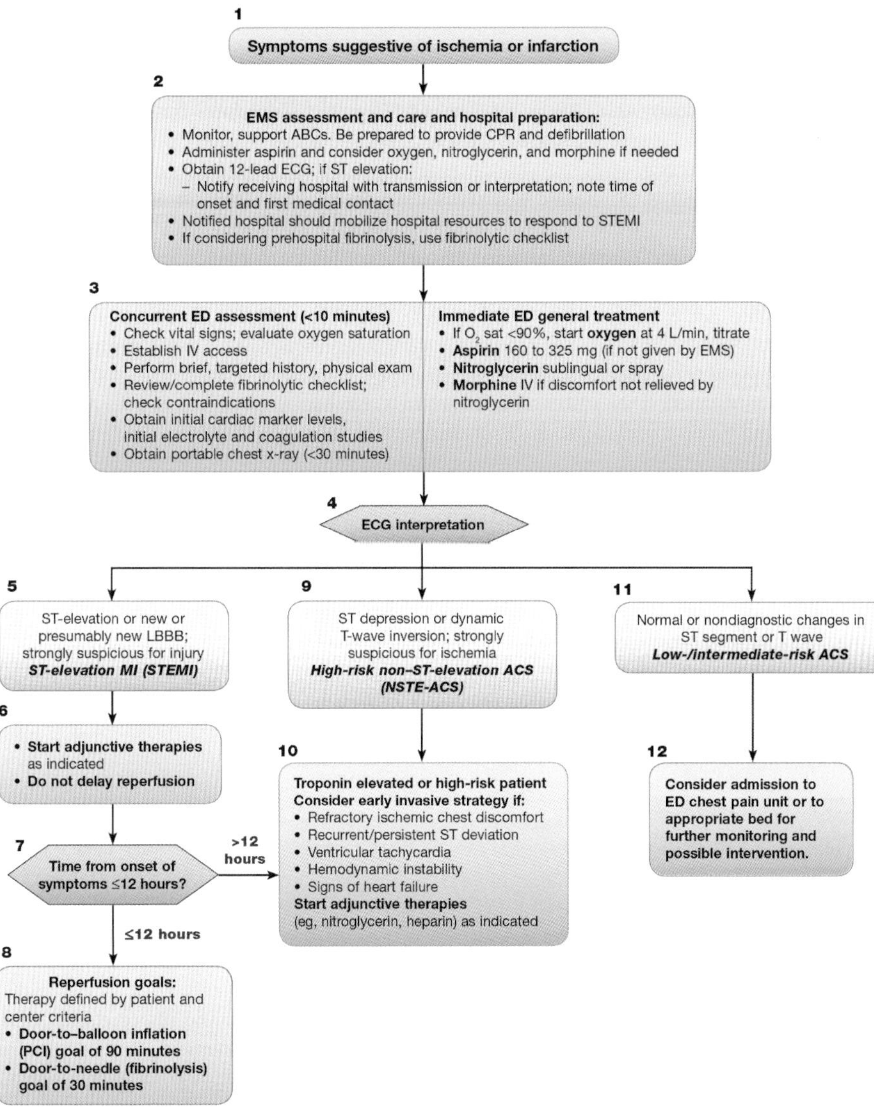

Fig. **3.32** (Reprinted with permission. *Web-Integrated 2010 & 2015 American Heart Association guidelines for CPR & ECC Part 9: Acute coronary syndromes.* ECCguidelines.heart.org. © 2015 American Heart Association, Inc.)

REFERENCES

Amsterdam, E. A., Wenger, N. K., Brindis, R. G., Casey Jr, D. E., Ganiats, T. G., Holmes Jr., D. R., ... Zieman, S. J. (2014). 2014 AHA/ACC guideline for the management of patients with non-ST-elevation acute coronary syndromes. *Journal of the American College of Cardiology, 64*(24), 1–150.

Anderson, J. L. (2016). ST segment elevation acute myocardial infarction and complications of myocardial infarction. In L. Goldman & A. I. Schafer (Eds.), *Goldman-Cecil medicine* (25th ed., pp. 441–456). Philadelphia, PA: Saunders.

Blanc-Brude, O. (2011). Myocardial cell death and regeneration. In P. Théroux (Ed.), *Acute coronary syndromes: A companion to Braunwald's heart disease* (2nd ed., pp. 66–80). Philadelphia, PA: Saunders.

Boden, W. E. (2016). Angina pectoris and stable ischemic heart disease. In L. Goldman & A. I. Schafer (Eds.), *Goldman-Cecil medicine* (25th ed., pp. 420–431). Philadelphia, PA: Saunders.

Boothroyd, L. J., Segal, E., Bogaty, P., Nasmith, J., Eisenberg, M. J., Boivin, J. F., ... de Champlain, F. (2013). Information on myocardial ischemia and arrhythmias added by prehospital electrocardiograms. *Prehospital Emergency Care, 17*(2), 187–192.

Bosson, N., Sanko, S., Stickney, R. E., Niemann, J., French, W. J., Jollis, J. G., ... Eckstein, M. (2017). Causes of prehospital misinterpretations of ST elevation myocardial infarction. *Prehospital Emergency Care, 21*(3), 283–290.

Brashers, V. L. (2014). Alterations of cardiovascular function. In K. L. McCance, S. E. Huether, V. L. Brashers, & N. S. Rote (Eds.), *Pathophysiology: The biologic basis for disease in adults and children* (7th ed., pp. 1129–1193). St. Louis: Mosby.

Brown, D. F. (2013). Acute coronary syndrome. In J. G. Adams (Ed.), *Emergency medicine* (2nd ed., pp. 452–468). Philadelphia, PA: Saunders.

Chen, C., Wei, J., AlBadri, A., Zarrini, P., & Bairey Merz, C. N. (2016). Coronary microvascular dysfunction—Epidemiology, pathogenesis, prognosis, diagnosis, risk factors and therapy. *Circulation Journal, 81*(1), 3–11.

Chien, S. C., Gregg, R., & Wen, M.-S. (2016). The relationship between ST depression in standard 12-leads and the ST elevation in extended leads. *Journal of Electrocardiology, 49*(6), 926–926.

Cinquegrani, M. P. (2016). Coronary heart disease. In I. J. Benjamin, R. C. Griggs, E. J. Wing, & J. G. Fitz (Eds.), *Andreoli and Carpenter's Cecil essentials of medicine* (9th ed., pp. 87–109). Philadelphia, PA: Saunders.

Crea, F., Camici, P. G., & Bairey Merz, C. N. (2014). Coronary microvascular dysfunction: An update. *European Heart Journal, 35*(17), 1101–1111.

Damjanov, I. (2017). The cardiovascular system. In *Pathology for the health professions* (5th ed., pp. 133–164). St. Louis, MO: Elsevier.

Davis, D. P., Graydon, C., Stein, R., Wilson, S., Buesch, B., Berthiaume, S., ... Leahy, D. R. (2007). The positive predictive value of paramedic versus emergency physician interpretation of the prehospital 12-lead electrocardiogram. *Prehospital Emergency Care, 11*(4), 399–402.

Falk, E., & Bentzon, J. F. (2017). New and emerging insights into the pathobiology of acute myocardial infarction. In D. A. Morrow (Ed.), *Myocardial infarction: A companion to Braunwald's heart disease* (pp. 22–33). St. Louis, MO: Elsevier.

Giugliano, R. P., Cannon, C. P., & Braunwald, E. (2015). Non-ST-elevation acute coronary syndromes. In D. L. Mann, D. P. Zipes, P. Libby, R. O. Bonow, & E. Braunwald (Eds.), *Braunwald's heart disease: A textbook of cardiovascular medicine* (10th ed., pp. 1155–1181). Philadelphia, PA: Saunders.

Glickman, S. W., Shofer, F. S., Wu, M. C., Scholer, M. J., Ndubuizu, A., Peterson, E. D., ... Glickman, L. T. (2012). Development and validation of a prioritization rule for obtaining an immediate 12-lead electrocardiogram in the emergency department to identify ST-elevation myocardial infarction. *American Heart Journal, 163*(3), 372–382.

Goktas, M. U., Sogut, O., Yigit, M., & Kaplan, O. (2017). A novel electrocardiographic sign of an ST-segment elevation myocardial infarction-equivalent: De Winter syndrome. *Cardiology Research, 8*(4), 165–168.

Goldstein, J. A. (2012). Acute right ventricular infarction. *Cardiology Clinics, 30*(2), 219–232.

Halim, S. A., Newby, K., & Ohman, E. M. (2010). Diagnosis of acute myocardial ischemia and infarction. In M. H. Crawford, J. P. DiMarco, & W. J. Paulus (Eds.), *Cardiology* (3rd ed., pp. 345–360). Philadelphia, PA: Elsevier.

Karve, A. M., Bossone, E., & Mehta, R. H. (2007). Acute ST-segment elevation myocardial infarction: critical care perspective. *Critical Care Clinics, 23*(4), 685–707.

Kaski, J. C., & Arroyo-Espliguero, R. (2010). Variant angina pectoris. In M. H. Crawford, J. P. DiMarco, & W. J. Paulus (Eds.), *Cardiology* (3rd ed., pp. 301–309). Philadelphia, PA: Elsevier.

Kawano, H., Motoyama, T., Yasue, H., Hirai, N., Waly, H. M., Kugiyama, K., & Ogawa, H. (2002). Endothelial function fluctuates with diurnal variation in the frequency of ischemic episodes in patients with variant angina. *Journal of the American College of Cardiology, 40*(2), 266–270.

Kumar, V., Abbas, A. K., & Aster, J. C. (2018). Heart. In V. Kumar, A. K. Abbas, & J. C. Aster (Eds.), *Robbins basic pathology* (10th ed.). Philadelphia, PA: Elsevier.(pp. 399–441).

Kurz, M. C., Mattu, A., & Brady, W. J. (2014). Acute coronary syndrome. In J. A. Marx, R. S. Hockberger, & R. M. Walls (Eds.), *Rosen's emergency medicine* (8th ed., pp. 997–1033). Philadelphia, PA: Saunders.

Lange, R. A., & Hillis, L. D. (2016). Acute coronary syndrome: Unstable angina and non-ST elevation myocardial infarction. In L. Goldman & A. I. Schafer (Eds.), *Goldman-Cecil medicine* (25th ed., pp. 432–441). Philadelphia, PA: Saunders.

Löffler, A. I., & Bourque, J. (2016). Coronary microvascular dysfunction, microvascular angina, and management. *Current Cardiology Reports, 18*(1). https://doi.org/10.1007/s11886-015-0682-9.

Mao, L., Jian, C., Wei, W., Tianmin, L., Changzhi, L., & Dan, H. (2013). For physicians: Never forget the specific ECG T-wave changes of Wellens' syndrome. *International Journal of Cardiology, 167*(1), e20-e21.

Martínez-Losas, P., & Fernández-Jiménez, R. (2016). de Winter syndrome. *Canadian Medical Association Journal, 188*(7), 528–528.

McSweeney, J. C., Cody, M., O'Sullivan, P., Elberson, K., Moser, D. K., & Garvin, B. J. (2003). Women's early warning symptoms of acute myocardial infarction. *Circulation, 108*(21), 2619–2623.

Morris, F., & Brady, W. J. (2002). Acute myocardial infarction—Part I. *British Medical Journal, 324*(7341), 831–834.

Morrow, D. A., & Boden, W. E. (2015). Stable ischemic heart disease. In D. L. Mann, D. P. Zipes, P. Libby, R. O. Bonow, & E. Braunwald (Eds.), *Braunwald's heart disease: A textbook of cardiovascular medicine* (10th ed., pp. 1182–1244). Philadelphia, PA: Saunders.

Naderi, S., & Cho, L. (2016). Sex and ethnicity issues in interventional cardiology. In E. J. Topol & P. S. Teirstein (Eds.), *Textbook of interventional cardiology* (7th ed.)(pp. 141–150). Philadelphia, PA: Elsevier.

O'Connor, R. E., Al Ali, A. S., Brady, W. J., Ghaemmaghami, C. A., Menon, V., Welsford, M., & Shuster, M. (2015a). *2015 American Heart Association guidelines for CPR & ECC.* Retrieved from American Heart Association. Web-based Integrated Guidelines for Cardiopulmonary Resuscitation and Emergency Cardiovascular Care – Part 9: Acute Coronary Syndromes: Eccguidelines.heart.org.

O'Connor, R. E., Al Ali, A. S., Brady, W. J., Ghaemmaghami, C. A., Menon, V., Welsford, M., & Shuster, M. (2015b). Part 9: Acute coronary syndromes: 2015 American Heart Association guidelines update for cardiopulmonary resuscitation and emergency cardiovascular care. *Circulation, 132*(18 Suppl 2), 483–500.

O'Gara, P. T., Kushner, F. G., Ascheim, D. D., Casey Jr, D. E., Chung, M. K., de Lemos, J. A., ... Zhao, D. X. (2013). 2013 ACCF/AHA guideline for the management of ST-elevation myocardial infarction. *Journal of the American College of Cardiology, 61*(4), e78–e140.

Schoen, F. J., & Mitchell, R. N. (2015). The heart. In V. Kumar, A. K. Abbas, & J. C. Aster (Eds.), *Robbins and Cotran pathologic basis of disease* (9th ed., pp. 523–578). Philadelphia, PA: Saunders.

Scirica, B. M., & Morrow, D. A. (2015). ST-elevation myocardial infarction: Pathology, pathophysiology, and clinical features. In D. L. Mann, D. P. Zipes, P. Libby, R. O. Bonow, & E. Braunwald (Eds.), *Braunwald's heart disease: A textbook of cardiovascular medicine* (10th ed., pp. 1068–1094). Philadelphia: Saunders.

Seo, D. W., Sohn, C. H., Ryu, J. M., Yoon, J. C., Ahn, S., & Kim, W. (2011). ST elevation measurements differ in patients with inferior myocardial infarction and right ventricular infarction. *American Journal of Emergency Medicine, 29*(9), 1067–1073.

Sovari, A. A., Assadi, R., Lakshminarayanan, B., & Kocheril, A. G. (2007). Hyperacute T wave, the early sign of myocardial infarction. *American Journal of Emergency Medicine, 25*(7), 859. e1–859.e7.

Stub, D., Smith, K., Bernard, S., Nehme, Z., Stephenson, M., & Bray, J. E., on behalf of the AVOID investigators. (2015). Air versus oxygen in ST-segment elevation myocardial infarction. *Circulation, 131*(24), 2143–2150.

Thygesen, K., Alpert, J. S., Jaffe, A. S., Simoons, M. L., Chaitman, B. R., & White, H. D. (2012). Third universal definition of myocardial infarction. *Circulation, 126*(16), 2020–2035.

Tobin, K., & Eagle, K. (2017). Angina pectoris. In E. T. Bope & R. D. Kellerman (Eds.), *Conn's current therapy 2017* (pp. 85–91). Philadelphia, PA: Elsevier.

Wagner, G. S., Macfarlane, P., Wellens, H., Josephson, M., Gorgels, A., Mirvis, D. M., ... Gettes, L. S. (2009). AHA/ACCF/HRS recommendations for the standardization and interpretation of the electrocardiogram: Part VI: Acute ischemia/infarction; a scientific statement from the American Heart Association Electrocardiography and Arrhythmias Committee. *Journal of the American College of Cardiology, 53*(11), 1003–1011.

QUICK REVIEW

1. When observed in two or more anatomically contiguous leads, STE is considered significant if it is elevated 2 mm or more at the J point in all leads other than V_2 and V_3 in a patient who is experiencing an ACS.
   a. True
   b. False

2. 2. A 66-year-old man is experiencing chest discomfort that he rates 9/10. His 12-lead ECG reveals STE in leads II, III, and aVF and ST-segment depression in leads I and aVL. These ECG findings suggest that
   a. a lateral NSTE-ACS is present; the STE reflects reciprocal changes.
   b. an anterior NSTE-ACS is present; the STE reflects reciprocal changes.
   c. an inferior STEMI is present; the ST-segment depression reflects reciprocal changes.
   d. a posterior STEMI is present; the ST-segment depression reflects reciprocal changes.

3. A patient has been diagnosed with an extensive anterior STEMI. When examining this patient's 12-lead ECG, you should expect to see indicative ECG changes in which of the following leads?
   a. V_7 through V_9
   b. II, III, and aVF
   c. V_1 through V_4, and V_4R
   d. I, aVL, and V_1 through V_6

4. Reciprocal changes of a high lateral infarction can usually be viewed in leads
   a. II and aVR.
   b. V_1 through V_3.
   c. II, III, and aVF.
   d. V_2 through V_4.

5. An 80-year-old woman presents with a sudden onset of difficulty breathing. The patient's 12-lead ECG shows STE in leads I, aVL, and V_2 through V_4. Troponin levels are elevated 4 hours after symptom onset. On the basis of this information, you suspect
   a. STEMI.
   b. NSTEMI.
   c. unstable angina.
   d. variant angina.

PRACTICE ECGS

To help you master the concepts introduced in this chapter, 12-lead ECGs have been included for practice (see Figs. 3.33 through 3.41). We recommend the following approach when reviewing a 12-lead ECG:

1. ***Identify the rate and underlying rhythm.*** Determining rate and rhythm is the first priority when interpreting the ECG. If baseline wander or artifact is present to any significant degree, note it. If the presence of either of these conditions interferes with the assessment of any lead, use a modifier such as "possible" or "apparent" in your interpretation.
2. ***Analyze waveforms, segments, and intervals.*** Select one good representative waveform or complex in each lead. Each lead, with the exception of aVR, should be examined for the presence of indicative changes, with special emphasis on ST-segment displacement (elevation or depression). If displacement is present, express it in millimeters. Examine the T waves for any changes in orientation, shape, and size. Note the presence of tall, peaked T waves or T-wave inversion. Examine all leads for pathologic Q waves. An abnormal (i.e., pathologic) Q wave is more than 0.03 second in duration or more than 30% of the height of the following R wave in that lead, or both (Anderson, 2016).
3. ***Examine for evidence of an ACS.*** If ST-segment displacement is present, assess the areas of ischemia or injury by assessing lead groupings. If an ACS is suspected, mentally picture the cardiac anatomy to localize the area at risk and predict which coronary artery is occluded.
4. ***Estimate the QRS axis.*** Using leads I and aVF, estimate the QRS axis.
5. ***Interpret your findings.*** On the basis of your examination, categorize the 12-lead ECG into one of the previously described groups: (1) STE, (2) ST-segment depression, or (3) normal or nondiagnostic ECG.

Our interpretation of each ECG is included at the end of this chapter. Please note that the interpretation of each lead and tracing includes only the material discussed in this text. Therefore, experienced electrocardiographers will note the presence of some conditions or findings that are not listed in the interpretation.

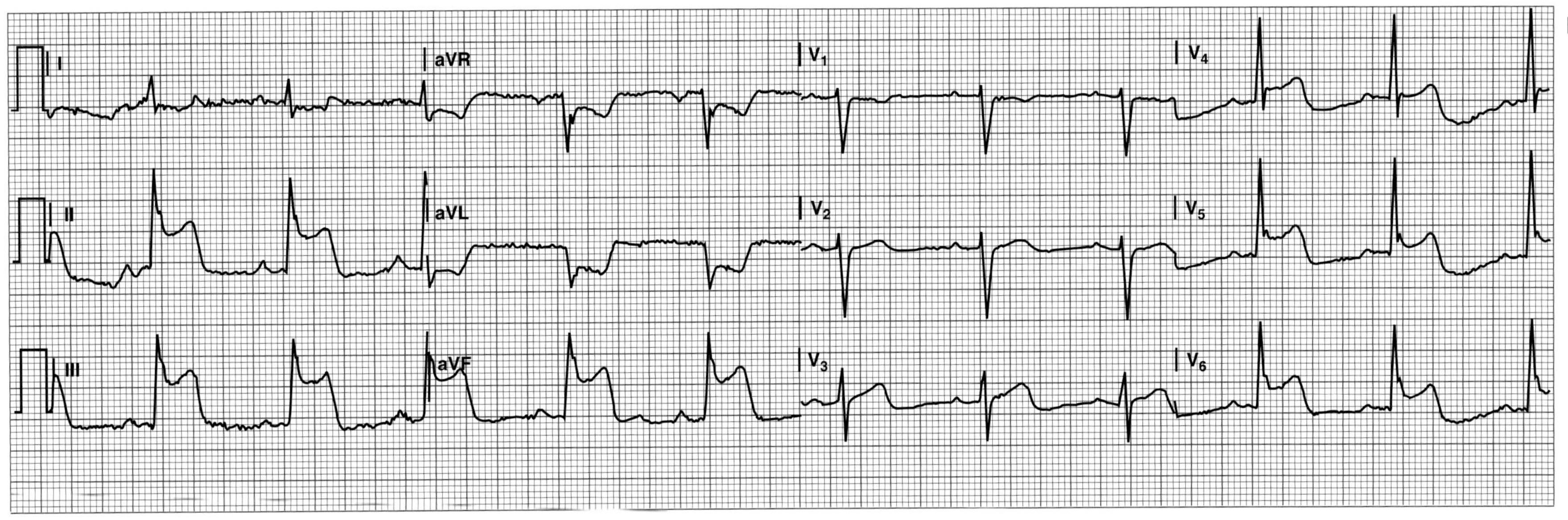

Fig. 3.33

I Lateral	aVR ---------	V_1 Septum	V_4 Anterior
II Inferior	aVL Lateral	V_2 Septum	V_5 Lateral
III Inferior	aVF Inferior	V_3 Anterior	V_6 Lateral

Rate and rhythm? ______________________ STE? ______________________ ST depression? ______________________

T-wave changes? ______________________ Pathologic Q waves? ______________________ Axis? ______________________

Interpretation: ____

Fig. 3.34

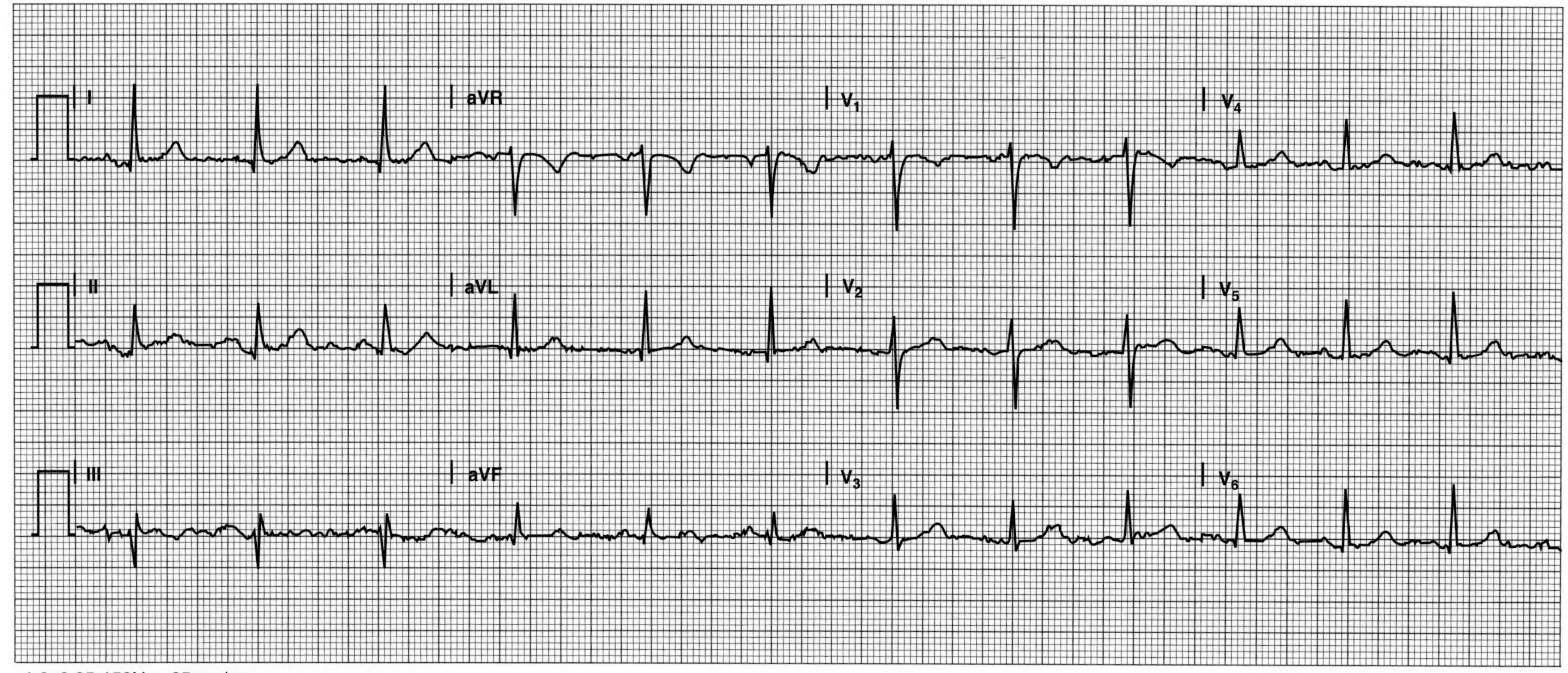

I Lateral	aVR ---------	V_1 Septum	V_4 Anterior
II Inferior	aVL Lateral	V_2 Septum	V_5 Lateral
III Inferior	aVF Inferior	V_3 Anterior	V_6 Lateral

Rate and rhythm? ______________ STE? ______________ ST depression? ______________

T-wave changes? ______________ Pathologic Q waves? ______________ Axis? ______________

Interpretation: ____

Fig. 3.35

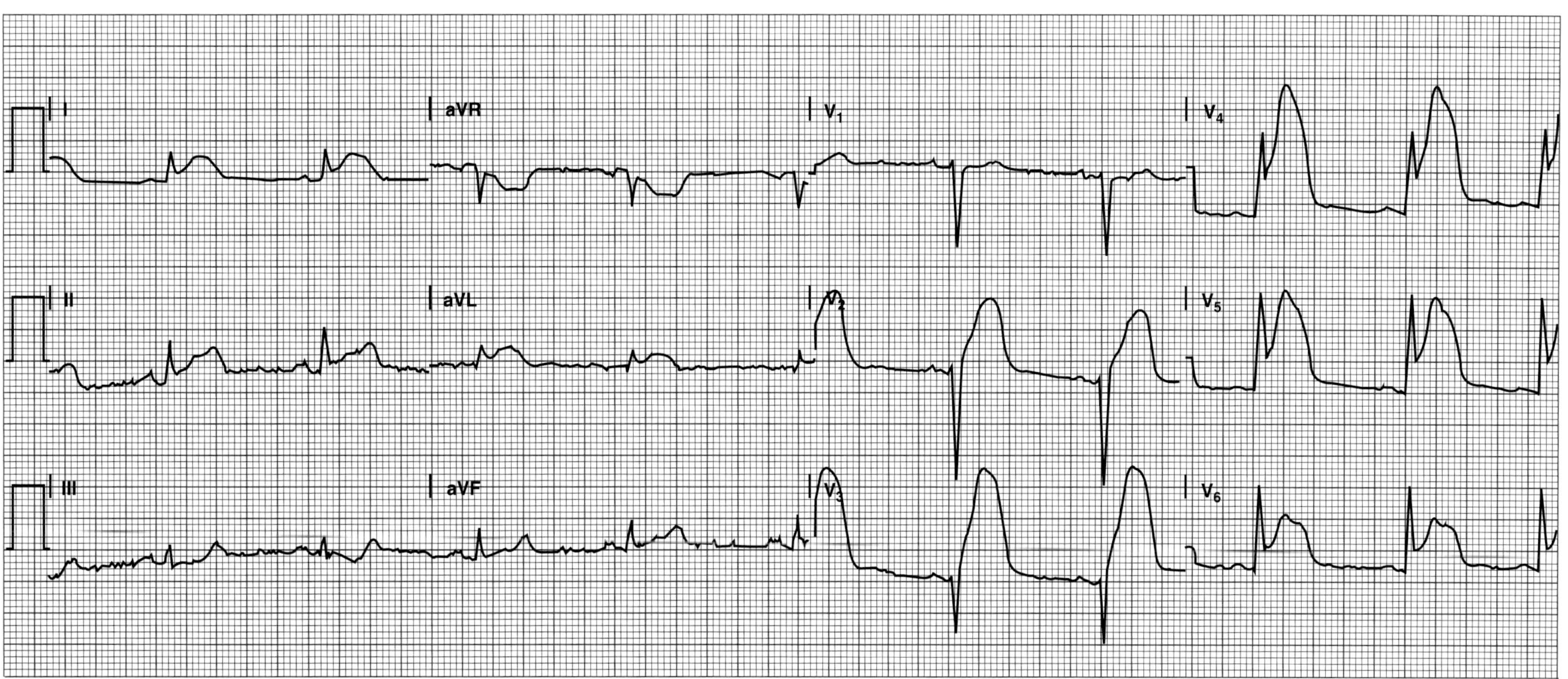

I Lateral	aVR ---------	V_1 Septum	V_4 Anterior
II Inferior	aVL Lateral	V_2 Septum	V_5 Lateral
III Inferior	aVF Inferior	V_3 Anterior	V_6 Lateral

Rate and rhythm? ______________________ STE? ______________________ ST depression? ______________________

T-wave changes? ______________________ Pathologic Q waves? ______________________ Axis? ______________________

Interpretation: ____

Fig. 3.36

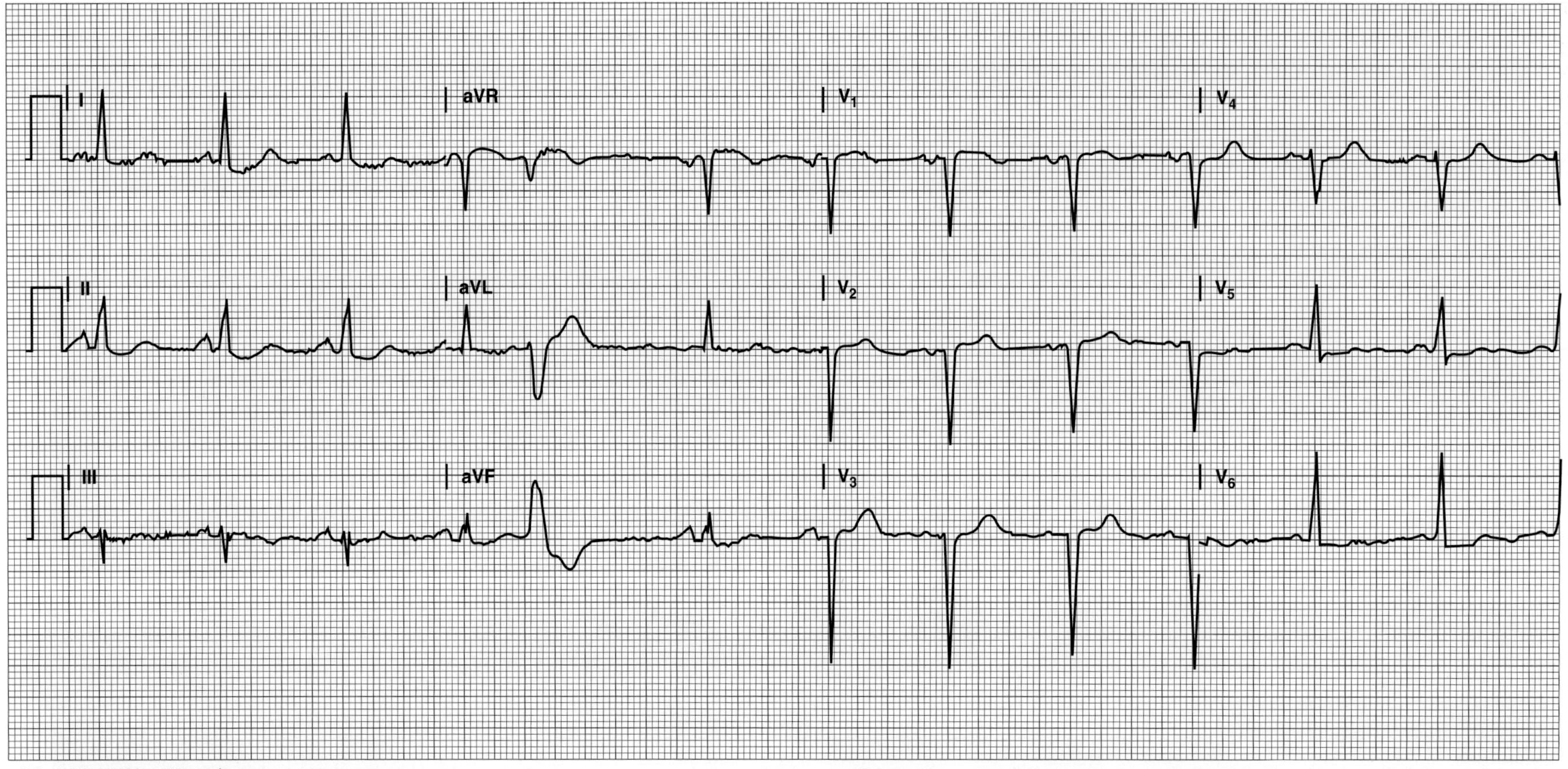

I Lateral	aVR ---------	V_1 Septum	V_4 Anterior
II Inferior	aVL Lateral	V_2 Septum	V_5 Lateral
III Inferior	aVF Inferior	V_3 Anterior	V_6 Lateral

Rate and rhythm? ______________________ STE? ______________________ ST depression? ______________________

T-wave changes? ______________________ Pathologic Q waves? ______________________ Axis? ______________________

Interpretation: ____

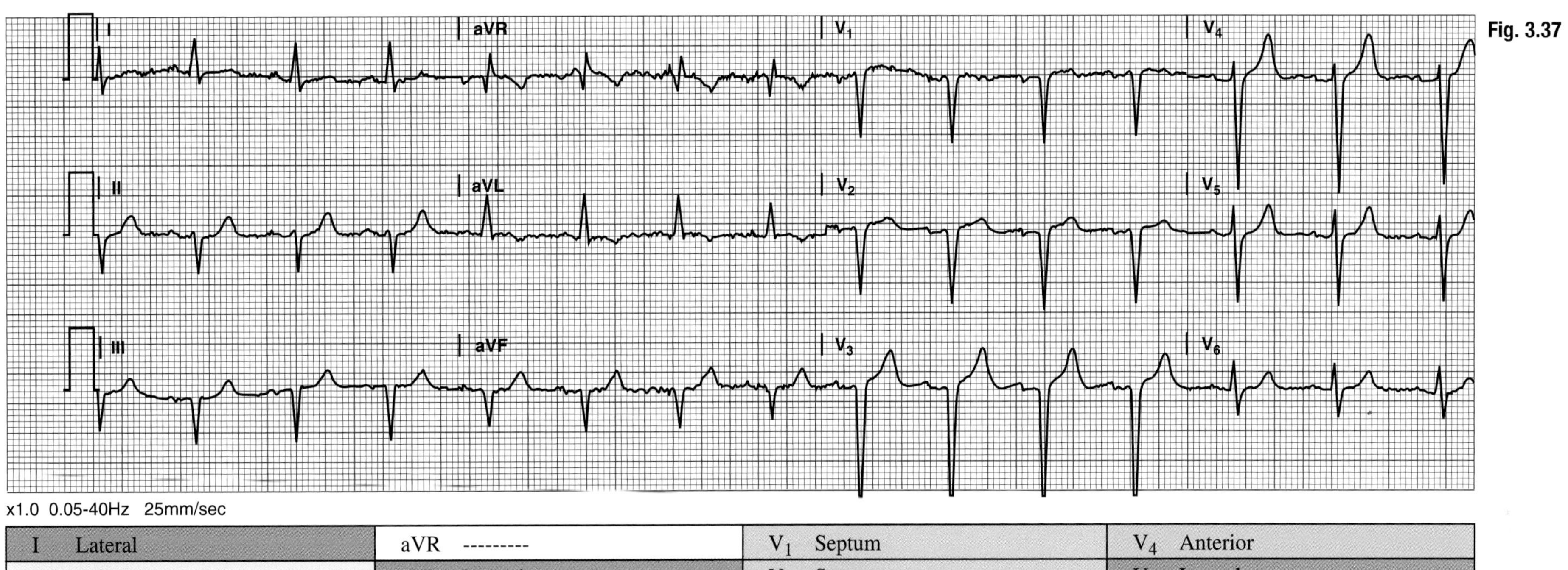

Fig. 3.37

I Lateral	aVR ---------	V_1 Septum	V_4 Anterior
II Inferior	aVL Lateral	V_2 Septum	V_5 Lateral
III Inferior	aVF Inferior	V_3 Anterior	V_6 Lateral

Rate and rhythm? ______________________ STE? ______________________ ST depression? ______________________

T-wave changes? ______________________ Pathologic Q waves? ______________________ Axis? ______________________

Interpretation: ____

Fig. 3.38

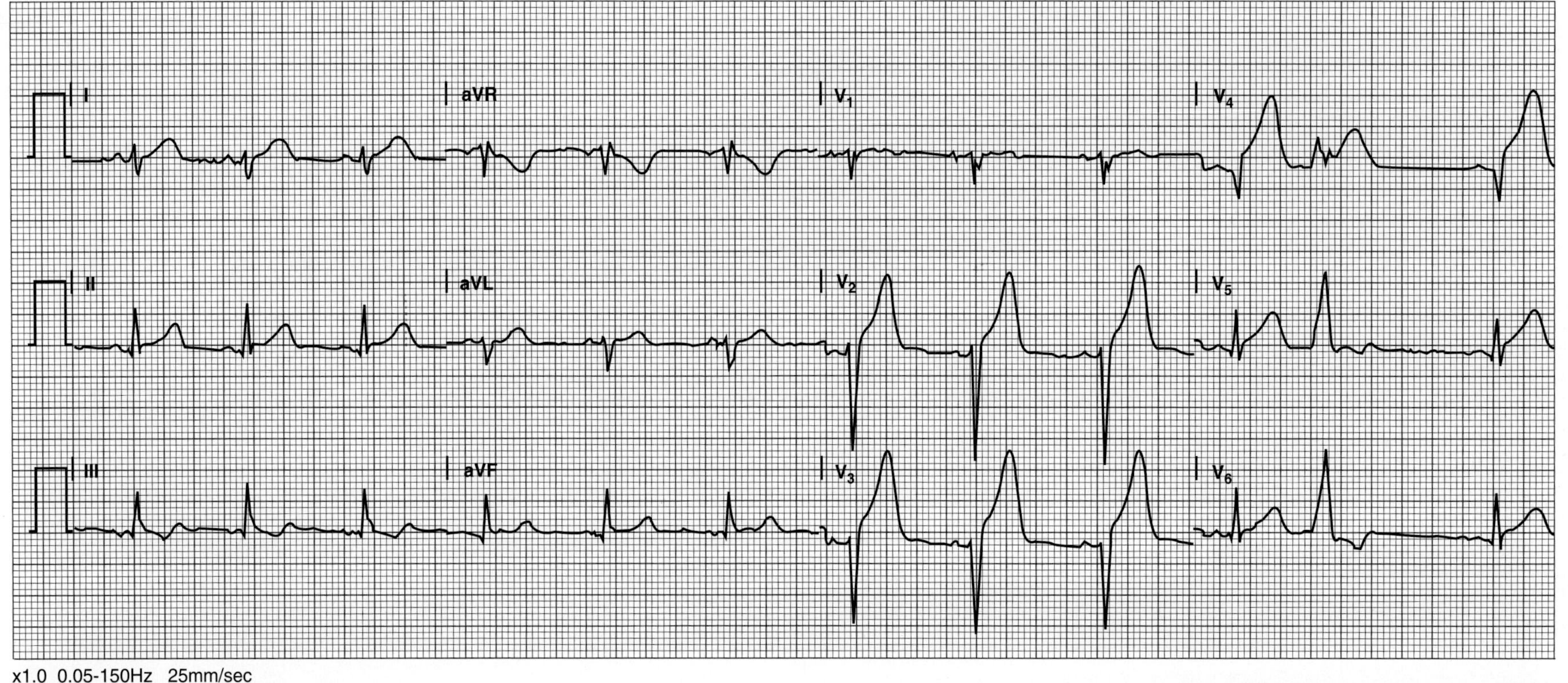

I Lateral	aVR ---------	V_1 Septum	V_4 Anterior
II Inferior	aVL Lateral	V_2 Septum	V_5 Lateral
III Inferior	aVF Inferior	V_3 Anterior	V_6 Lateral

Rate and rhythm? ______________________ STE? ______________________ ST depression? ______________________

T-wave changes? ______________________ Pathologic Q waves? ______________________ Axis? ______________________

Interpretation: ____

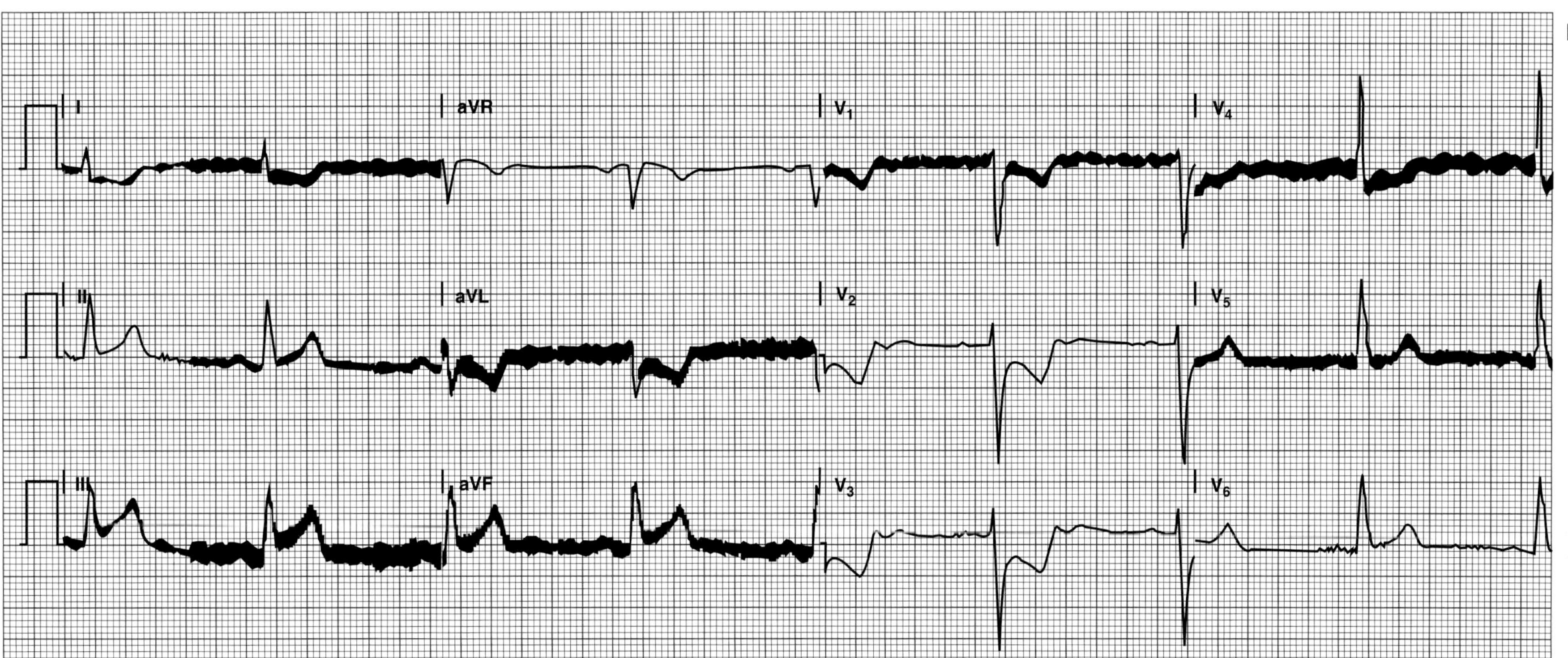

Fig. 3.39

x1.0 0.05-150Hz 25mm/sec

I Lateral	aVR ---------	V_1 Septum	V_4 Anterior
II Inferior	aVL Lateral	V_2 Septum	V_5 Lateral
III Inferior	aVF Inferior	V_3 Anterior	V_6 Lateral

Rate and rhythm? ______________ STE? ______________ ST depression? ______________

T-wave changes? ______________ Pathologic Q waves? ______________ Axis? ______________

Interpretation: ______________

Fig. 3.40

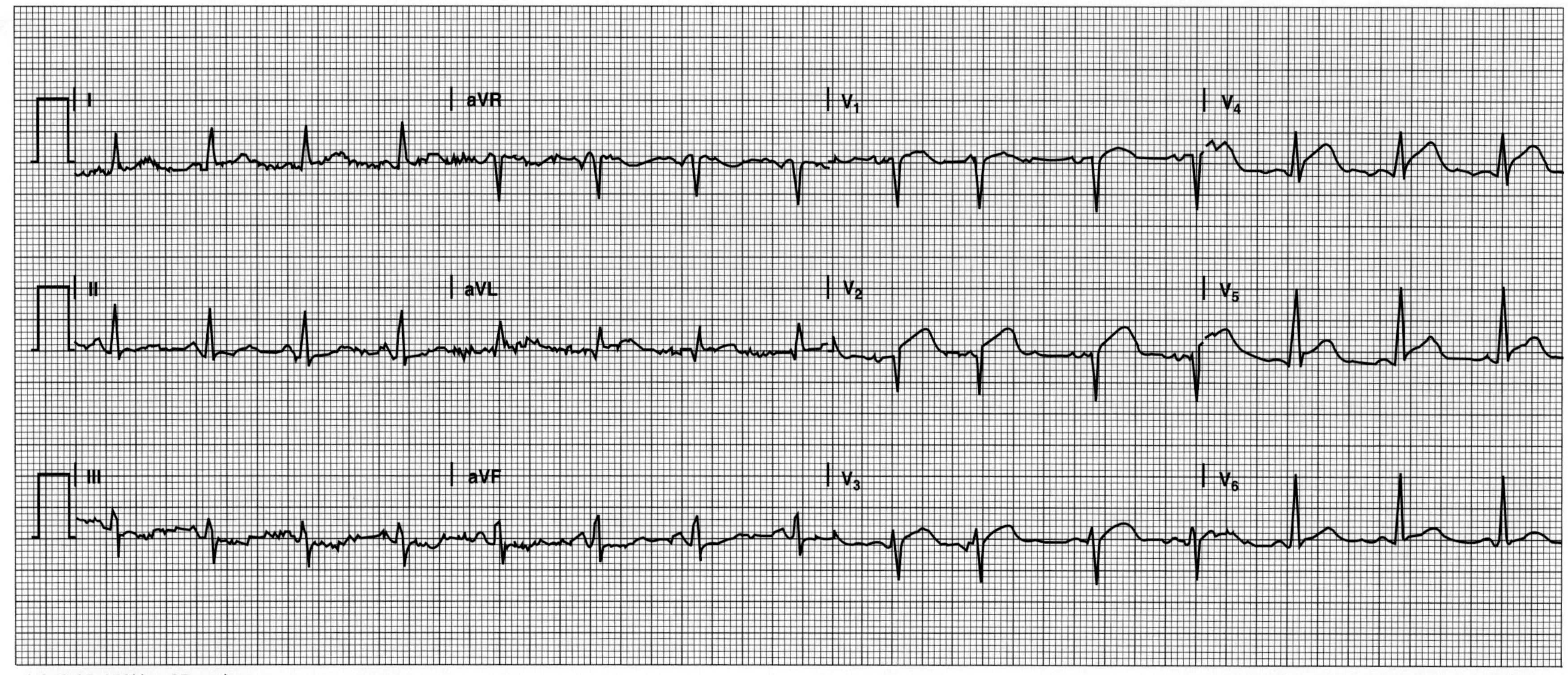

I Lateral	aVR ---------	V_1 Septum	V_4 Anterior
II Inferior	aVL Lateral	V_2 Septum	V_5 Lateral
III Inferior	aVF Inferior	V_3 Anterior	V_6 Lateral

Rate and rhythm? ______________________ STE? ______________________ ST depression? ______________________

T-wave changes? ______________________ Pathologic Q waves? ______________________ Axis? ______________________

Interpretation: ____

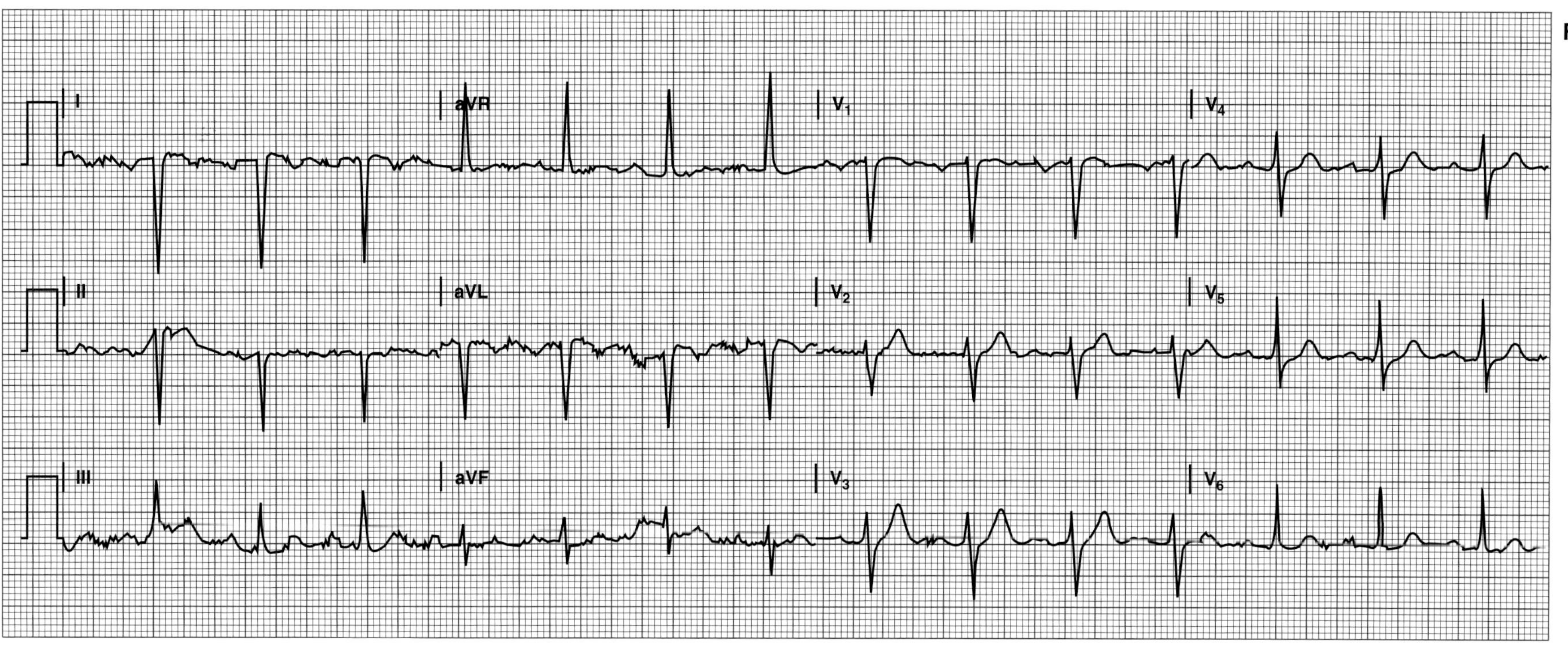

Fig. 3.41

I Lateral	aVR ---------	V_1 Septum	V_4 Anterior
II Inferior	aVL Lateral	V_2 Septum	V_5 Lateral
III Inferior	aVF Inferior	V_3 Anterior	V_6 Lateral

Rate and rhythm? ______________________ STE? ______________________ ST depression? ______________________

T-wave changes? ______________________ Pathologic Q waves? ______________________ Axis? ______________________

Interpretation: ____

CASE STUDIES

For each of the following case studies, carefully evaluate the description of the patient's clinical presentation, systematically analyze each 12-lead ECG, and formulate a treatment plan on the basis of the information provided.

CASE STUDY 3.1

A 51-year-old woman presents with a sudden onset of shortness of breath, fatigue, and tingling of her left hand. She denies chest pain or discomfort. The patient reports that she was outside gardening when her symptoms began about 2 hours ago. She has no significant medical history and has no known medication allergies. Her medications include a baby aspirin and a multivitamin daily, as well as melatonin that she uses as a sleep aide.

Physical examination reveals that the patient is alert and oriented to person, place, time, and event. Her skin is pink, warm, and dry, and her breath sounds are clear. Her SpO_2 is 96% on room air. Her blood pressure is 128/58 mm Hg, pulse 68 beats/min, and ventilations 18/min. The patient has been placed on a cardiac monitor. Vascular access has been established and a 12-lead ECG has been obtained (Fig. 3.42). Review the patient's ECG and describe your initial interventions for this patient.

Fig. 3.42

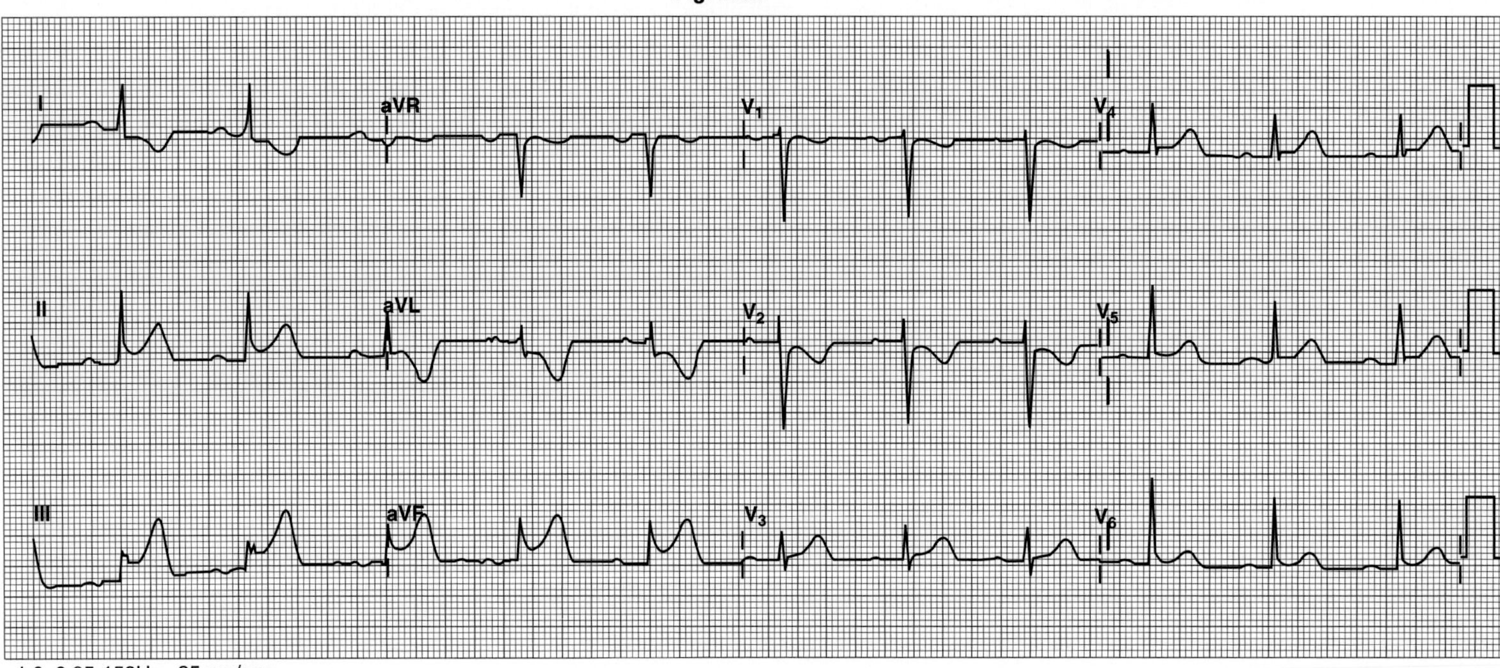

CASE STUDY 3.2

A 58-year-old man presents with crushing substernal chest pain with radiation to his left arm that he rates 10/10. He denies nausea, vomiting, and shortness of breath. The patient states he was putting away dishes when his symptoms began about 45 minutes ago. He has a history of asthma and had a pulmonary embolism 1 year ago, at which time an inferior vena cava umbrella filter was surgically placed. Current medications include warfarin and albuterol. He is allergic to penicillin.

Physical examination reveals the patient is alert and oriented to person, place, time, and event. His skin is pink, warm, and moist. Breath sounds are clear. His SpO_2 is 98% on room air. His blood pressure is 130/70 mm Hg, pulse 53 beats/min, and ventilations 20/min. The patient has been placed on a cardiac monitor. Vascular access has been established and a 12-lead ECG has been obtained (Fig. 3.43). Review the patient's ECG and describe your initial interventions for this patient.

Fig. 3.43

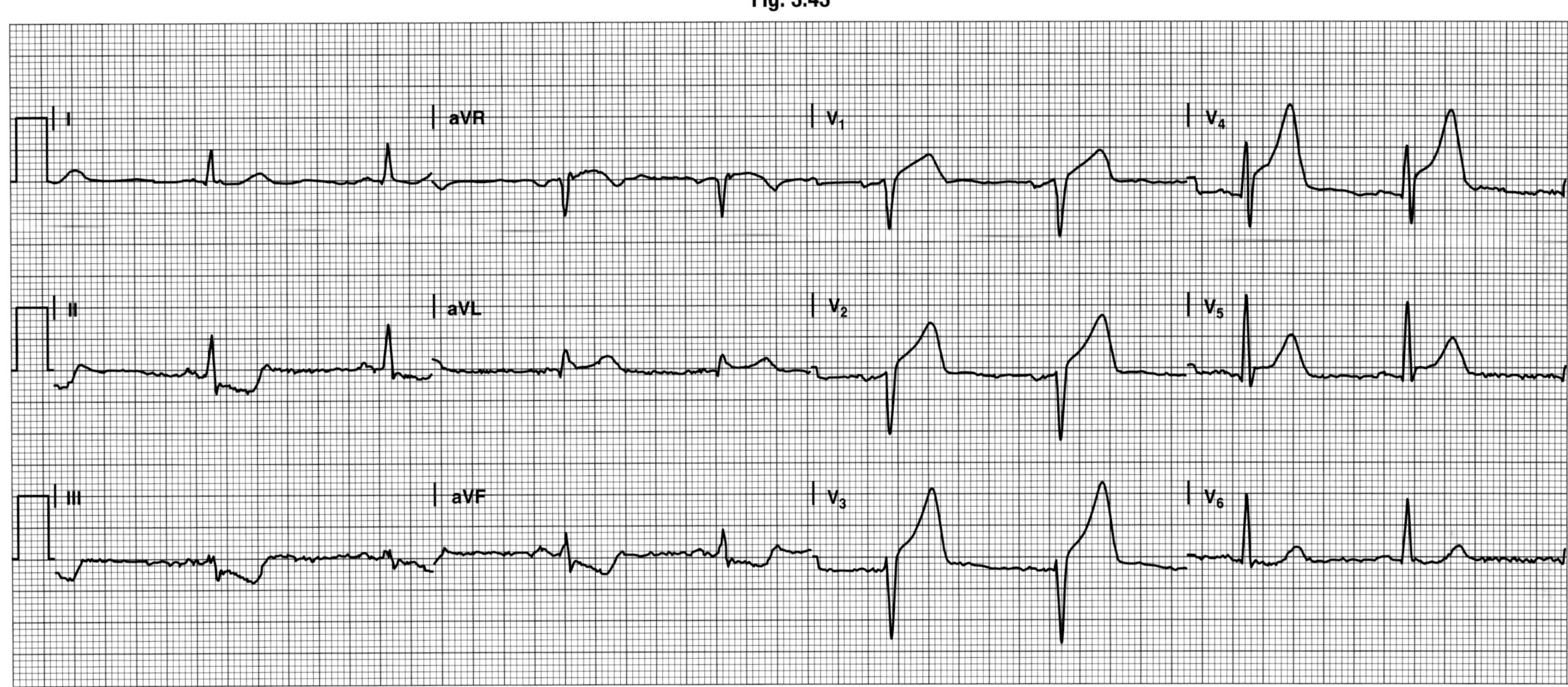

ANSWERS

1. **B**. When observed in two or more anatomically contiguous leads, STE is considered significant if it is elevated 1 mm or more at the J point in all leads other than V_2 and V_3 in a patient who is experiencing an ACS. For leads V_2 and V_3, STE is considered significant if it is elevated 2 mm or more in men older than 40 years or elevated 1.5 mm or more in women.

2. **C**. An inferior STEMI is present (as evidenced by the STE in leads II, III, and aVF); the ST-segment depression in leads I and aVL reflects reciprocal changes.

3. **D**. The term *extensive anterior MI* is used when an infarction involves the anterior wall, septum, and lateral walls. ECG changes should be visible in leads V_1 through V_6, as well as leads I and aVL.

4. **C**. The term *high lateral infarction* is used to describe ST changes viewed in leads I and aVL. Reciprocal changes of a high lateral infarction can usually be seen in leads II, III, and aVF.

5. **A.** The patient's ECG findings and elevated troponin levels confirm an anterolateral STEMI. Biomarkers are not elevated with angina because there is no tissue death.

INTERPRETATION OF PRACTICE ECGS

Fig. 3.33

Rate and rhythm: Sinus rhythm at 65 beats/min
STE: II, III, aVF, V_3, V_4, V_5, V_6
ST depression: I, aVL
Axis: Normal
Interpretation: Suspected inferolateral STEMI. Obtain V_4R to assess for RVI. Artifact in I, III.

Fig. 3.34

Rate and rhythm: Sinus arrhythmia at 75 beats/min
Axis: Normal
Interpretation: Normal ECG. Artifact in I, II, III, aVL, aVF, V_3.

Fig. 3.35

Rate and rhythm: Sinus bradycardia at 59 beats/min
STE: I, aVL, V_2 through V_6
T-wave changes: Tall in V_2, V_3, V_4, V_5
Axis: Normal
Interpretation: Suspected anterolateral STEMI. Baseline wander in II, III.

Fig. 3.36

Rate and rhythm: Sinus rhythm at 75 beats/min with occasional premature ventricular complexes (PVCs)
ST depression: I, II, aVF, V_5, V_6
Axis: Normal
Interpretation: No evidence of STEMI. Artifact in III.

Fig. 3.37

Rate and rhythm: Sinus rhythm at 90 beats/min
STE: V_1 through V_4; borderline in III and aVF
T-wave changes: Inverted in aVL
Pathologic Q waves: V_1 through V_3
Axis: Left
Interpretation: Possible inferior, anteroseptal STEMI. STE in V_1 through V_4. Borderline STE in III, aVF. Poor R-wave progression. Left axis deviation. Artifact in aVR, aVL, and V_1. Obtain V_4R to assess for RVI.

Fig. 3.38

Rate and rhythm: Sinus rhythm at 73 beats/min with occasional PVCs
STE: V_2, V_3, V_4, V_5, V_6
ST depression: III
T-wave changes: Tall, peaked in V_2, V_3, V_4
Axis: Normal
Interpretation: Suspected anterior STEMI.

Fig. 3.39

Rate and rhythm: Unable to determine
Interpretation: Data quality prohibits interpretation; artifact in I, II, III, aVL, aVF, V_1 through V_6.

Fig. 3.40

Rate and rhythm:	Sinus rhythm at 92 beats/min with occasional supraventricular premature complexes
STE:	V_2 through V_4; borderline in V_1 and V_5
ST depression:	II, III, aVF
Pathologic Q waves:	V_1, V_2
Axis:	Normal
Interpretation:	Suspected anteroseptal STEMI. Artifact in I, III, aVL, aVF.

Fig. 3.41

Rate and rhythm:	89 beats/min
Interpretation:	Arm leads reversed (negative PQRST waveforms in I, positive PQRST waveforms in aVR). No further interpretation possible.

INTERPRETATION OF CASE STUDIES

CASE STUDY 3.1

Although this patient is not complaining of chest pain or discomfort, she is presenting with anginal equivalent symptoms (e.g., sudden onset of shortness of breath, fatigue). Because chest pain or discomfort can develop at any time, be sure to ask her if these symptoms are present when obtaining repeat vital signs, and ask her to notify you if they occur.

The patient's 12-lead ECG shows evidence of an inferior STEMI (STE in leads II, III, and aVF and reciprocal ST depression in I and aVL). You should obtain a right-sided 12-lead ECG and determine if an RVI is present. Because borderline STE is present in leads V_3 through V_6, closely evaluate subsequent 12-lead ECGs for the development of a lateral infarction. Be alert for the development of complications of inferior infarction, such as bradydysrhythmias and AV blocks.

Select a reperfusion strategy: pharmacologic reperfusion (i.e., fibrinolytic therapy) or mechanical reperfusion (i.e., PCI). Minimize the time to reperfusion by working quickly and efficiently. While completing a fibrinolytic checklist, obtain a portable chest radiograph and draw initial laboratory tests including cardiac biomarkers, electrolytes, and coagulation studies.

CASE STUDY 3.2

If there are no contraindications, give aspirin as soon as possible. An anteroseptal STEMI is suspected on the basis of this patient's 12-lead ECG. Quickly screen the patient for indications and contraindications to fibrinolytic therapy and PCI. Select a reperfusion strategy, obtain a portable chest radiograph, and draw initial laboratory studies.

Relief of the patient's chest pain is a priority. Recall that up to three doses of sublingual or aerosol NTG can be given at 3- to 5-minute intervals for patients with ischemic chest discomfort until the discomfort is relieved or the presence of hypotension limits its use. Closely monitor the patient's vital signs and ECG after each dose. Morphine is the preferred analgesic for STEMI patients with ischemic chest discomfort that is unresponsive to nitrates.

Six minutes after administering a sublingual NTG tablet to this patient, he rated his chest pain 9/10. Within 2 minutes of giving a second tablet, he rated his pain 6/10 and said, "I feel funny." Reassessment revealed a blood pressure of 90/60 mm Hg, a heart rate of 92 beats/min, and pale, clammy skin. After placing the patient in a supine position and administration of 200 mL of normal saline, his blood pressure was 120/74 mm Hg, his heart rate was 78 beats/min, and his skin was pink, warm, and dry. However, his chest pain increased to 10/10. He was taken to the cardiac catheterization laboratory for immediate PCI.

ST-Elevation Variants

4

CHAPTER

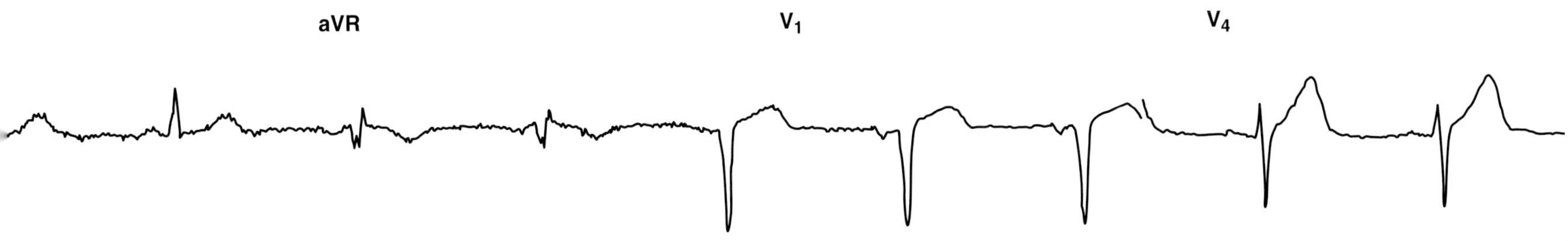

LEARNING OBJECTIVES

After reading this chapter, you should be able to:

1. Recognize that many conditions other than infarction may produce ST-segment elevation (STE).
2. Identify the electrocardiographic (ECG) criteria for left ventricular hypertrophy (LVH), bundle branch block (BBB), ventricular rhythms, benign early repolarization (BER), and pericarditis.
3. Recognize the manner in which the ST segment is displaced by LVH, left bundle branch block (LBBB), and ventricular rhythms.
4. Review the anatomy of the intraventricular conduction system.
5. Develop an approach to differentiating right bundle branch block (RBBB) from LBBB.
6. Describe the clinical presentation of pericarditis.

KEY TERMS

bundle branch block: A disruption in impulse conduction from the bundle of His through either the right or left bundle branch to the Purkinje fibers.

cardiac enlargement: Situations in which one or more of the heart's chambers becomes bigger because of an increase in its cavity volume, wall thickness, or both.

terminal force: The final portion of the QRS complex.

INTRODUCTION

Thus far, most examples of ST-segment elevation (STE) provided in this text have been the result of myocardial infarction (MI). This strategy was used to encourage your familiarity with the pattern(s) of MI. However, if every instance of STE were interpreted as MI, gross overdiagnosis would result. MI produces STE because the infarction affects ventricular repolarization, ventricular depolarization, or both. Likewise, any condition that affects ventricular repolarization and/or depolarization can also produce STE. This chapter focuses on the following five conditions that can produce STE: left ventricular hypertrophy (LVH), bundle branch block (BBB), ventricular rhythms (including paced ventricular rhythms), benign early repolarization (BER), and pericarditis (Fig. 4.1).

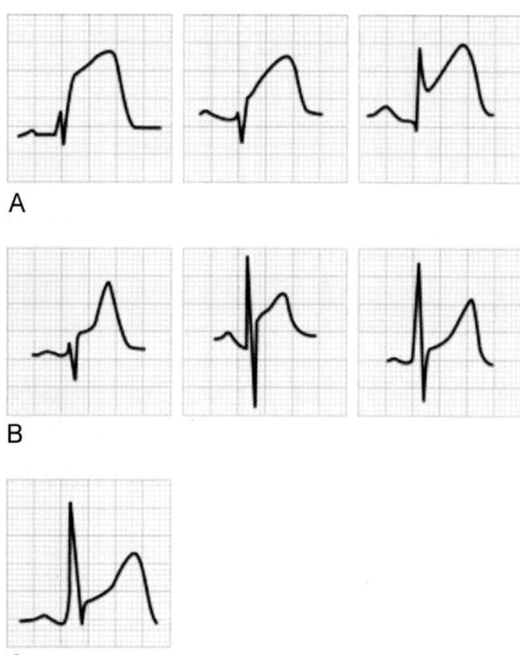

Fig. **4.1** Analysis of ST segment–T wave morphology in acute myocardial infarction (AMI), benign early repolarization (BER), and acute pericarditis. An analysis of the ST segment–T wave morphology (from the beginning at the J point to the end at the apex of the T wave) may be particularly helpful in distinguishing among the various causes of ST-segment elevation (STE) and identifying the AMI case. **A,** The initial upsloping portion of the ST segment is usually either flat (horizontally or obliquely) or convex in the patient with AMI. This morphologic observation, however, should be used only as a guideline; it is not infallible. **B,** Non-AMI causes of STE are seen here with concavity of the ST segment–T wave (left BER, middle pericarditis, right BER). **C,** Patients with STE related to AMI may demonstrate concavity of this portion of the waveform. (From Walls, R.M., Hockberger, R. S., & Gausche-Hill, M. [2018]. *Rosen's emergency medicine.* [9th ed.]. Philadelphia, PA: Elsevier.)

VENTRICULAR HYPERTROPHY

Cardiac enlargement refers to situations in which one or more of the heart's chambers becomes bigger because of an increase in its cavity volume, wall thickness, or both (Goldberger, Goldberger, & Shvilkin, 2018). When enlargement occurs, the number of heart muscle fibers does not increase, rather the individual muscle fibers become larger (i.e., hypertrophied) (Goldberger et al., 2018). Hypertrophy is commonly accompanied by dilation. With dilation, the heart muscle cells typically become longer (Goldberger et al., 2018). Dilation may be acute or chronic. When enlargement occurs because of increased wall thickness, the heart muscles cells tend to become wider (Goldberger et al., 2018). When evaluating the electrocardiogram (ECG) for the presence of chamber enlargement, it is particularly important to check the calibration marker to ensure that it is 10 mm (1 mV) tall.

Right Ventricular Hypertrophy

With right ventricular hypertrophy (RVH), current travels between hypertrophied cells and moves through the enlarged right ventricle, producing higher-than-normal voltages on the body surface (Mirvis & Goldberger, 2015) (Fig. 4.2). Because the right ventricle is normally considerably smaller than the left, it must become extremely enlarged before changes are visible on the ECG.

Several criteria have been proposed for detecting RVH on the ECG, most of which involve assessing the amplitude of R and S waveforms in leads I, V_1, and V_6 (Box 4.1, Fig. 4.3). The sensitivity of the ECG criteria for RVH is generally low (Hancock et al., 2009).

Evidence of right atrial abnormality may be seen. Right atrial abnormality produces changes in the initial part of the P wave. The P wave is tall (more than 2.5 mm in height), peaked, and usually of normal duration (Hancock et al., 2009). Causes of RVH include pulmonary hypertension and chronic pulmonary diseases, valvular heart disease, and congenital heart disease.

Left Ventricular Hypertrophy

LVH is primarily recognized on the ECG by increased QRS amplitude accompanied by changes in the ST segment and T wave (see Fig. 4.2). Typically, R waves in leads I, aVL, V_5, and V_6 are taller than normal, and S waves in leads V_1 and V_2 are deeper than normal (Mirvis & Goldberger, 2015). The QRS duration is often increased in LVH and may be attributed to the longer time required to activate the thickened wall of the left ventricle (Hancock et al., 2009) and the slower-than-normal conduction within the working myocardium (Mirvis & Goldberger, 2015). Causes of LVH include systemic hypertension, hypertrophic cardiomyopathy, aortic stenosis, and aortic insufficiency. LVH may be accompanied by left axis deviation.

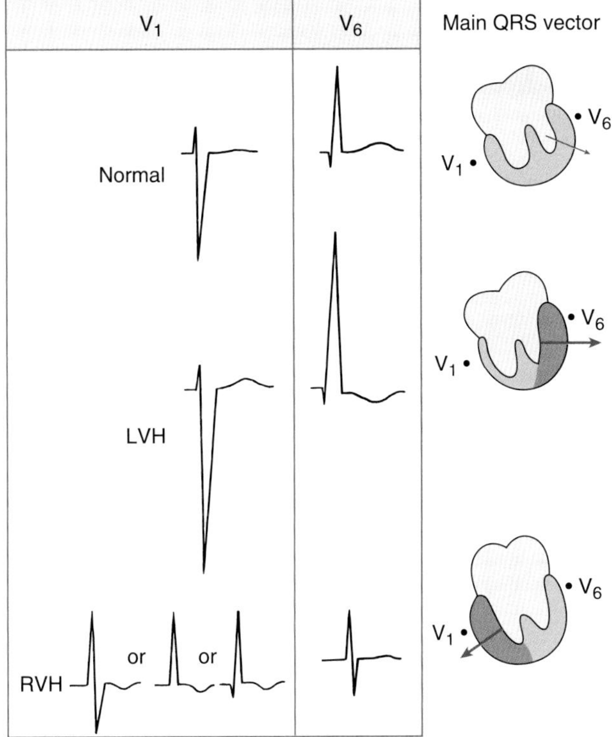

Fig. 4.2 Left ventricular hypertrophy (LVH) increases the amplitude of electrical forces directed to the left and posteriorly. In addition, repolarization abnormalities can cause ST-segment depression and T-wave inversion in leads with a prominent R wave. Right ventricular hypertrophy (RVH) can shift the QRS vector to the right, usually with an RS, R, or qR complex in lead V_1, especially when caused by severe pressure overload. T-wave inversion may be present in the right chest leads. (From Mirvis, D., & Goldberger, A. L. [2015]. Electrocardiography. In: Mann, D. L., Zipes, D. P., Libby, P., & Bonow, R. O. [eds.]. *Braunwald's heart disease: A textbook of cardiovascular medicine* [10th ed.]. Philadelphia, PA: WB Saunders/Elsevier.)

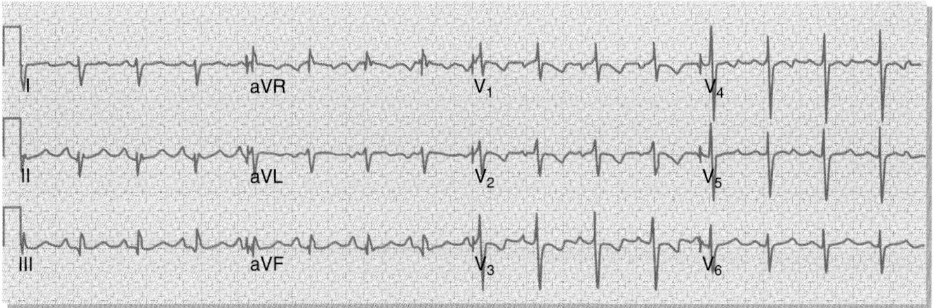

Fig. 4.3 Right ventricular hypertrophy with tall R wave in right chest leads, downsloping ST depression in the chest leads, right axis deviation, and evidence of right atrial enlargement. (From Andreoli, T. E., Griggs, R., Wing, W., & Fitz, J. G. [2016]. *Andreoli and Carpenter's Cecil essentials of medicine* [9th ed.]. Philadelphia, PA: Saunders.)

Several formulas exist to assist in LVH recognition (Box 4.2). When applying the criteria for LVH on the basis of QRS amplitude, keep in mind that several factors other than the size or mass of the left ventricle can influence QRS voltages. Examples of these factors include age, gender, race, body habitus (i.e., obesity), and the sites of ECG electrode placement (Hancock et al., 2009).

An example of LVH is shown in Fig. 4.4. Note the STE in leads V_1, V_2, and V_3 and the ST-segment depression in leads V_5 and V_6. These ECG findings conform to a pattern shared by LVH, left bundle branch block (LBBB), and ventricular rhythms in which the QRS complex and the T wave are oppositely directed. In other words, when the QRS complex points down, the T wave points up and vice versa. This phenomenon would hardly be noteworthy in a discussion of infarction except for one important fact: the T wave often "drags" the ST segment along with it. Thus, when the QRS complex is primarily negative, the T wave will be positively deflected, and it can drag the ST segment up with it. This is how LVH, LBBB, and ventricular rhythms can masquerade as an infarction. Additionally, the negative deflection may produce

Box 4.1 Examples of ECG Criteria for Right Ventricular Hypertrophy Recognition

- Tall R waves (7 mm or more) in V_1
- qR pattern in V_1
- Deeper-than-normal S waves (7 mm or more) in leads V_5 or V_6
- Right axis deviation usually present

Box 4.2 Examples of ECG Criteria for Left Ventricular Hypertrophy Recognition

- R wave in lead aVL is 11 mm or more
- R wave in lead aVF is 20 mm or more
- R wave in lead I + the S wave in III is 25 mm or more
- S wave in lead III is 20 mm or more
- S wave in lead V_1 or V_2 is 30 mm or more
- R wave in lead I + S wave in lead III is 25 mm or more
- S wave in lead V_3 + R wave in lead aVL is 20 mm or more in women, 28 mm or more in men
- S wave in V_1 + height of the tallest R wave in V_5 or V_6 is 35 mm or more

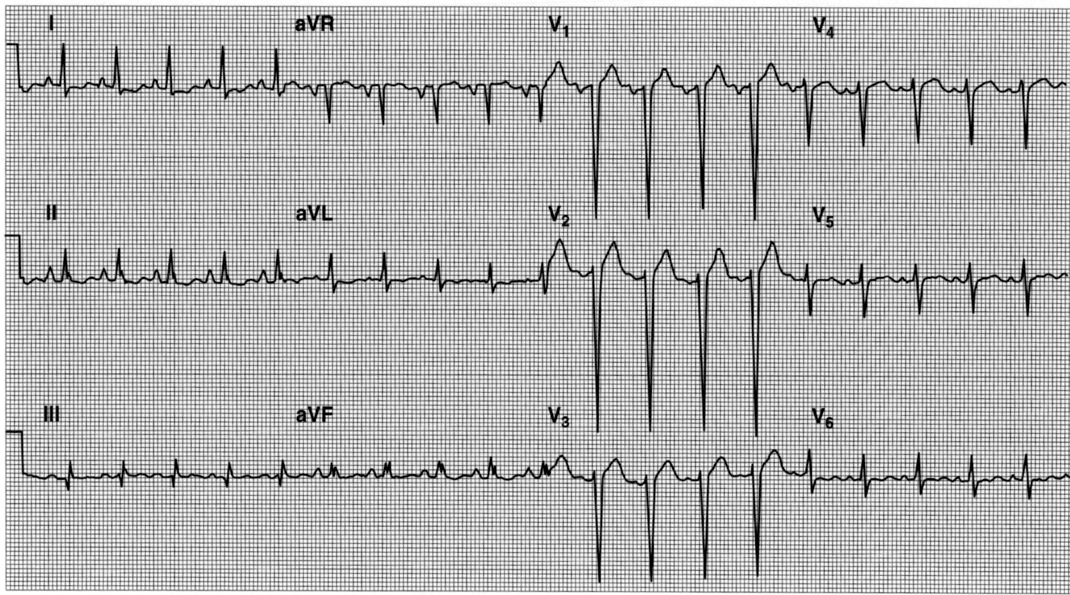

Fig. 4.4 Left ventricular hypertrophy. Note the ST-segment elevation in leads V_1, V_2, and V_3.

a Q wave or QS complex equal to 40 ms or more in duration. This further clouds the interpretation by giving the appearance of pathologic Q waves. Careful correlation of the patient's ECG, his or her clinical presentation, and the results of other diagnostic studies is essential.

A 12-lead ECG's interpretive algorithm checks for the presence of LVH using preprogrammed criteria, including formulas, to measure voltage. If the 12-lead machine determines that an ECG meets the criteria for LVH, a message is displayed, such as "Meets voltage criteria for left ventricular hypertrophy." In contrast, a message such as "Possible criteria for left ventricular hypertrophy with repolarization abnormality" does *not* mean the same thing.

BUNDLE BRANCH BLOCKS

Structures of the Intraventricular Conduction System

After passing through the AV node, the electrical impulse enters the bundle of His, which is normally the only electrical connection between the atria and the ventricles. It is located in the upper portion of the interventricular septum and connects the AV node with the two bundle branches (Fig. 4.5). A **BBB** is a disruption in impulse conduction from the bundle of His through either the right or left bundle

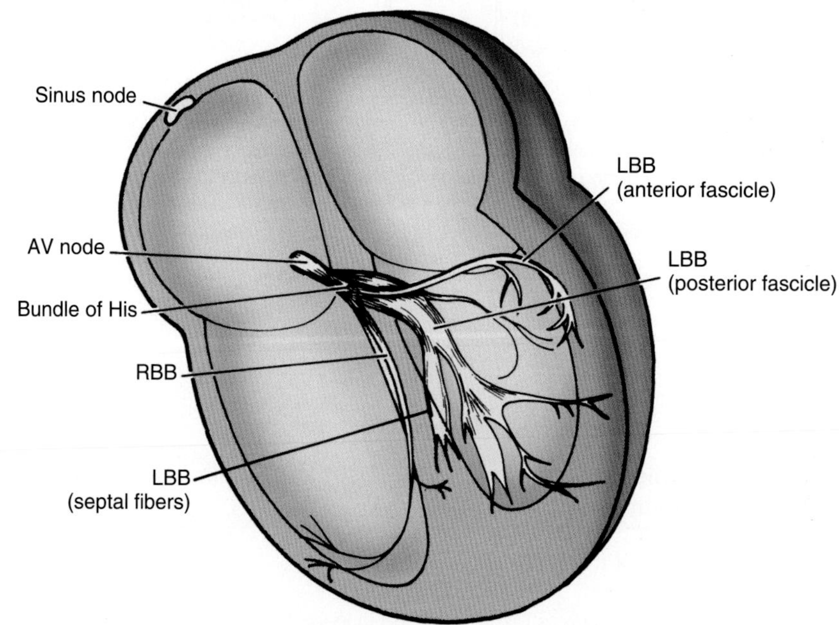

Fig. 4.5 Cardiac conduction system. AV, atrioventricular; LBB, left bundle branch; RBB, right bundle branch. (From Conover, M. B. [1995]. *Understanding electrocardiography* [7th ed.]. St. Louis, MO: Mosby.)

branch to the Purkinje fibers. A BBB may be intermittent or permanent, complete or incomplete.

The right bundle branch travels down the right side of the interventricular septum to conduct the electrical impulse to the right ventricle. Structurally, the right bundle branch is long, thin, and more fragile than the left. Because of its structure, a relatively small lesion in the right bundle branch can result in delays or interruptions in electrical impulse transmission.

The left bundle branch begins as a single structure that is short and thick (the left common bundle branch or main stem) and then divides into two subdivisions that are called the *anterior fascicle* and the *posterior fascicle*. The fascicles branch into networks of Purkinje fibers. The anterior fascicle receives its blood supply from septal branches of the left anterior descending (LAD) artery. This fascicle spreads the electrical impulse to the anterior and lateral portions of the left ventricle (Surawicz & Knilans, 2008). This fascicle is thin and vulnerable to disruptions in electrical impulse transmission. The posterior fascicle relays the impulse to the inferior and posterior portions of the left ventricle (Surawicz & Knilans, 2008). It is short, thick, and rarely disrupted because of its structure and dual blood supply from both the LAD and the right coronary artery. In some people, a third fascicle, called the *medial fascicle* or *septal fascicle*, emerges from the left bundle itself or its posteroinferior division (Latcu & Nadir, 2010).

Bundle Branch Activation

The wave of normal ventricular depolarization moves from the endocardium to the epicardium. The left side of the interventricular septum, which is stimulated by the left posterior fascicle, is stimulated first. The electrical impulse (i.e., wave of depolarization) then traverses the septum to stimulate the right side. The left and right ventricles are then depolarized at the same time (Fig. 4.6).

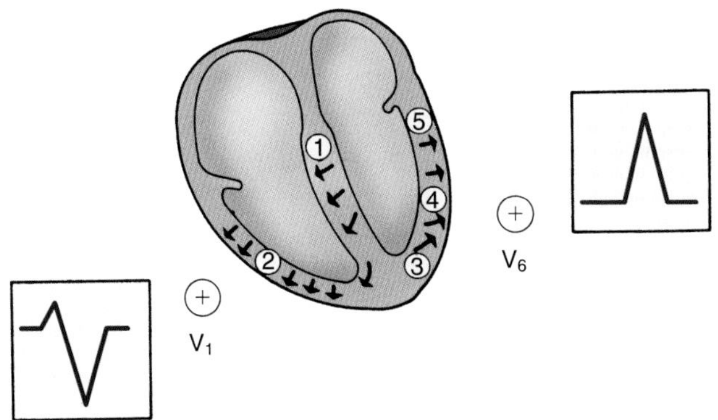

Fig. 4.6 Sequence of normal ventricular depolarization and resulting QRS complex, as seen in leads V_1 and V_6. (From Urden, L. D., Stacy, K. M., & Lough, M. E. [2018]. *Critical care nursing* [8th ed.]. St. Louis, MO: Mosby.)

A delay or block can occur in any part of the intraventricular conduction system. If a delay or block occurs in one of the bundle branches, the ventricles will not be depolarized at the same time. The electrical impulse travels first down the unblocked branch and stimulates that ventricle. Because of the block, the impulse must then travel from cell to cell through the myocardium, rather than through the normal conduction pathway, to stimulate the other ventricle. The ventricle with the blocked bundle branch is the last to be depolarized.

Significance of Bundle Branch Block

Because the LAD artery supplies much of the bundle branches, patients experiencing septal and anteroseptal infarctions are most likely to develop BBB. Of course, an infarcting patient presenting with BBB may have had it as a preexisting condition. Unless a previous ECG is available for comparison or the BBB develops during the infarction, it can be difficult to determine which came first, the infarct or the BBB. When BBB is caused by an infarction, it can progress to a complete atrioventricular (AV) block with a slow ventricular rate. LBBB is significant because of its ability to produce STE and wide Q waves that resemble infarction, thereby complicating the ECG recognition of acute MI.

Electrocardiographic Criteria

When one of the bundles becomes blocked, the impulse normally conducted by that bundle branch is interrupted and does not depolarize the intended ventricle. Meanwhile, the other bundle branch is conducting its impulse and depolarizing its respective ventricle. How does the other ventricle depolarize? Very slowly. For the second ventricle to depolarize, the electrical impulses must trudge through myocardial cells, which are not specialized for electrical conduction. Thus, the impulses from one ventricle must be transmitted, cell by cell, to the other ventricle. Because the impulses are wading through the muck and mire, and not travelling down the normal conduction pathway, ventricular depolarization takes longer to occur. This delay is evidenced in the form of a wide QRS complex.

Consider This

Whereas bundle branch block increases the *width* of the QRS complex, LVH increases the *amplitude* because of the increase in electrical activity due to the thicker ventricle.

Essentially, two conditions must exist to suspect BBB (Box 4.3). First, the QRS complex must have an abnormal duration (i.e., 120 ms or more in duration if a complete BBB), and second, the QRS complex must arise as the result of supraventricular activity (this excludes paced beats and beats that originate from the ventricles). If these two conditions are met, delayed ventricular conduction is assumed to be present, and BBB is the most common (but not the only) cause of this abnormal conduction.

Box 4.3 ECG Criteria for Bundle Branch Block Recognition

To be considered a BBB, the following ECG criteria must be met:

- QRS duration of 120 ms or more in adults (if a *complete* RBBB or LBBB); if a BBB pattern is discernible and the QRS duration is between 110 and 119 ms in adults, it is called an *incomplete* right or left BBB (Surawicz, Childers, Deal, & Gettes, 2009). (If the QRS is wide but there is no BBB pattern, the term *wide QRS* or *intraventricular conduction delay* is used to describe the QRS.)
- Visible QRS complexes are produced by supraventricular activity (i.e., the QRS complex is not a paced beat, and it does not originate in the ventricles).

Variation in QRS duration from lead to lead is often seen and may produce confusion about whether the complex is or is not wide. Some complexes appear narrow in some leads but, when measured, are just as wide as the other leads. Therefore, *measure the QRS complex duration. Do not trust only your eyes.* As a rule, use the widest QRS complex to determine width. Try to pinpoint the exact beginning and end of the QRS complex. This can be difficult to do and is sometimes impossible. Therefore, *when measuring for BBB, select the widest QRS complex with a discernible beginning and end.*

The criteria for BBB recognition may be found in any lead of the ECG. However, when differentiating right bundle branch block (RBBB) from LBBB, pay attention to the QRS morphology (i.e., shape) in specific leads. Lead V_1 is probably the single best lead to use when differentiating between RBBB and LBBB.

Differentiating RBBB From LBBB

Once the presence of BBB is suspected, an examination of V_1 can reveal whether the block affects the right or the left bundle branch. Following are descriptions of how each type of block affects the direction of electrical current and produces its own distinct QRS morphology.

Right Bundle Branch Block

In RBBB, the electrical impulse travels through the AV node and down the left bundle branch into the interventricular septum. The septum is activated by the left posterior fascicle and is depolarized in a left-to-right direction (Fig. 4.7). Thus, septal depolarization moves in a left-to-right direction, which is toward V_1, and produces an initial small R wave. As the left bundle continues to conduct impulses, the entire left ventricle is depolarized from right to left. This produces movement away from V_1 and results in a negative deflection (i.e., an S wave). Now the impulses that depolarized the left ventricle conduct through the myocardial cells and depolarize the right ventricle. This depolarization creates a movement of electrical activity in the direction of V_1, and so a second positive deflection is recorded (R′). The rSR′ pattern is characteristic of RBBB.

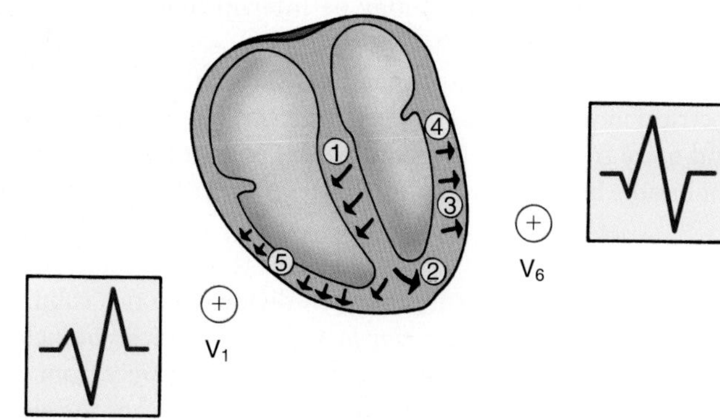

Fig. 4.7 Sequence of ventricular depolarization for a right bundle branch block and resulting QRS complex, as seen in leads V_1 and V_6. (From Urden, L. D., Stacy, K. M., & Lough, M. E. [2018]. *Critical care nursing* [8th ed.]. St. Louis, MO: Mosby.)

The rSR′ pattern is sometimes referred to as an "M" or "rabbit ear" pattern. *Whenever the two criteria for BBB have been met, and V_1 displays an RSR′ pattern, suspect RBBB* (Fig. 4.8).

RBBB can occur in individuals with no underlying heart disease. Acute RBBB may occur secondary to an acute anteroseptal infarction, acute heart failure, acute pericarditis or myocarditis, or acute pulmonary embolism. Chronic RBBB may be caused by coronary artery disease, cardiac surgery, degenerative disease of the heart's conduction system, or congenital cardiac disorders.

Left Bundle Branch Block

In LBBB, the septum is depolarized by the right bundle branch as is the right ventricle. The septum is part of the left ventricle and is normally depolarized by the left bundle branch. Because the left bundle branch is blocked, depolarization of the septum by the right bundle branch occurs in an abnormal direction (i.e., from right to left); thus, the wave of myocardial depolarization begins with the net movement of current going away from V_1 and is recorded as an initial negative deflection (Fig. 4.9). The right ventricle is depolarized next. Because the wave of depolarization moves briefly toward the positive electrode in lead V_1, a small upright notch in the QRS complex is seen on the ECG. As the remainder of the left ventricle is depolarized, the QRS complex is inscribed in lead V_1 as a deep negative deflection (i.e., an S wave), which reflects the left ventricle's large muscle mass. Sometimes, depolarization of the left ventricle overshadows that of the right ventricle on the ECG. When this occurs, a QS deflection is inscribed in lead V_1, and the small upright notch that is usually seen with right ventricular depolarization is absent. *When BBB is known to exist and a QS pattern is seen in V_1, suspect LBBB* (Fig. 4.10).

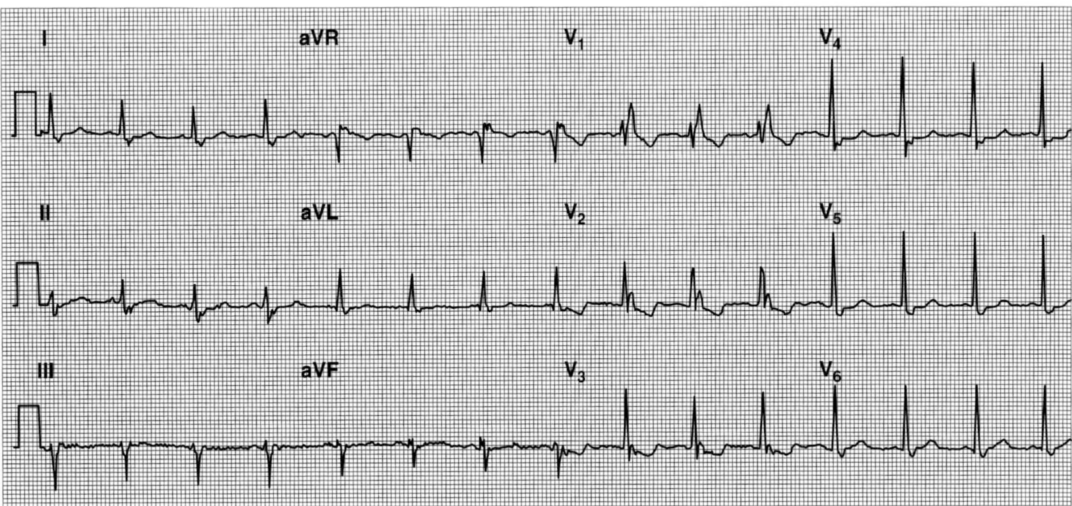

Fig. 4.8 Right bundle branch block.

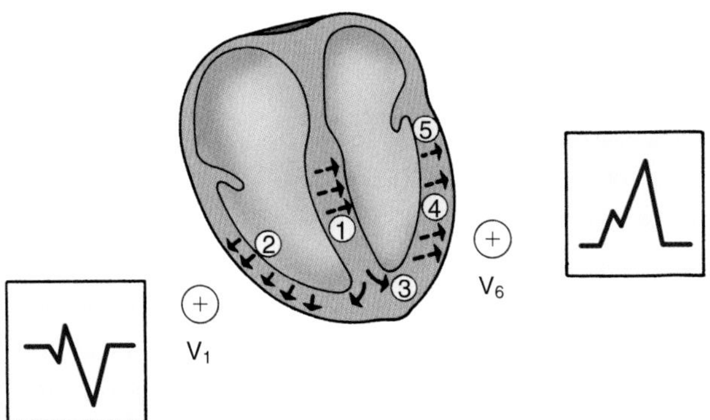

Fig. 4.9 Sequence of ventricular depolarization for a left bundle branch block and resulting QRS complex, as seen in leads V_1 and V_6. (From Urden, L. D., Stacy, K. M., & Lough, M. E. [2018]. *Critical care nursing* [8th ed.]. St. Louis, MO: Mosby.)

Unfortunately, not every BBB presents with a clear RSR′ or QS pattern in V_1. Often, the pattern more closely resembles a qR pattern or an rS pattern (Fig. 4.11), making the differentiation less clear.

LBBB may be acute or chronic. Acute LBBB may occur secondary to an anteroseptal MI, acute heart failure, acute pericarditis or myocarditis, or acute cardiac trauma. Chronic LBBB may occur because of hypertensive heart disease, severe coronary artery disease, and aortic stenosis. Nonischemic diseases, such as Lev's disease and Lenègre's disease, are also capable of producing a BBB. Lev's disease produces BBB through a calcification of the heart's fibrous skeleton. The fibrous skeleton is the infrastructure to which the muscles and valves are attached. Portions of the conduction system are located near the fibrous skeleton or may pass through it. If the fibrous skeleton begins to calcify, part of the electrical conduction system may become "pinched," resulting in a block. Lenègre's disease is a more diffuse sclerodegenerative disease that tends to affect the distal portions of the conduction system, but it may affect the more proximal portions as well. This process occurs with age, is not related to ischemic heart disease, and is sometimes referred to as the "graying" of the electrical conduction system.

An Easier Way

Remember that in the setting of BBB, the ventricles are not depolarized in their normal simultaneous manner. Instead, they are depolarized sequentially. The last ventricle to be depolarized is, of course, the ventricle with the blocked bundle branch. Therefore, if it is possible to determine the ventricle that was depolarized last, it becomes possible to determine the bundle branch that was blocked. For example, if the right ventricle was depolarized last, it is because the impulse travelled down the left bundle branch, depolarized the left ventricle first, then marched through and depolarized the right ventricle.

It stands to reason that if one ventricle is depolarized late, its depolarization makes up the later portion of the QRS complex. The final portion of the QRS complex is referred to as the **terminal force**. Examination of the terminal force of the QRS complex reveals the ventricle that was depolarized last and, therefore, the bundle that was blocked.

To identify the terminal force, first locate the J point. From the J point, move backward into the QRS and determine if the last electrical activity produced an upward or downward deflection. An example of the terminal force in both RBBB and LBBB is illustrated in Fig. 4.12. If the right bundle branch is blocked, then the right ventricle will be depolarized last and the current will be moving from the left ventricle to the right. This

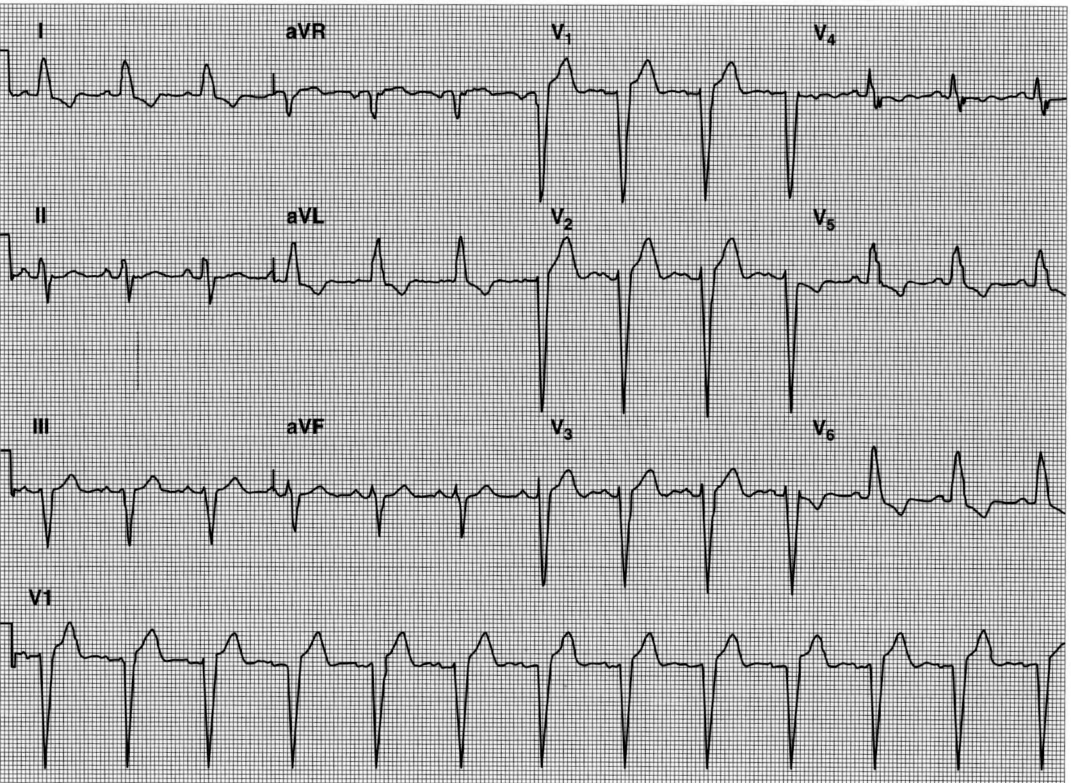

Fig. **4.10** Left bundle branch block.

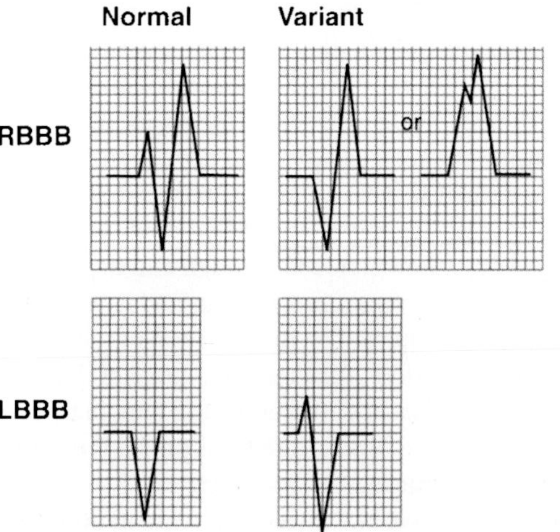

Fig. **4.11** Variant patterns of bundle branch block as seen in lead V_1. *LBBB,* Left bundle branch block; *RBBB,* right bundle branch block.

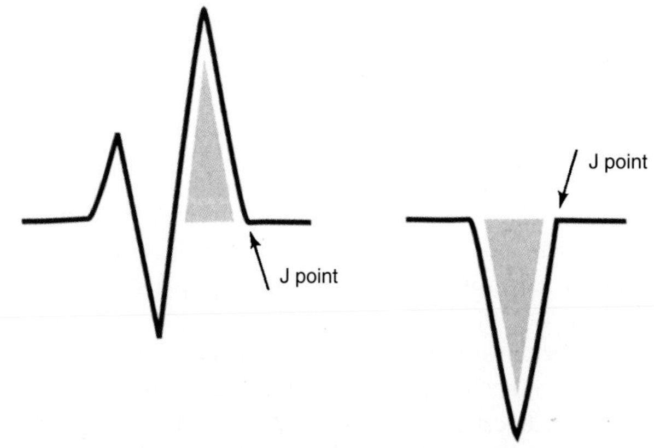

Fig. **4.12** Determining the direction of the terminal force. In lead V_1, move from the J point into the QRS complex and determine whether the terminal portion (last 0.04 second) of the QRS complex is a positive (upright) or negative (downward) deflection. If the two criteria for BBB are met and the terminal portion of the QRS is positive, right bundle branch block is most likely present. If the terminal portion of the QRS is negative, left bundle branch block is most likely present.

will create a positive deflection in the terminal force of the QRS complex in V_1. If the left bundle branch is blocked, the left ventricle will be depolarized last, and the current will flow from right to left. This will produce a negative deflection in the terminal force of the QRS complex seen in V_1. Therefore, to differentiate RBBB from LBBB, look at V_1 and determine whether the terminal force of the QRS complex is directed upward or downward. If it is directed upward, an RBBB is present (i.e., the current is moving toward the right ventricle and toward V_1). An LBBB is present when the terminal force of the QRS complex is directed downward (i.e., the current is moving away from V_1 and toward the left ventricle). This rule is especially helpful when RSR′ and QS variants are present.

A simple way to remember this rule has been suggested by Mike Taigman and Syd Canan and is demonstrated in Fig. 4.13. They recognized the similarity between this rule and the turn indicator on a car. When a right turn is made, the turn indicator is lifted up. Likewise, when an RBBB is present, the terminal force of the QRS complex points up. Conversely, left turns and LBBB are directed downward.

Concordance

When analyzing a BBB, *concordance* refers to ST segments and T waves that deflect in the same direction as the terminal (last) portion of the QRS complex. Normally, a BBB produces *discordant* ST segments and T waves. In other words, the ST segments and T waves are in the opposite direction of the terminal portion of the QRS complex. Concordant STE is almost always abnormal with a BBB.

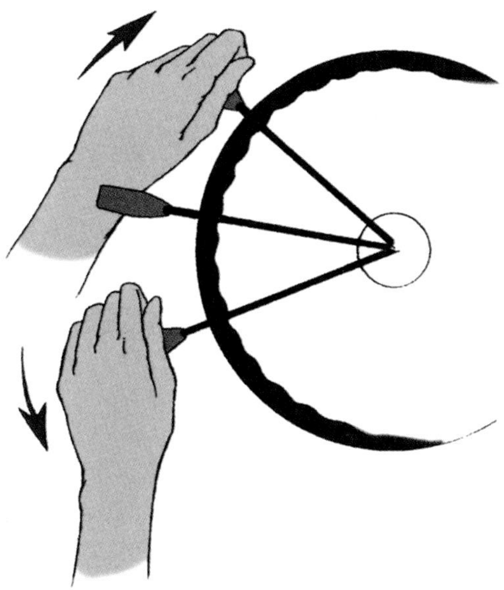

Fig. **4.13** Differentiating between right and left bundle branch blocks. The "turn signal" theory is that right is up and left is down.

Sgarbossa Criteria

In 1996, Elena Sgarbossa and colleagues published the results of a study that tested ECG criteria for the diagnosis of acute MI in the presence of LBBB (Sgarbossa et al., 1996). These ECG criteria include the following:

1. STE of 1 mm or more that is concordant with (i.e., in the same direction as) the QRS complex in any lead (5 points)
2. ST-segment depression of 1 mm or more in lead V_1, V_2, or V_3 (3 points)
3. STE of 5 mm or more that is discordant with (i.e., in the opposite direction from) the QRS complex in any lead. (2 points)

Research has shown that a score of 3 or higher has a specificity of 98% but a sensitivity of only 20% for the diagnosis of acute MI (Tabas, Rodriguez, Seligman, & Goldschlager, 2008). The third criterion (i.e., STE of 5 mm or more) has been shown to add little diagnostic or prognostic value.

To improve diagnostic accuracy, the Sgarbossa criteria have been modified; specifically, the 5-mm discordant STE requirement has been replaced with a proportion. The modified Sgarbossa criteria include the following (Smith, Dodd, Henry, Dvorak, & Pearce, 2012):

1. STE of 1 mm or more that is concordant with the QRS complex in any lead
2. Concordant ST-segment depression of 1 mm or more in lead V_1, V_2, or V_3
3. Proportionally excessive discordant STE, as defined by 25% or more of the depth of the preceding S wave

The modified Sgarbossa criteria does not use a point system; if any of the modified ECG criteria are met, the result is considered positive and the cardiac catheterization laboratory should be activated.

Consider This

New or presumed new LBBB has been considered a STEMI equivalent (O'Gara et al., 2013). Experts have recommended that these patients undergo early reperfusion therapy with fibrinolytics or percutaneous coronary intervention (O'Connor et al., 2015). A 2011 study by Kontos et al. showed that early reperfusion treatment may not be appropriate for all patients with new LBBB because only a minority are diagnosed with MI (Kontos et al., 2011). These researchers found that concordant ST changes were the most important predictor of MI and an independent predictor of death; new or presumably new LBBB was neither (Kontos et al., 2011).

Exceptions

Two notable exceptions must be mentioned to complete the discussion of BBB. The first involves the criteria used to recognize BBB, whereas the second relates to differentiating LBBB from RBBB.

The criteria used to recognize BBB are valid but lack some sensitivity and specificity. The sensitivity can be limited by junctional rhythms because there may be no discernible

P waves when the AV junction is the pacemaker site. The AV junction is a supraventricular pacemaker, but this presents as an exception to the two-part rule of BBB recognition. Specificity is limited by Wolff-Parkinson-White (WPW) syndrome and other conditions that produce wide QRS complexes resulting from atrial activity. If the characteristic delta wave and shortened PR interval are recognized (Fig. 4.14), WPW syndrome should be suspected. This exception should not present too great a concern because the incidence of WPW syndrome is low. Similarly, hyperkalemia and other conditions that can widen the QRS are relatively infrequent.

As for differentiating LBBB from RBBB, a third category exists: nonspecific intraventricular conduction delay (NSIVCD). These blocks do not display the typical V_1 morphologies generally produced by BBB. Their origin may not be due to a complete BBB but is often the result of several factors, of which incomplete BBB may be one. Atypical patterns of BBB can be attributed to NSIVCD.

Consider This

The patient's clinical presentation is of little value in recognizing BBB because a ventricular conduction delay itself does not produce any clinical signs or symptoms. The underlying cause of the presence of a BBB may present with specific symptoms, but it does not help to identify the presence of a BBB. Therefore, rely on the ECG criteria to recognize the presence of BBB.

	Normal conduction	WPW
A		Delta or
B		Delta or

Fig. 4.14 Characteristic findings with the Wolff-Parkinson-White (WPW) pattern (short PR interval, QRS widening, and delta wave) compared with normal conduction. **A,** The usual appearance of WPW in leads where the QRS complex is mainly upright. **B,** The usual appearance of WPW when the QRS is predominantly negative. Negative delta waves may simulate pathologic Q waves—mimicking myocardial infarction. (From Grauer, K. [1998]. *A practical guide to ECG interpretation* [2nd ed.]. St Louis, MO: Mosby.)

Fascicular Blocks

A block in only one of the fascicles of the bundle branches is called a *monofascicular block*. A block in any two divisions of the bundle branches is called a *bifascicular block*. Although this term can be used to describe a block in both the anterior and posterior branches of the left bundle branch, it is more commonly used to describe a combination of a RBBB and either a left anterior fascicular block (LAFB) or a left posterior fascicular block (LPFB).

Left Anterior Fascicular Block

LAFB, also called *left anterior hemiblock*, is relatively common. With an LAFB, the septum is depolarized in a left to right direction, which is normal. Impulse conduction occurs normally down the right bundle branch and into the right ventricle. Because conduction in the anterior fascicle of the left bundle branch is impaired, the posterior fascicle of the left ventricle is activated first. The electrical impulse then spreads in an upward and leftward direction to depolarize the anterior and lateral walls of the left ventricle. Despite the change in the sequence of ventricular activation, the overall conduction time (i.e., the QRS duration) is usually less than 120 ms because only a portion of the left bundle branch is affected.

ECG characteristics of LAFB include the following (Surawicz et al., 2009):

- Left axis deviation between −45° and −90°
- qR pattern in lead aVL
- QRS duration less than 120 ms

To quickly identify LAFB, look at leads I and aVF (Fig. 4.15). If the QRS is positive in lead I and negative in aVF, left axis deviation is present. Next, look at lead aVL for a qR pattern (i.e., small Q waves with tall R waves). This pattern may also be seen in lead I. An rS pattern (i.e., small R waves with deep S waves) may be seen in the inferior leads (i.e., II, III, and aVF). Finally, measure the QRS duration. With LAFB, the QRS duration is typically less than 120 ms.

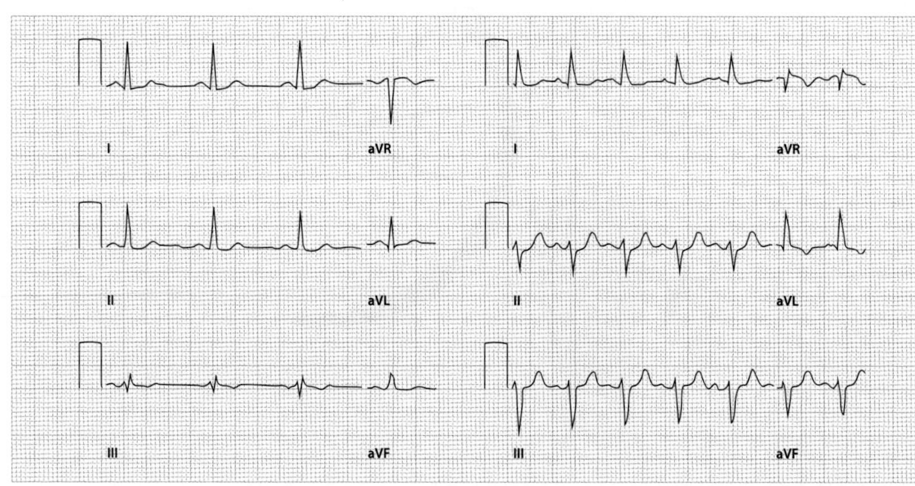

Fig. 4.15 Two electrocardiograms of a 50-year-old man are recorded 1 day apart, before and after development of left anterior fascicular block. (From Surawicz, B., & Knilans, T. K. [2008]. *Chou's electrocardiography in clinical practice* [6th ed.]. Philadelphia, PA: Saunders.)

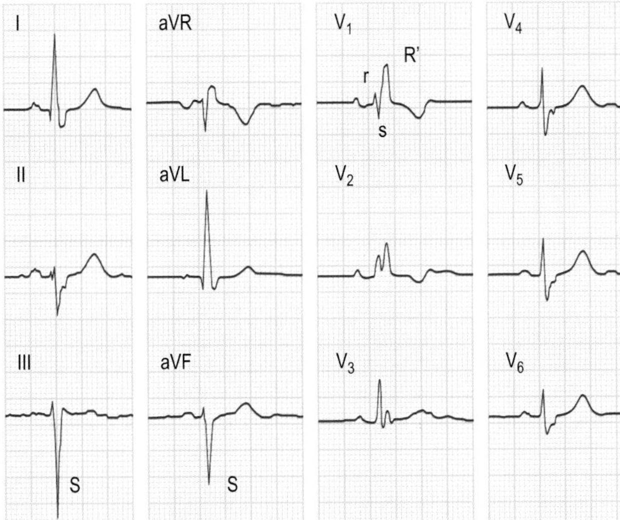

Fig. 4.16 Right bundle branch block with left anterior fascicular block (bifascicular block). The chest leads show a typical right bundle branch block pattern. Notice the rSR′ and tall R′ in leads V_1 and V_2, and rS in leads I, V_5, and V_6. The limb leads show left axis deviation, consistent with left anterior fascicular block. (From Kumar, P., & Clark, M. [2017]. *Kumar and Clark's clinical medicine* [9th ed.]. The Netherlands: Elsevier.)

LAFB is sometimes associated with RBBB (Fig. 4.16). LAFB may be seen in patients with aortic valve disease, coronary disease, hypertension, and age-related degenerative disease. The ECG pattern associated with this type of block can simulate LVH in leads I and aVL, and it can also hide signs of inferior ischemia (Issa, Miller, & Zipes, 2012).

Left Posterior Fascicular Block

LPFB, also called *left posterior hemiblock*, rarely occurs by itself. It more commonly occurs with RBBB (Fig. 4.17). With LPFB, impulse conduction occurs normally down the right bundle branch and into the right ventricle. In the left ventricle, the anterior fascicle is activated first, depolarizing the anterior and lateral walls. The impulse then spreads in a downward and rightward direction, resulting in right axis deviation. The posterior wall of the left ventricle and, ultimately, the interventricular septum are then depolarized. As with LAFB, the QRS duration is usually less than 120 ms because only a portion of the left bundle branch is affected.

ECG characteristics of LPFB include the following (Surawicz et al., 2009):

- Right axis deviation between 90° and 180°
- rS pattern in leads I and aVL
- qR pattern in leads III and aVF
- QRS duration less than 120 ms

LPFB most often occurs in patients who have coronary artery disease but can occur in patients who have hypertension and valvular disease. Experts recommend that a diagnosis of LPFB be made only after other causes of right axis deviation have been ruled out, such as normal variants, mechanical shifts associated with inspiration or emphysema, RVH, chronic obstructive pulmonary disease, and acute or chronic pulmonary thromboembolism.

Trifascicular Block

The term *trifascicular block* is used to describe a conduction delay in the right bundle branch and either the main left bundle branch or both the left anterior fascicle and left posterior fascicle (Issa et al., 2012). ECG documentation of this type of block is uncommon. ECG characteristics of trifascicular block include the following (Issa et al., 2012):

- Third-degree AV block with a slow ventricular escape rhythm
- Alternating RBBB and LBBB
- Fixed RBBB with alternating LAFB and LPFB

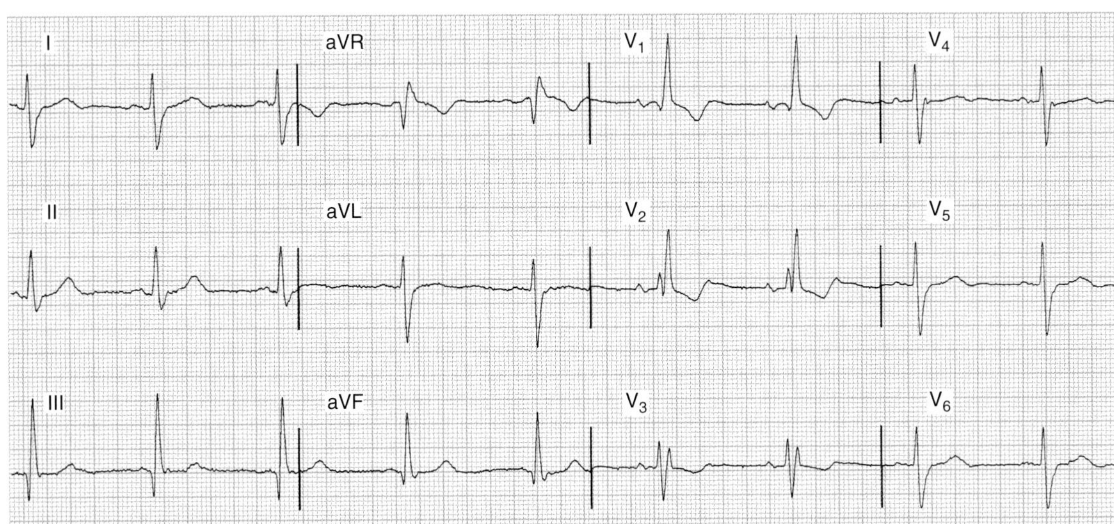

Fig. 4.17 Bifascicular block (right bundle branch block [RBBB] with left posterior fascicular block). The chest leads show a typical RBBB pattern, while the limb leads show prominent right axis deviation (RAD). The combination of these two findings (in the absence of other more common causes of RAD such as right ventricular hypertrophy or lateral myocardial infarction) is consistent with chronic bifascicular block due to left posterior fascicular block in concert with the RBBB. This elderly patient had severe coronary artery disease. The prominent Q waves in leads III and aVF suggest underlying inferior wall MI. (From Goldberger, A. L., Goldberger, Z. D., & Shvilkin, A. [2018]. *Goldberger's clinical electrocardiography: A simplified approach* [9th ed.]. Philadelphia, PA: Elsevier.)

VENTRICULAR RHYTHMS

Impulses originating in the ventricles may be the result of either natural pacemaker sites or implanted pacemakers. Just as with BBB, ventricular rhythms may exhibit STE not related to any infarct-related causes. This imitation STE is seen when the QRS complex is negatively deflected.

Ventricular Paced Rhythm

In many ways, a ventricular paced beat is a manmade LBBB. Consider that, when LBBB occurs, the electrical impulse travels down the right bundle branch and depolarizes the right ventricle, and the impulse spreads through the myocardium to depolarize the left ventricle. Pacemakers are most often introduced into the right ventricle attached to the right ventricular wall. When a pacemaker fires, it sends its impulse into the right ventricle, which depolarizes, and the impulse is spread through the myocardium to depolarize the left ventricle. An example of a ventricular paced rhythm producing STE is shown in Fig. 4.18.

Similarly, spontaneous impulses originating in the ventricles can produce STE, which is often seen accompanying a negatively deflected premature ventricular complex. If a ventricular rhythm is present, the ECG may show STE in the leads that are negatively deflected.

The 12-lead ECG machine does an excellent job of measuring QRS width. A QRS of normal duration results when the ventricles contract simultaneously. A QRS of prolonged duration results when the ventricles contract sequentially. Both BBB and ventricular rhythms widen the QRS complex. If the QRS is of normal duration, no complete BBB or ventricular rhythm exists.

Consider This

Expect to see discordant ST segments and T waves (ST segments and T waves in the opposite direction of the last portion of the QRS complex) in ventricular rhythms and ventricular paced rhythms because ventricular depolarization is abnormal.

BENIGN EARLY REPOLARIZATION

BER produces an infarct-like pattern on the ECGs of healthy asymptomatic patients. BER is a normal electrocardiographic variant that does not imply, or exclude, ACS or coronary artery disease (Kurz, Mattu, & Brady, 2014).

Electrocardiographic Criteria

Like the other conditions discussed in this chapter, BER produces STE (Box 4.4, Fig. 4.19). J-point elevation is usually less than 3.5 mm, and the concave ST segment is usually elevated less than 2 mm in the chest leads and 0.5 mm in the limb leads (Kurz et al., 2014). In general, maximal STE in BER is seen in leads V_2 to V_5. Additionally, BER produces tall, symmetric T waves resembling those seen in the hyperacute phase of MI. This combination creates a pattern on the ECG that closely resembles that of anterior or anterolateral infarction.

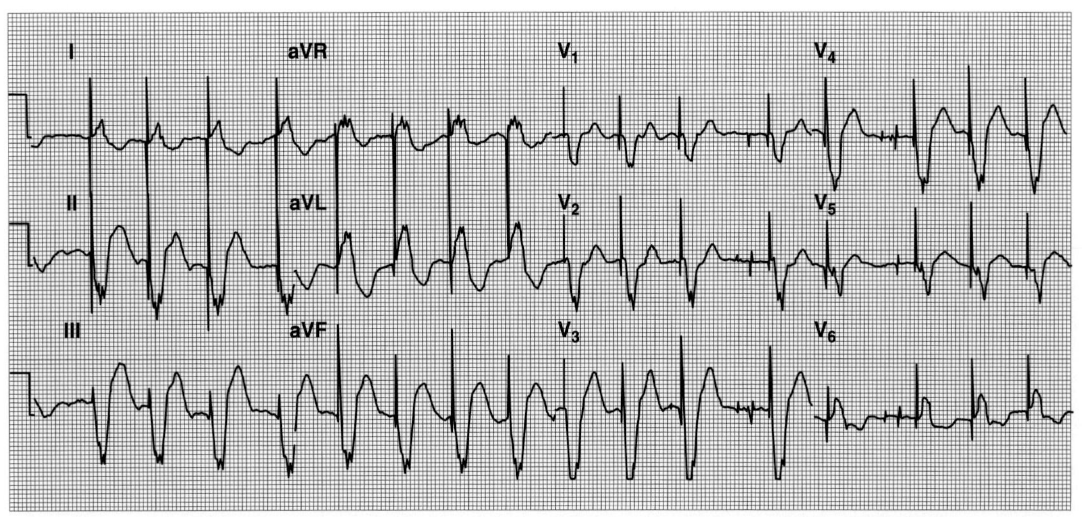

Fig. 4.18 Example of a ventricular paced rhythm producing paced ST-segment elevation.

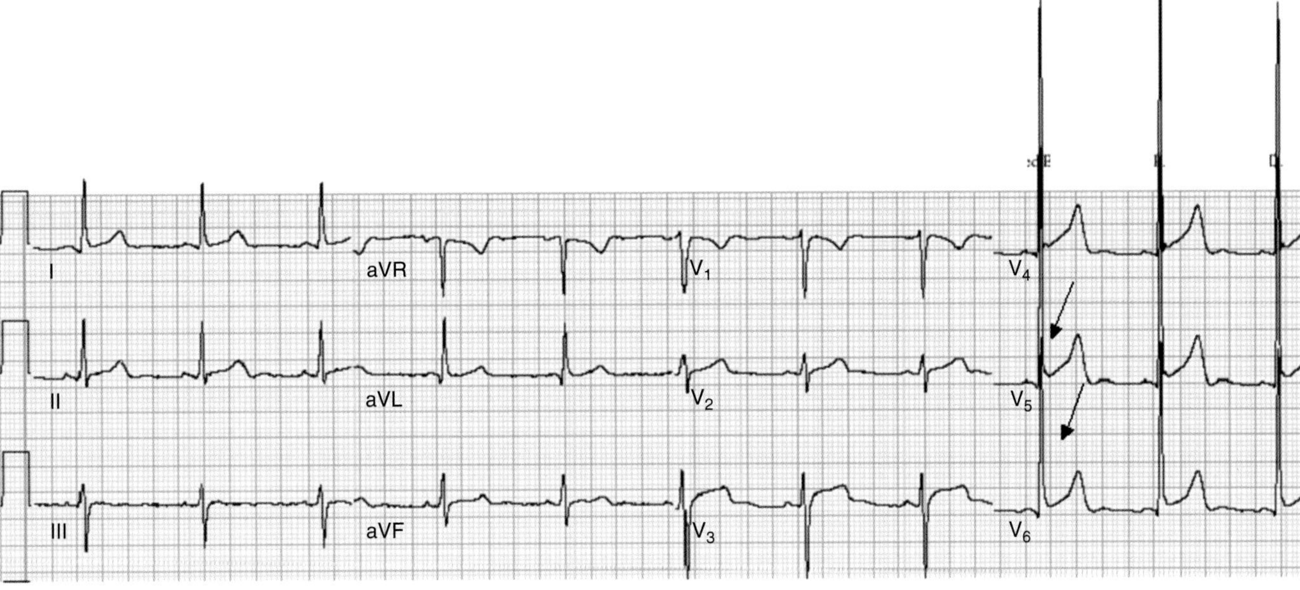

Fig. **4.19** Benign early repolarization. Note the upwardly concave ST-segment elevation, best seen in leads V_4 to V_6. The T waves are relatively large in the same leads. Subtle notching is also seen at the J point in leads V_4 and V_5.

Box 4.4 Typical ECG Characteristics of Benign Early Repolarization

STE with upward concavity of the initial portion of the ST segment
Notching at the J point
Symmetric T waves of large amplitude
Diffuse STE

J-point elevation in BER is usually accompanied by a slur, oscillation, or notch at the end of the QRS just before and including the J point. Just as with pericarditis, a notch at the J point causes one to consider noninfarct conditions as possible explanations for the STE. In general, R wave and T wave voltages are large in BER.

Clinical Presentation

BER is a normal finding. Enhanced parasympathetic activity and increased cardiovascular fitness are the most common explanations for these ECG changes (Lombardi, 2013).

Consider This

Benign early repolarization can appear to meet the voltage criteria for LVH, but often, this is not true pathologic hypertrophy but rather the result of a young or athletic heart.

Whereas BER is a normal finding, Brugada syndrome (BrS) is a repolarization abnormality that can predispose the patient to cardiac dysrhythmias, including polymorphic ventricular tachycardia and ventricular fibrillation. BrS is an inherited condition caused by mutations in one of several genes. It is more prevalent in Asian countries than in North America or Western Europe and predominantly affects males (Shen et al., 2017).

One of three patients diagnosed with BrS is identified after an episode of syncope (Adler et al., 2016). Dysrhythmias may occur at rest, during sleep, or after a large meal, presumably because of high vagal tone (Brugada, Campuzano, Sarquella-Brugada, Brugada, & Brugada, 2014). Fever has been shown to be an important trigger for ECG changes (Mizusawa & Wilde, 2012). Some patients have no symptoms; it is only detected on an ECG. For many, cardiac arrest may be the first manifestation of BrS.

Originally, three ECG patterns were described regarding BrS. Type I Brugada pattern consists of RBBB and coved (downsloping) STE of 2 mm or more and inverted T waves in more than one right chest lead (i.e., V_1 to V_3) (Fig. 4.20). With type 2 Brugada pattern, there is an RBBB pattern and STE, but the STE is followed by a positive or biphasic T wave that results in a saddleback configuration (Brugada et al., 2014). With type 3 Brugada pattern, there is an RBBB and STE in V_1 to V_3 that is 1 mm or less with a coved-type configuration, a saddleback configuration, or both (Brugada et al., 2014; Mizusawa & Wilde, 2012). Type 2 and type 3 are not considered diagnostic. In some patients, ECG changes can be provoked by medications such as class I antiarrhythmics and beta-blockers, among many others.

At present, there is no cure for BrS. Although several pharmacologic therapies are being tried, the only treatment proved to prevent sudden cardiac death in patients with BrS is the use of an implantable cardioverter-defibrillator.

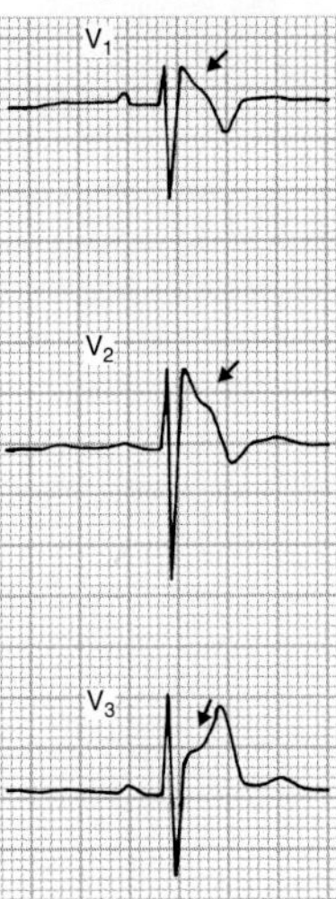

Fig. **4.20** Brugada pattern showing characteristic ST-segment elevation *(arrows)* in leads V_1 to V_3. (From Goldberger, A. L., Goldberger, Z. D., & Shvilkin, A. [2018]. *Goldberger's clinical electrocardiography: A simplified approach* [9th ed.]. Philadelphia, PA: Elsevier.)

PERICARDITIS

Another cause of STE is pericarditis. In this case, portions of the pericardium become inflamed, as does the adjoining epicardial surface of the heart. When STE occurs as the result of that inflammation, it is not the result of coronary artery disease. Anyone can develop pericarditis, but post-MI and post–cardiac surgery patients are especially susceptible.

Electrocardiographic Criteria

Pericarditis can produce several changes in the ECG. Because the STE is related to scattered patches of inflammation around the pericardium and is not caused by an occluded coronary artery, STE is usually diffuse and not strictly grouped into leads that are anatomically contiguous. During the first hours to days of illness, STE is usually present in leads I, II, III, aVL, aVF, and V_2 through V_6 (Jouriles, 2014). Reciprocal ST depression may be seen in leads aVR and V_1 (Jouriles, 2014).

Pericarditis can also produce PR-segment depression. When the ST segment is compared with a depressed PR segment, it can give the appearance of STE. Using the TP segment to establish the isoelectric line will minimize this illusion. The frequent presence of PR-segment elevation in lead aVR, with reciprocal PR-segment depression in other leads, is an important ECG clue in recognizing acute pericarditis (Mirvis & Goldberger, 2015).

Another change that pericarditis may bring to the ECG is a notching of the J point. Although not exclusive to pericarditis, J-point notching signifies the possibility of a noninfarct cause of STE. Fig. 4.21 illustrates how some leads show examples of true STE, whereas other leads appear elevated because of PR-segment depression, and a few display J-point notching.

Clinical Presentation

Chest pain is commonly the chief complaint in pericarditis. The pain is often described as "sharp" (the term *sharp* is intended to convey a knifelike pain, not to convey intensity) or "stabbing," unlike the more typical "pressure" or "heaviness" accompanying infarction. The pain of pericarditis can often be localized with one finger. In contrast, the discomfort associated with acute MI is typically over a larger area that cannot be localized with one finger. The pain of pericarditis tends to be affected by movement, ventilation, and position. The patient may state that the pain is minimized by leaning forward and intensified by lying supine. If pain radiation occurs, the patient may report that it is felt about the base of the neck or the area between the shoulder blades.

The recognizable ECG features of pericarditis are subtle and can easily be overlooked or misinterpreted. Therefore, it is often the clinical presentation of pericarditis that is first recognized. Once pericarditis is suspected, the ECG can be closely examined (or re-examined) for substantiating evidence. Table 4.1 compares the ECG and clinical features of MI and pericarditis.

Although BER and pericarditis can cause STE, neither condition is particularly good at causing reciprocal changes. If STE is present on the ECG and clear, obvious reciprocal changes are present, it is reasonable to scratch BER and pericarditis from the list of possible causes of STE.

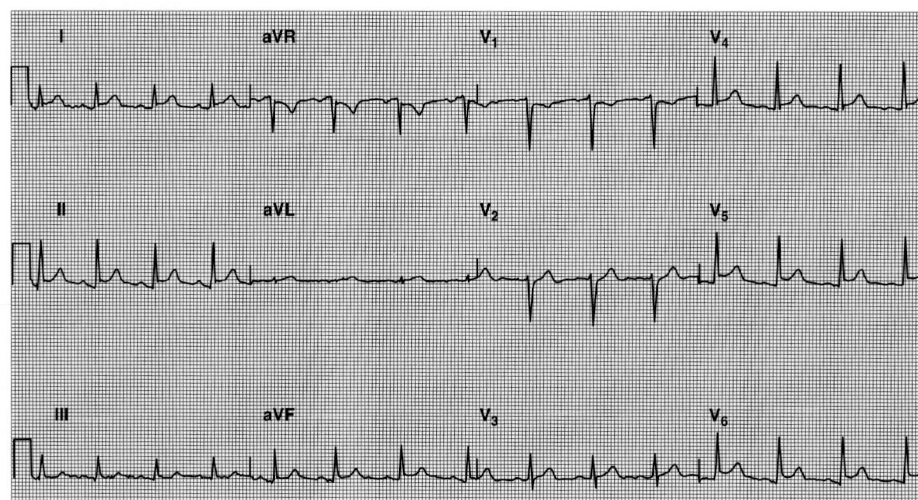

Fig. **4.21** The pattern of pericarditis. Note the diffuse pattern of ST-segment elevation, PR-segment depression in lead II, and J-point notching in leads II, V_5, and V_6.

TABLE 4.1 Clinical Presentation of Acute Myocardial Infarction and Pericarditis

Finding	Myocardial Infarction	Pericarditis
Chest pain (nature)	Pressure	Sharp, stabbing
Chest pain (radiation)	Left arm, shoulder, jaw	Base of neck, trapezius area
Chest pain (aggravation)	Unaffected by movement	Affected by movement, ventilation, swallowing, etc. May improve when leaning forward
ST-elevation (STE)	Appears in anatomically contiguous leads	Diffuse across ECG, may occur in leads not grouped anatomically
PR-segment depression	Uncommon	Common, may give appearance of STE

WHAT SHOULD YOU DO NOW?

At times, it is very difficult to differentiate between infarct and noninfarct causes of STE. Some cases can be decided only after hours of observation, serial ECGs, and extensive testing. Therefore, it is not reasonable to expect that a single ECG will always provide enough information to determine the cause of STE.

Remember that the ECG is simply a recording of electrical current on the patient's skin. For this reason, the ECG is not always sensitive enough to detect subtle changes and is not always specific enough to differentiate between certain conditions. While the clinical presentation can be very helpful in differentiating between the causes of STE in some cases, it does not always settle the matter.

How then can the ECG best be used when treating cardiac patients in the early hours of chest pain? *A realistic initial goal is to recognize situations when STE could be the result of an MI or some other condition.* For example, LBBB can very closely simulate the ECG pattern of an anterior wall infarction. However, you need not attempt to determine if the cause of the STE is an infarction or an STE variant. In these instances, simply note the presence of STE, recognize that it could be attributed to infarct or an STE variant, and bring it to the attention of the emergency department (ED) provider for review. When the patient's clinical presentation is suspicious enough to motivate you to obtain a 12-lead ECG, the presence of an STE variant should prompt an immediate review by the ED provider.

The ED provider can determine if the patient should be worked up as a cardiac patient. Outside of the hospital, the paramedic should transmit the ECG for interpretation by an ED provider. If transmission is not possible, objective findings can be relayed via radio or phone. For example, one may state, "There is 4 to 5 mm of STE in V_1 through V_3, and a LBBB pattern is present." Given that information, the ED provider will immediately realize the interpretive predicament. He or she can determine whether the paramedic should proceed with reperfusion therapy screening, aspirin, and multiple intravenous lines.

In some ways, this approach may seem inappropriate, but it is not. In fact, sometimes, the phrase "I don't know" is the most intelligent response that you can give. In situations in which there is simply not enough information to make a reasonable interpretation, it is far better to defer to the ED provider than to assign an interpretation without sufficient evidence. Often, the provider will not have an immediate answer either. It may be only after comparative and serial ECGs are available, cardiac biomarkers are analyzed, and the patient is observed over time that the provider will feel comfortable applying a definitive interpretation. Therefore, do not be disheartened by this predicament. Table 4.2 presents a summary of the five STE variants discussed in this chapter and how they mimic infarction.

TABLE 4.2 Summary of Five Common STE Variants

Condition	Infarction Resemblance	Recognition
LVH	• STE in the negatively deflected leads, usually V_1–V_3	• Add S-wave amplitude in lead V_3 and R-wave amplitude in lead aVL • Suspect LVH if total greater than 20 mm (2 mV) in women and 28 mm or more (2.8 mV) in men
LBBB	• STE in the negatively deflected leads, usually V_1–V_3 • QS complexes in the negatively deflected leads, usually V_1–V_3	• QRS complex 120 ms or more • QRS complex produced by supraventricular activity • QS complex or negative terminal force in V_1
Ventricular rhythms	• STE in the negatively deflected leads • QS complexes in the negatively deflected leads	• Wide QRS complex following pacer spikes (if noticeable) • Negative terminal force in V_1 (right ventricle paced)

Continued

TABLE 4.2 Summary of Five Common STE Variants—Cont'd

Condition	Infarction Resemblance	Recognition
Benign early repolarization	• STE, particularly in anterior or anterolateral leads • Tall T waves	• STE with upward concavity of the initial portion of the ST segment • Symmetric T waves of large amplitude • Notching at the J point • Patient may be asymptomatic • Highest prevalence in athletic individuals
Pericarditis	• STE in multiple leads	• STE not in anatomical grouping • STE usually present leads I, II, III, aVL, aVF, and V_2 through V_6 • Reciprocal ST depression in aVR and V_1 • PR-segment elevation in aVR, with PR-segment depression in other leads • Notching of the J point

LBBB, Left bundle branch block; *LVH*, left ventricular hypertrophy; *STE*, ST-elevation.

REFERENCES

Adler, A., Rosso, R., Chorin, E., Havakuk, O., Antzelevitch, C., & Viskin, S. (2016). Risk stratification in Brugada syndrome: Clinical characteristics, electrocardiographic parameters, and auxiliary testing. *Heart Rhythm*, *13*(1), 299–310.

Brugada, R., Campuzano, O., Sarquella-Brugada, G., Brugada, J., & Brugada, P. (2014). Brugada syndrome. *Methodist Debakey Cardiovascular Journal*, *10*(1), 25–28.

Goldberger, A. L., Goldberger, Z. D., & Shvilkin, A. (2018). Atrial and ventricular enlargement. In *Goldberger's clinical electrocardiography: A simplified approach* (9th ed., pp. 50–60). Philadelphia, PA: Elsevier.

Hancock, E. W., Deal, B. J., Mirvis, D. M., Okin, P., Kligfield, P., & Gettes, L. S. (2009). AHA/ACCF/HRS recommendations for the standardization and interpretation of the electrocardiogram: Part V: Electrocardiogram changes associated with cardiac chamber hypertrophy. *Journal of the American College of Cardiology*, *53*(11), 992–1002.

Issa, Z. F., Miller, J. M., & Zipes, D. P. (2012). Intraventricular conduction abnormalities. In Z. F. Issa, J. M. Miller, & D. P. Zipes (Eds.), *Clinical arrhythmology and electrophysiology: A companion to Braunwald's heart disease* (2nd ed., pp. 194–211). Philadelphia, PA: Saunders.

Jouriles, N. J. (2014). Pericardial and myocardial disease. In J. A. Marx, R. S. Hockberger, & R. M. Walls (Eds.), *Rosen's emergency medicine* (8th ed., pp. 1091–1105). Philadelphia: Saunders.

Kontos, M. C., Aziz, H. A., Chau, V. Q., Roberts, C. S., Ornato, J. P., & Vetrovec, G. W. (2011). Outcomes in patients with chronicity of left bundle-branch block with possible acute myocardial infarction. *American Heart Journal*, *161*(4), 698–704.

Kurz, M. C., Mattu, A., & Brady, W. J. (2014). Acute coronary syndrome. In J. A. Marx, R. S. Hockberger, & R. M. Walls (Eds.), *Rosen's emergency medicine* (8th ed., pp. 997–1033). Philadelphia, PA: Saunders.

Latcu, D.-G., & Nadir, S. (2010). Atrioventricular and intraventricular conduction disorders. In M. H. Crawford, J. P. DiMarco, & W. J. Paulus (Eds.), *Cardiology* (3rd ed., pp. 725–739). Philadelphia, PA: Elsevier.

Lombardi, F. (2013). Early repolarization: a benign electrocardiographic pattern or an ominous proarrhythmic sign? *Journal of the American College of Cardiology*, *61*(8), 870–871.

Mirvis, D. M., & Goldberger, A. L. (2015). Electrocardiography. In D. L. Mann, D. P. Zipes, P. Libby, R. O. Bonow, & E. Braunwald (Eds.), *Braunwald's heart disease: A textbook of cardiovascular medicine* (10th ed., pp. 114–154). Philadelphia, PA: Saunders.

Mizusawa, Y., & Wilde, A. A. (2012). Brugada syndrome. *Circulation: Arrhythmia and Electrophysiology*, *5*(3), 606–616.

O'Connor, R. E., Al Ali, A. S., Brady, W. J., Ghaemmaghami, C. A., Menon, V., Welsford, M., & Shuster, M. (2015). *2015 American Heart Association guidelines for CPR & ECC.* Retrieved from American Heart Association. Web-based Integrated Guidelines for Cardiopulmonary Resuscitation and Emergency Cardiovascular Care – Part 9: Acute Coronary Syndromes: Eccguidelines.heart.org

O'Gara, P. T., Kushner, F. G., Ascheim, D. D., Casey, Jr, D. E., Chung, M. K., de Lemos, J. A.,… Zhao, D. X. (2013). 2013 ACCF/AHA guideline for the management of ST-elevation myocardial infarction. *Journal of the American College of Cardiology*, *61*(4), e78–e140.

Sgarbossa, E. B., Pinski, S. L., Barbagelata, A., Underwood, D. A., Gates, K. B., Topol, E. J.,…Wagner, G. S. (1996). Electrocardiographic diagnosis of evolving acute myocardial infarction in the presence of left bundle-branch block. GUSTO-1 (Global Utilization of Streptokinase and Tissue Plasminogen Activator for Occluded Coronary Arteries) Investigators. *New England Journal of Medicine*, *334*(8), 481–487.

Shen, W. K., Sheldon, R. S., Benditt, D. G., Cohen, M. I., Forman, D. E., Goldberger, Z. D.,… Yancy, C. W. (2017). 2017 ACC/AHA/HRS guideline for the evaluation and management of patients with syncope. *Journal of the American College of Cardiology*, *70*(5), e39–e110.

Smith, S. W., Dodd, K. W., Henry, T. D., Dvorak, D. M., & Pearce, L. A. (2012). Diagnosis of ST-elevation myocardial infarction in the presence of left bundle branch block with the ST-elevation to S-wave ratio in a modified Sgarbossa rule. *Annals of Emergency Medicine*, *60*(6), 766–776.

Surawicz, B., Childers, R., Deal, B. J., & Gettes, L. S. (2009). AHA/ACCF/HRS Recommendations for the standardization and interpretation of the electrocardiogram: Part III: Intraventricular conduction disturbances: A scientific statement from the American Heart Association Electrocardiography and Arrhythmias Committee, *Journal of the American College of Cardiology*, *53*(11), 976–981.

Surawicz, B., & Knilans, T. K. (2008). Other intraventricular conduction disturbances. In *Chou's electrocardiography in clinical practice* (6th ed., pp. 108–123). Philadelphia, PA: Saunders.

Tabas, J. A., Rodriguez, R. M., Seligman, H. K., & Goldschlager, N. F. (2008). Electrocardiographic criteria for detecting acute myocardial infarction in patients with left bundle branch block: A meta-analysis. *Annals of Emergency Medicine*, *52*(4), 329–336.

QUICK REVIEW

1. Benign early repolarization (BER)
   a. is associated with an increased incidence of cardiogenic shock.
   b. is an electrocardiographic variant that most often occurs in elderly men.
   c. produces ST-segment depression that is typically seen in the limb leads.
   d. produces an electrocardiographic pattern resembling an anterior infarction.

2. Which of the following is characteristic of right bundle branch block?
   a. Pathologic Q waves
   b. An rSR′ pattern in lead V_1
   c. A broad R wave in leads I and V_6
   d. A deep S wave in lead V_1 and a tall R wave in leads I and V_6

3. Characteristics of left posterior fascicular block typically include
   a. left axis deviation.
   b. a qR pattern in lead aVL.
   c. an rS pattern in leads I and aVL.
   d. a QRS duration of 120 ms or more.

4. The primary ECG characteristic associated with left ventricular hypertrophy is
   a. increased QRS amplitude.
   b. deeper-than-normal S waves.
   c. the presence of tall T waves.
   d. prolongation of the PR interval.

5. Which of the following ECG changes may be observed with pericarditis?
   a. Diffuse STE, PR segment depression, J-point notching
   b. STE in the inferior leads, J-point notching, PR-segment elevation
   c. Tall P waves, diffuse ST-segment depression, prolonged PR intervals
   d. Notched P waves, increased QRS amplitude, ST-segment depression in the lateral leads

CASE STUDIES

For each of the following case studies, carefully evaluate the description of the patient's clinical presentation, systematically analyze each 12-lead ECG, and formulate a treatment plan on the basis of the information provided.

CASE STUDY 4.1

A 78-year-old man presents with a sudden onset of shortness of breath and "feeling faint." While speaking in sentences of four to five words, he relays that he was using a plunger to clear a clogged toilet when his symptoms began about 45 minutes ago. He denies chest pain. The patient has a history of asthma, for which he takes albuterol and ipratropium bromide. He has no known allergies.

Physical examination reveals that the patient is alert, anxious, and oriented to person, place, time, and event. His skin is pink, warm, and dry. There is no jugular vein distention. Bilateral inspiratory and expiratory wheezing is present. His blood pressure is 170/110 mm Hg, heart rate 100 beats/min, ventilations 24/min, and SpO_2 91% on room air.

The patient has been placed on a cardiac monitor, and supplemental oxygen is being administered. Vascular access has been established and a 12-lead ECG has been obtained (Fig. 4.22). Review the patient's ECG and describe your initial interventions for this patient.

Fig. 4.22

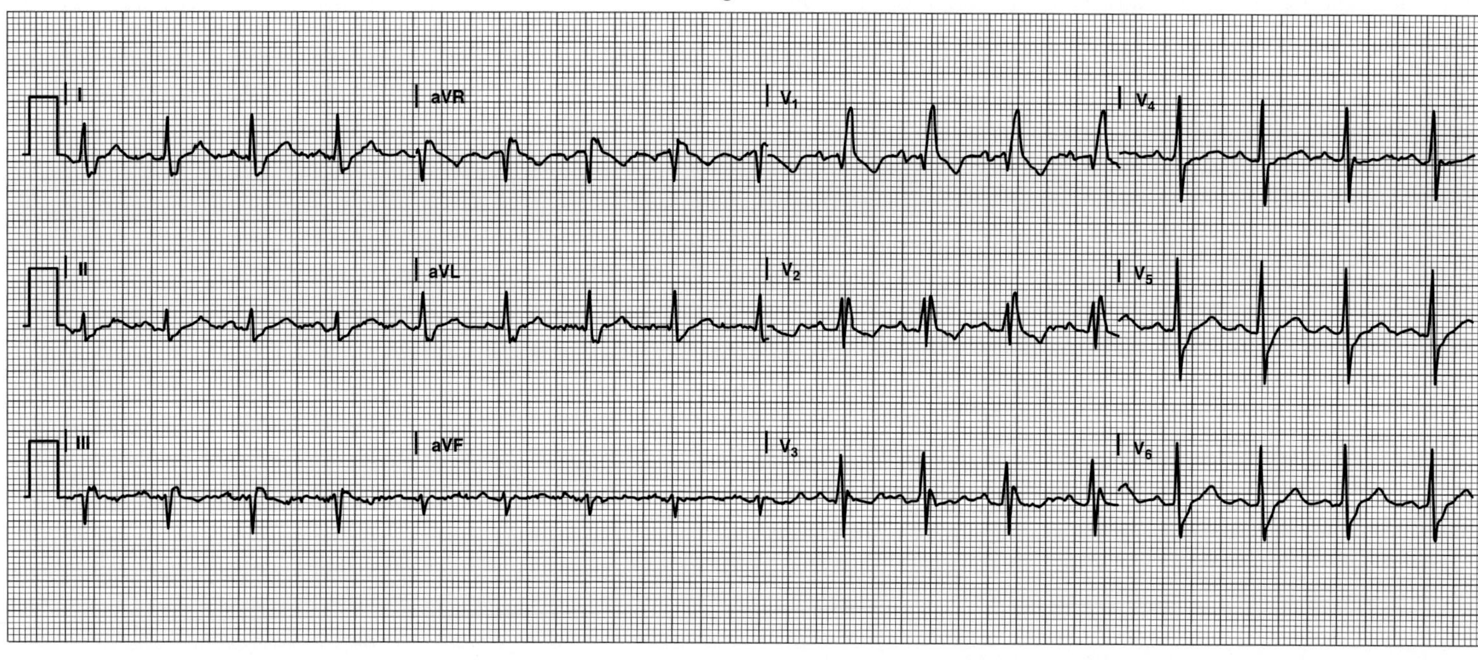

CASE STUDY 4.2

A 78-year-old man presents with a sudden onset of substernal chest pain and shortness of breath that began 3 hours ago while at rest. He rates his pain 9/10 and says it radiates to his left arm and back. The patient had a coronary artery bypass graft 4 years ago.

The patient regularly takes at least 20 medications, which he has brought with him. He is allergic to codeine. Physical examination reveals that the patient is alert, anxious, and oriented to person, place, time, and event. His skin is pink, warm, and moist. Breath sounds are clear. His SpO_2 is 98% on room air. His blood pressure is 178/82 mm Hg, pulse 120 beats/min, and ventilations 26/min.

The patient has been placed on a cardiac monitor and supplemental oxygen is being administered. Vascular access has been established and a 12-lead ECG has been obtained (Fig. 4.23). Review the patient's ECG and describe your initial interventions for this patient.

Fig. 4.23

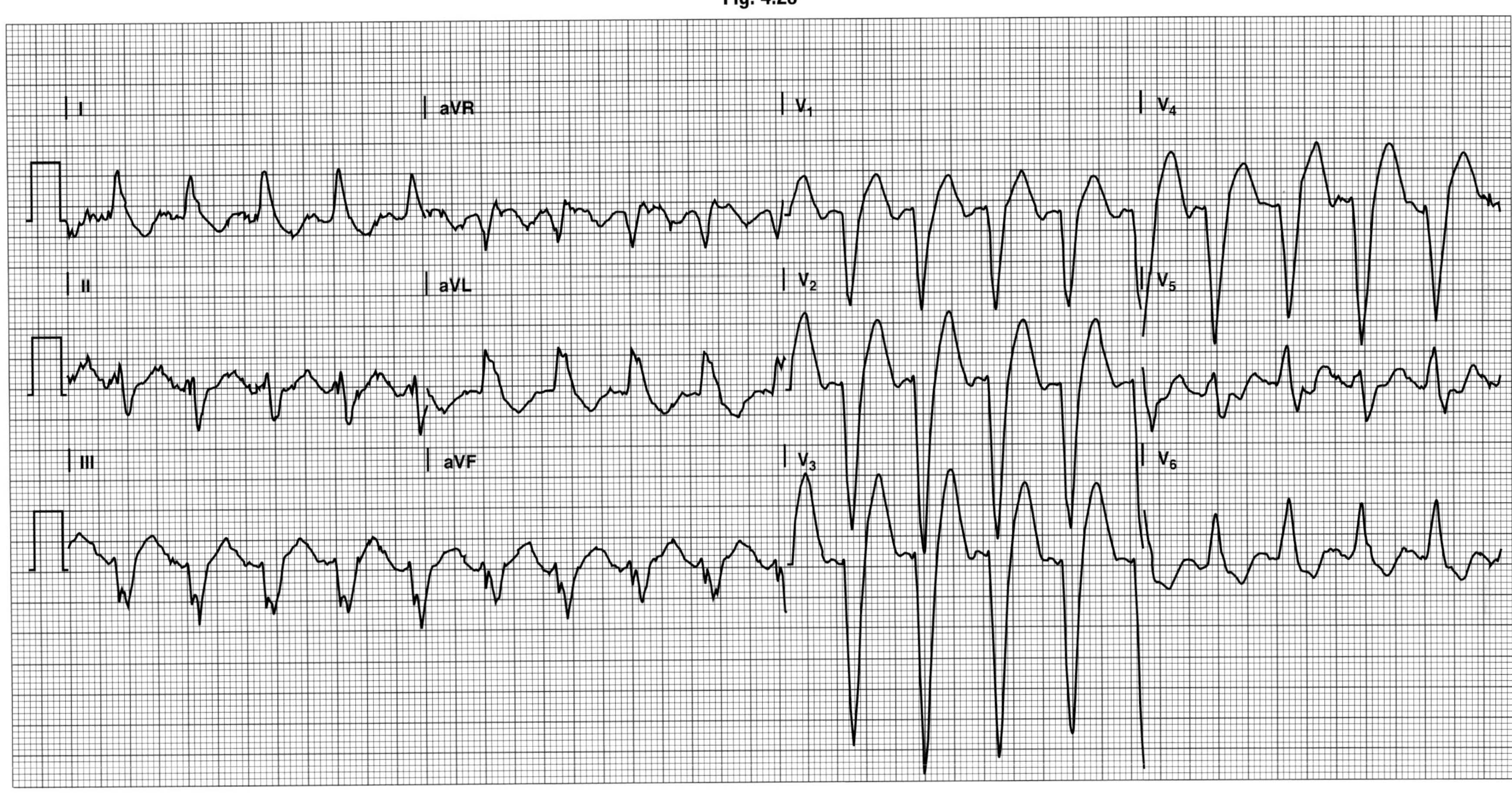

ANSWERS

1. **D**. BER is a normal electrocardiographic variant that produces a pattern resembling an anterior or anterolateral infarction on the ECGs of healthy asymptomatic patients. It is most often seen in young athletic individuals. BER produces STE that is generally maximal in leads V_2 to V_5.

2. **B**. An rSR′ pattern in lead V_1 is characteristic of RBBB.

3. **C**. The ECG characteristics of left posterior fascicular block include right axis deviation, an rS pattern in leads I and aVL, a qR pattern in leads III and aVF, and a QRS duration less than 120 ms.

4. **A**. Left ventricular hypertrophy is primarily recognized on the ECG by increased QRS amplitude accompanied by changes in the ST segment and T wave.

5. **A**. ECG changes that may be observed with pericarditis include diffuse STE, PR-segment depression, and J-point notching.

INTERPRETATION OF CASE STUDIES

CASE STUDY 4.1

Although this patient's symptoms are likely to be respiratory in origin, shortness of breath is also an anginal equivalent. Allow the patient to assume a position of comfort and measure his peak expiratory flow rate. Administer a bronchodilator and an inhaled corticosteroid and reassess. The patient's 12-lead ECG shows a sinus tachycardia with a RBBB, but no evidence of STEMI at this time.

Over a period of 2 hours in the ED, the patient's symptoms resolved. After evaluating the results of his chest radiograph, a second 12-lead ECG, and laboratory studies, the patient was discharged home with the addition of an inhaled corticosteroid to his asthma therapy regimen.

CASE STUDY 4.2

The patient's 12-lead ECG shows ECG changes consistent with an anteroseptal STEMI; however, a LBBB is present. LBBB can cause STE and T-wave changes, confounding the ECG diagnosis of STEMI. While none of the modified Sgarbossa criteria have been met, the shape of the ST segments here makes STEMI a strong consideration.

Give aspirin as soon as possible if not already done and if there are no contraindications. Quickly screen the patient for indications and contraindications to fibrinolytic therapy and PCI. At the same time, administer nitroglycerin (NTG) to address the patient's ischemic chest discomfort. Closely monitor the patient's vital signs and ECG after each dose. Select a reperfusion strategy, obtain a portable chest radiograph, and draw initial laboratory studies.

After one sublingual NTG tablet, the patient rated his chest pain 8/10. After a second tablet, 7/10, and after a third, 4/10. The patient was then given intravenous morphine and moved to the cardiac catheterization laboratory.

Practice ECGs

5

CHAPTER

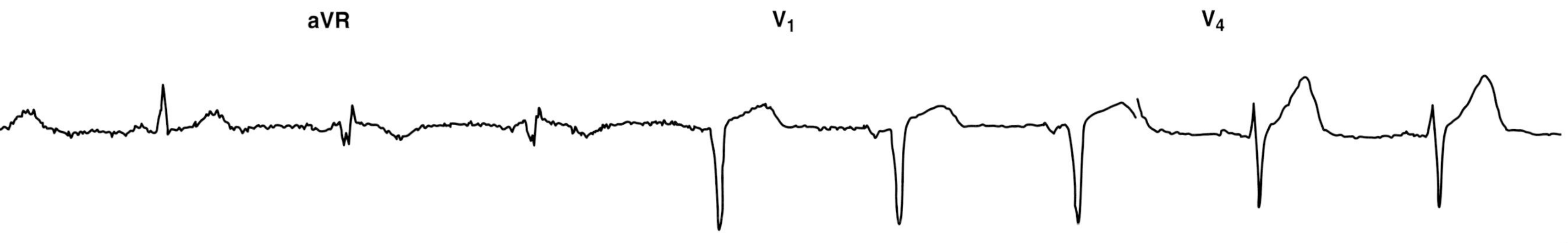

LEARNING OBJECTIVES

After reading this chapter, you should be able to:

1. Develop a systematic approach for infarct recognition on the electrocardiogram (ECG).
2. Gain familiarity with 12-lead ECG interpretation.

12-LEAD ANALYSIS

We began the discussion regarding the approach to reviewing a 12-lead ECG in Chapter 3. In this chapter, we expand that approach to include ST-elevation variants and the patient's clinical presentation.

1. Identify the rate and underlying rhythm.
2. Analyze waveforms, segments, and intervals. Examine each lead (except aVR), looking for the following:
    - *Pathologic Q waves*. Recall that a pathologic Q wave is more than 0.03 second in duration or more than 30% of the height of the following R wave in that lead, or both.
    - *R-wave progression*. Recall that when viewing the chest leads in a normal heart, the R wave typically becomes taller (i.e., increases in amplitude) and the S wave becomes smaller as the electrode is moved from right to left. In the area of leads V_3 and V_4, the amplitude of the R wave should begin to exceed the amplitude of the S wave and then gradually become smaller again through V_6. Use the phrase *poor R-wave progression* to describe R waves that decrease in size from V_1 to V_4.
    - *ST-segment displacement*. Looking at the J point, determine if ST-elevation (STE) or ST-segment depression is present.
    - *T-wave changes*. Examine the T waves for changes in orientation, shape, and size. Note if they are tall, peaked, inverted, biphasic, or notched.
3. Examine for evidence of an acute coronary syndrome (ACS). If ST-segment displacement is present, assess the areas of ischemia or injury by assessing lead groupings.
4. Ascertain if an STE variant is present that may account for ECG changes (Box 5.1).
    - Use one of several available formulas to rule out left ventricular hypertrophy (LVH) as a possible cause of STE.
    - Bundle branch blocks (BBBs) and ventricular rhythms can cause a wide QRS and mimic the infarct pattern on the ECG. If the QRS is of normal duration (110 ms or less), no *complete* BBB or ventricular rhythm exists and you can scratch BBB and ventricular rhythms from the list of STE variants.
    - Benign early repolarization (BER) and pericarditis can also cause STE, mimicking an infarct pattern on the ECG. However, neither BER nor pericarditis is particularly good at causing reciprocal changes. If STE is present on the ECG and clear, obvious, reciprocal changes are present, it is reasonable to scratch BER and pericarditis from the list of possible causes of STE.
    - The presence of an STE variant does not rule out myocardial infarction. Sometimes the ECG will show STE *and* meet the criteria for LVH. In this situation, it is possible that the STE is caused by LVH. However, it is also possible that the patient may have an enlarged left ventricle *and* simultaneously have a clot in a coronary artery. Similarly, it is possible that a patient may have a BBB *and* be experiencing an MI. In such cases, a physician should be consulted.
5. Estimate the QRS axis using leads I and aVF.
6. Interpret your findings. Categorize the 12-lead ECG into one of the following groups: (1) STE, (2) ST-segment depression, or (3) normal or nondiagnostic ECG.

Box 5.1 Examples of ST-Elevation Variants

- Left ventricular hypertrophy
- Left bundle branch block
- Ventricular rhythms
- Benign early repolarization
- Pericarditis

Clinical Presentation

Discovering the patient's clinical presentation is a priority. The inclusion of the clinical presentation at this point does not imply that it is the first time that you should obtain patient information. Rather, it is assumed that you will already have obtained the relevant subjective and objective information from the patient. The specific inclusion of the clinical presentation is included here to emphasize the importance of integrating the clinical presentation into the ECG interpretation. When incorporating the clinical picture into the ECG interpretation, remember that not all patients experiencing an ACS will present with substernal chest pain. A high index of suspicion is always warranted, especially when treating women, individuals with diabetes, or older adults.

Complicating the effort to recognize infarction is the fact that only a minority of nontraumatic chest pain is the result of infarction. Causes of noninfarction chest pain include pericarditis, aneurysm, musculoskeletal pain, a variety of pulmonary conditions, gastrointestinal disorders, and various emotional and psychologic states. Clearly, the task of early infarct recognition can be challenging. It is the physician's task to ultimately differentiate infarction from other conditions.

PRACTICE ECGs

Our interpretation of each ECG is included at the end of this chapter. Please note that the interpretation of each lead and tracing includes only the material discussed in this text. Therefore, experienced electrocardiographers will note the presence of some conditions or findings that are not listed in the interpretation.

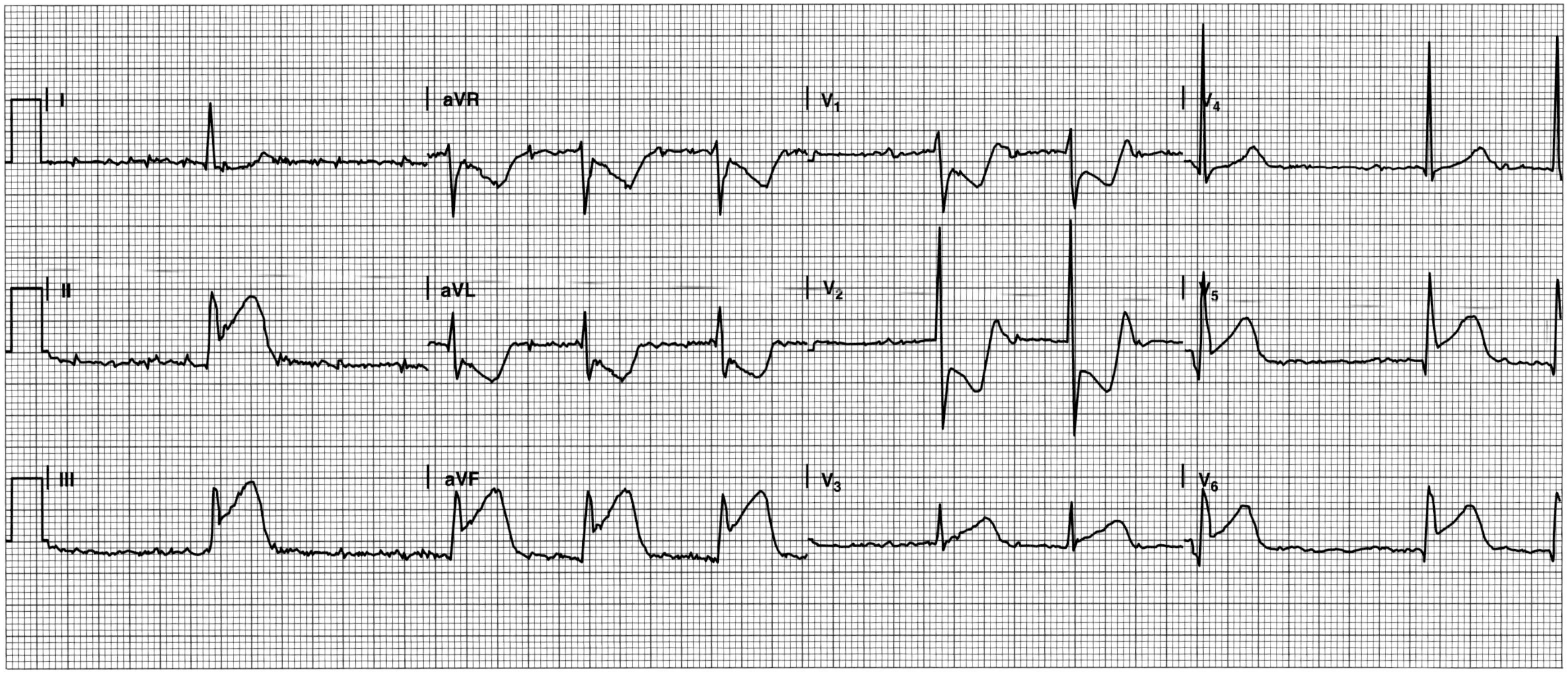

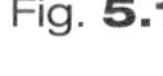

Fig. 5.1

x1.0 0.05-150Hz 25mm/sec

Rate and rhythm? ______ Pathologic Q waves? ______

STE? ______ ST depression? ______ T-wave changes? ______

Reciprocal changes? ______ Imposter present? ______ Axis? ______

Interpretation: ______

Inferior: II, III, aVF | **Septum: V_1, V_2** | **Anterior: V_3, V_4** | **Lateral: I, aVL, V_5, V_6**

Fig. **5.2**

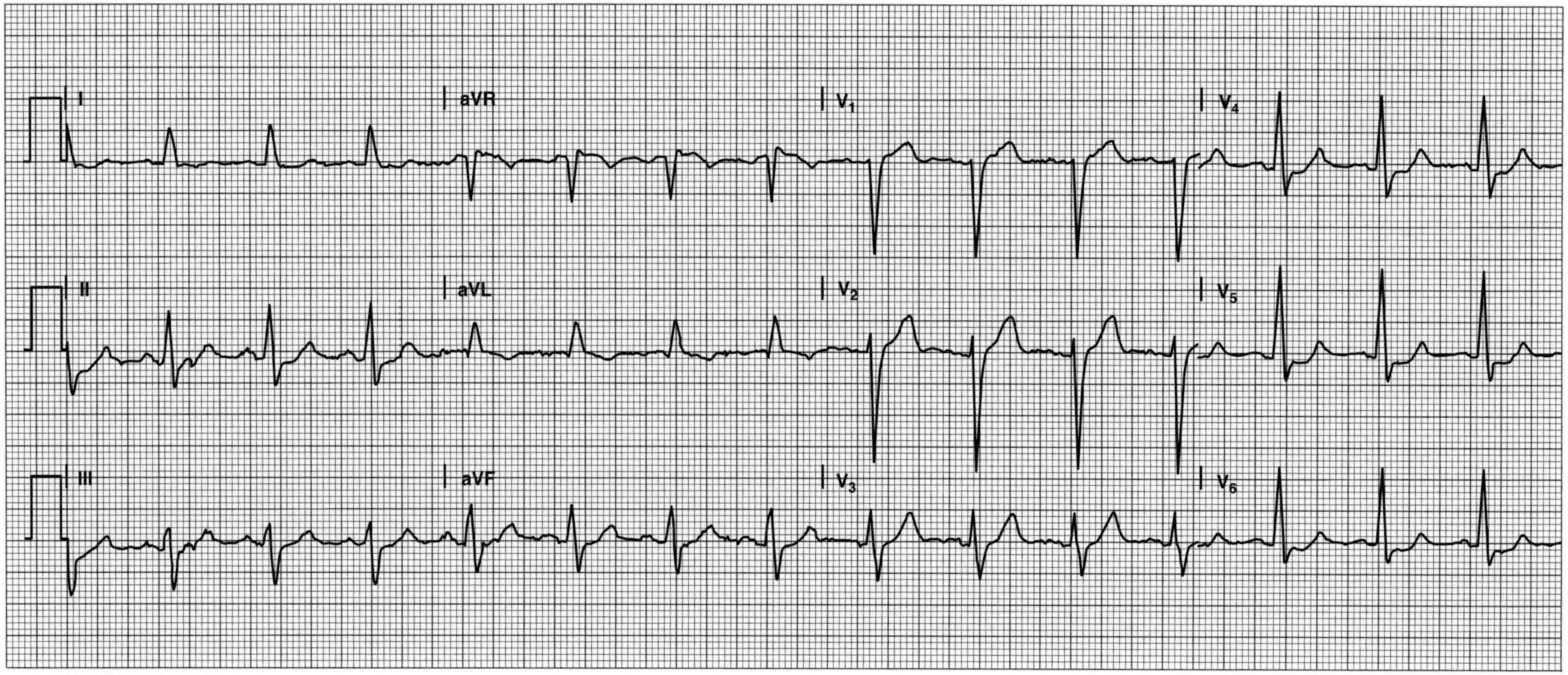

x1.0 0.05-150Hz 25mm/sec

Rate and rhythm? ____________________ Pathologic Q waves? ____________________

STE? ____________________ ST depression? ____________________ T-wave changes? ____________________

Reciprocal changes? ____________________ Imposter present? ____________________ Axis? ____________________

Interpretation: ____________________

Inferior: II, III, aVF | **Septum: V_1, V_2** | Anterior: V_3, V_4 | **Lateral: I, aVL, V_5, V_6**

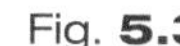

Fig. 5.3

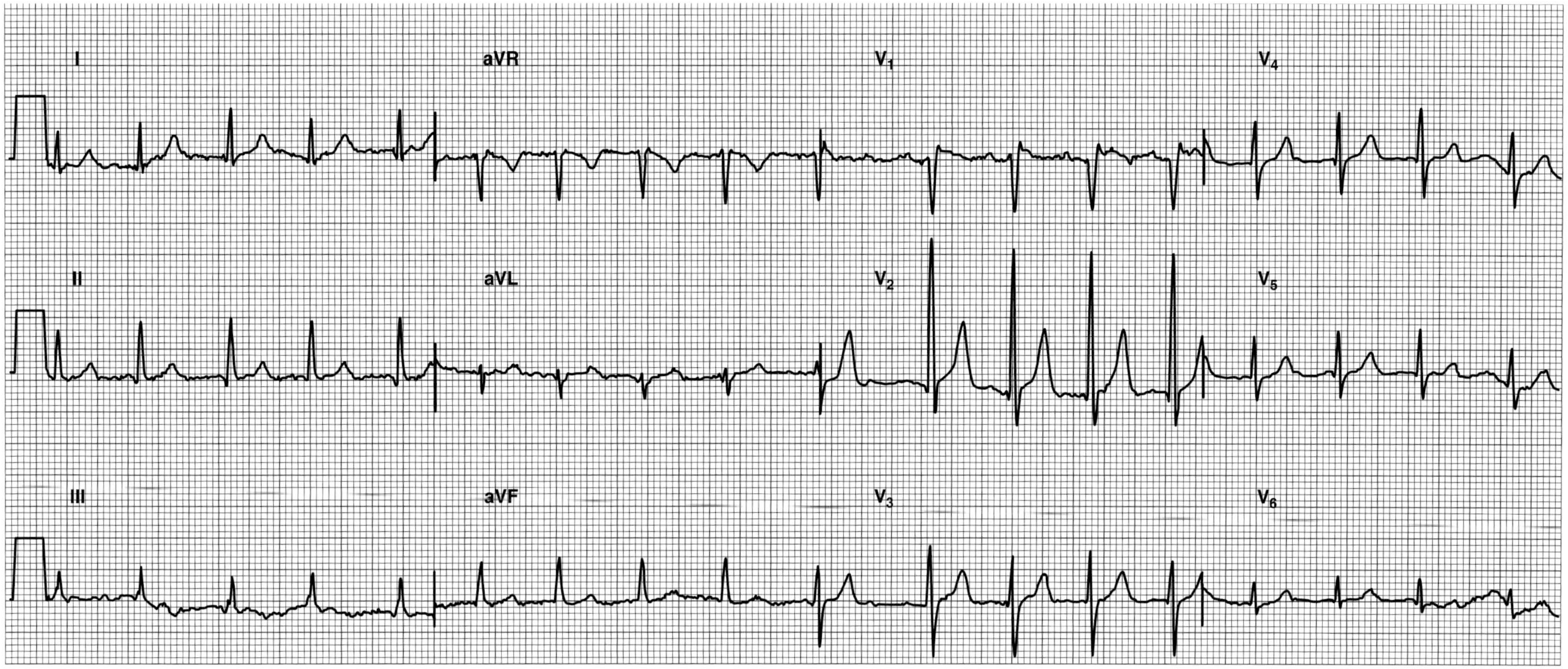

Rate and rhythm? ______________________ Pathologic Q waves? ______________________

STE? ______________________ ST depression? ______________________ T-wave changes? ______________________

Reciprocal changes? ______________________ Imposter present? ______________________ Axis? ______________________

Interpretation: ______________________

Inferior: II, III, aVF | **Septum: V_1, V_2** | **Anterior: V_3, V_4** | **Lateral: I, aVL, V_5, V_6**

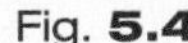

Fig. **5.4**

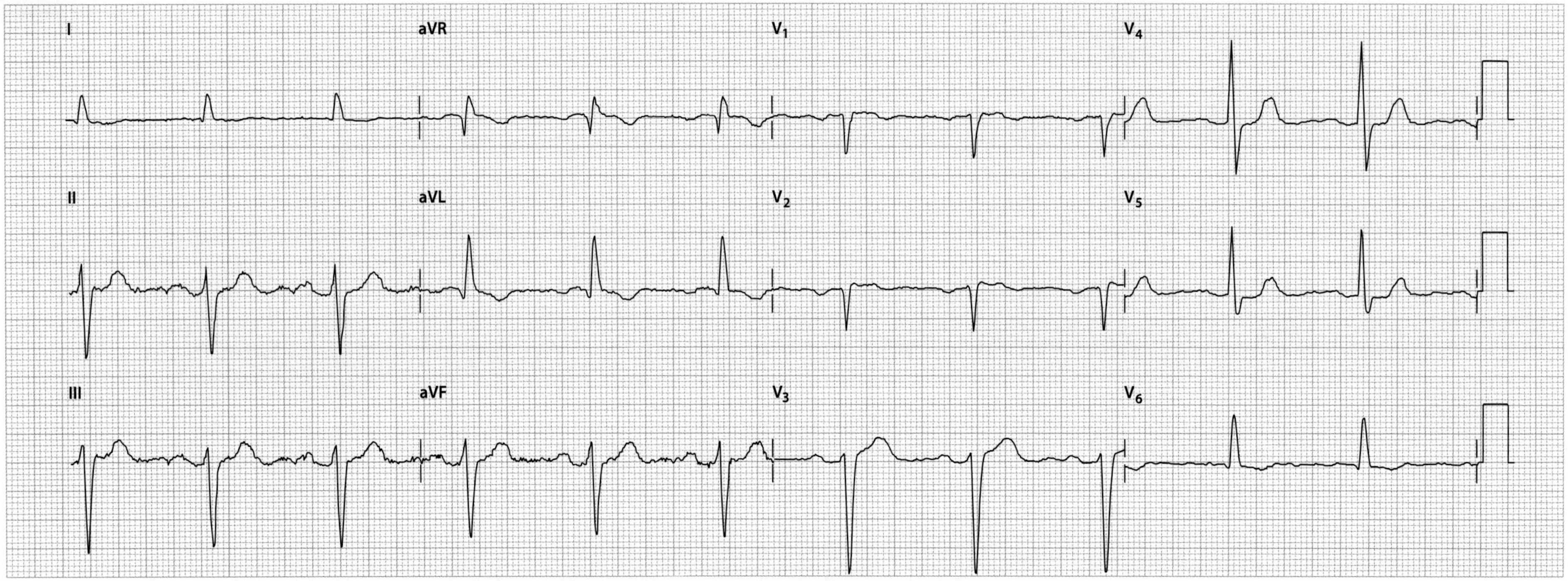

Rate and rhythm? ________________ Pathologic Q waves? ________________

STE? ________________ ST depression? ________________ T-wave changes? ________________

Reciprocal changes? ________________ Imposter present? ________________ Axis? ________________

Interpretation: ________________

Inferior: II, III, aVF | **Septum: V_1, V_2** | Anterior: V_3, V_4 | **Lateral: I, aVL, V_5, V_6**

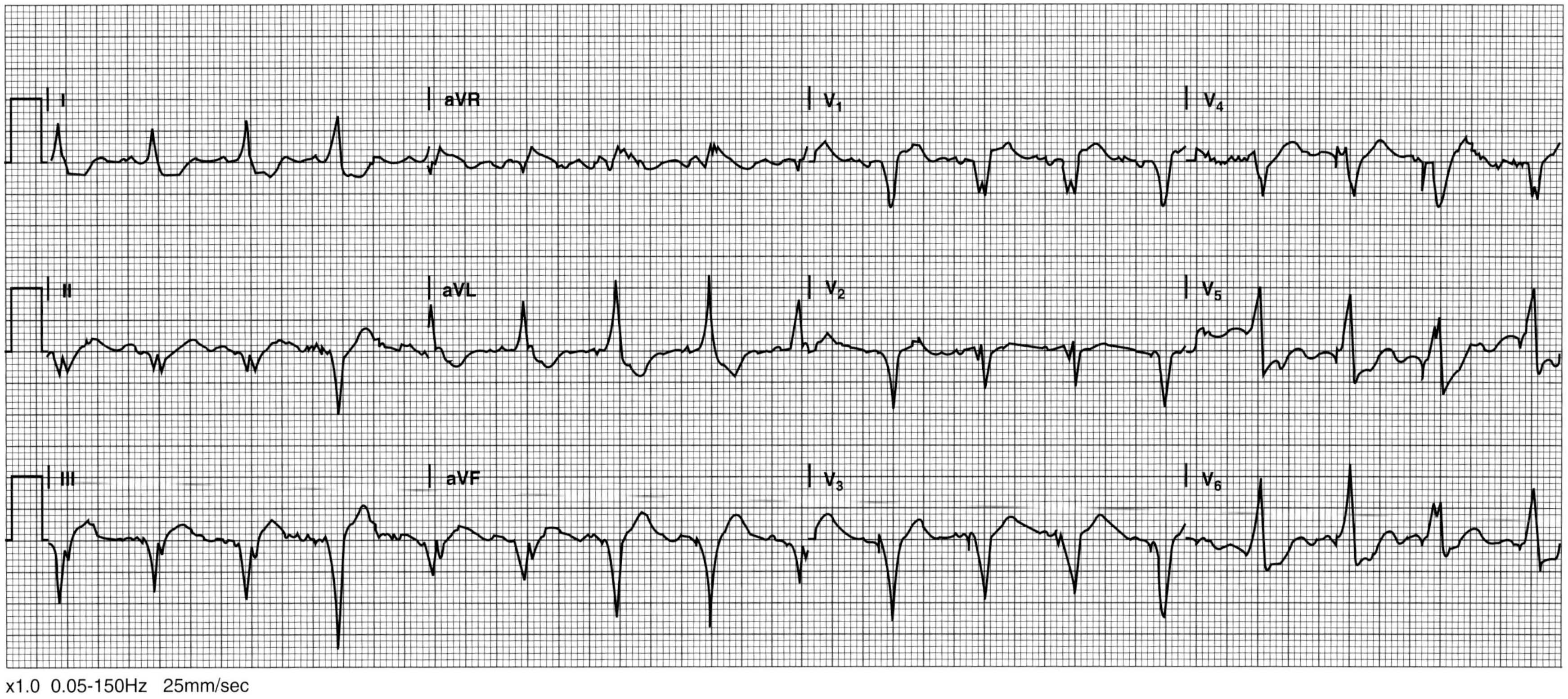

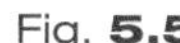
Fig. 5.5

x1.0 0.05-150Hz 25mm/sec

Rate and rhythm? ______________________ Pathologic Q waves? ______________________

STE? ______________________ ST depression? ______________________ T-wave changes? ______________________

Reciprocal changes? ______________________ Imposter present? ______________________ Axis? ______________________

Interpretation: ______________________

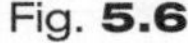

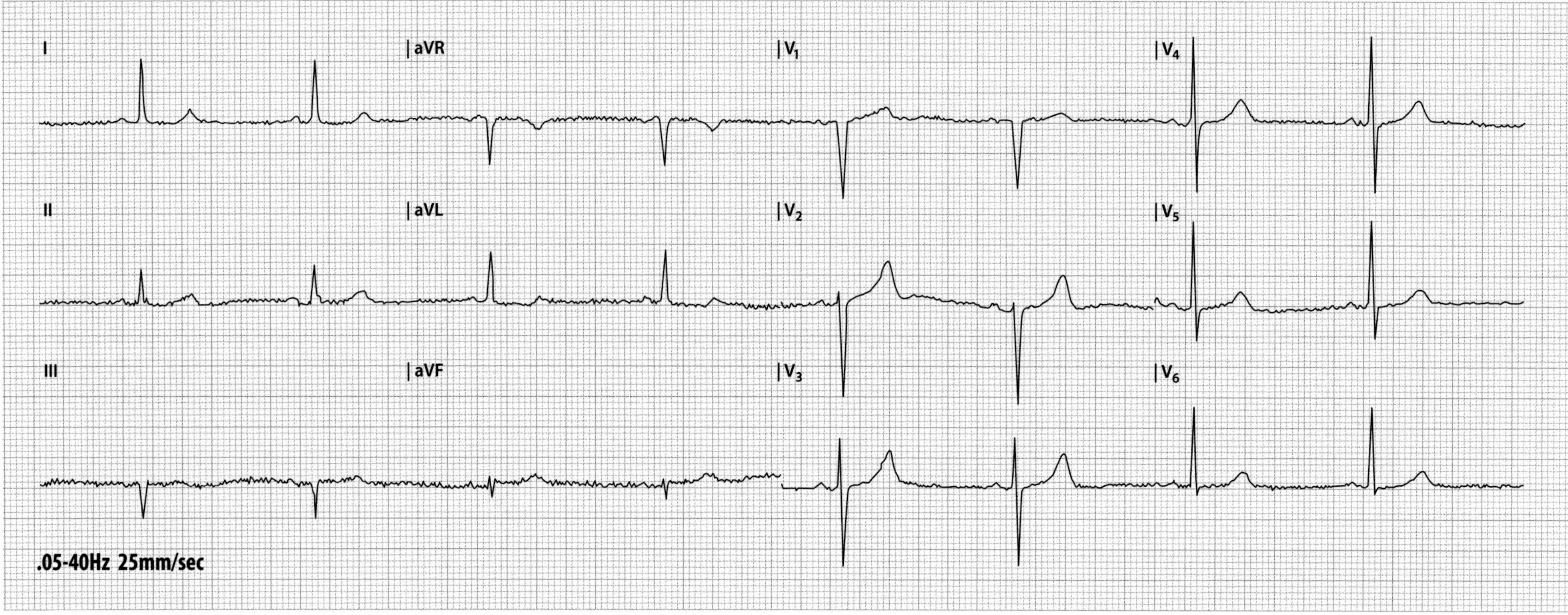

Fig. 5.6

Rate and rhythm? ______ Pathologic Q waves? ______

STE? ______ ST depression? ______ T-wave changes? ______

Reciprocal changes? ______ Imposter present? ______ Axis? ______

Interpretation: ______

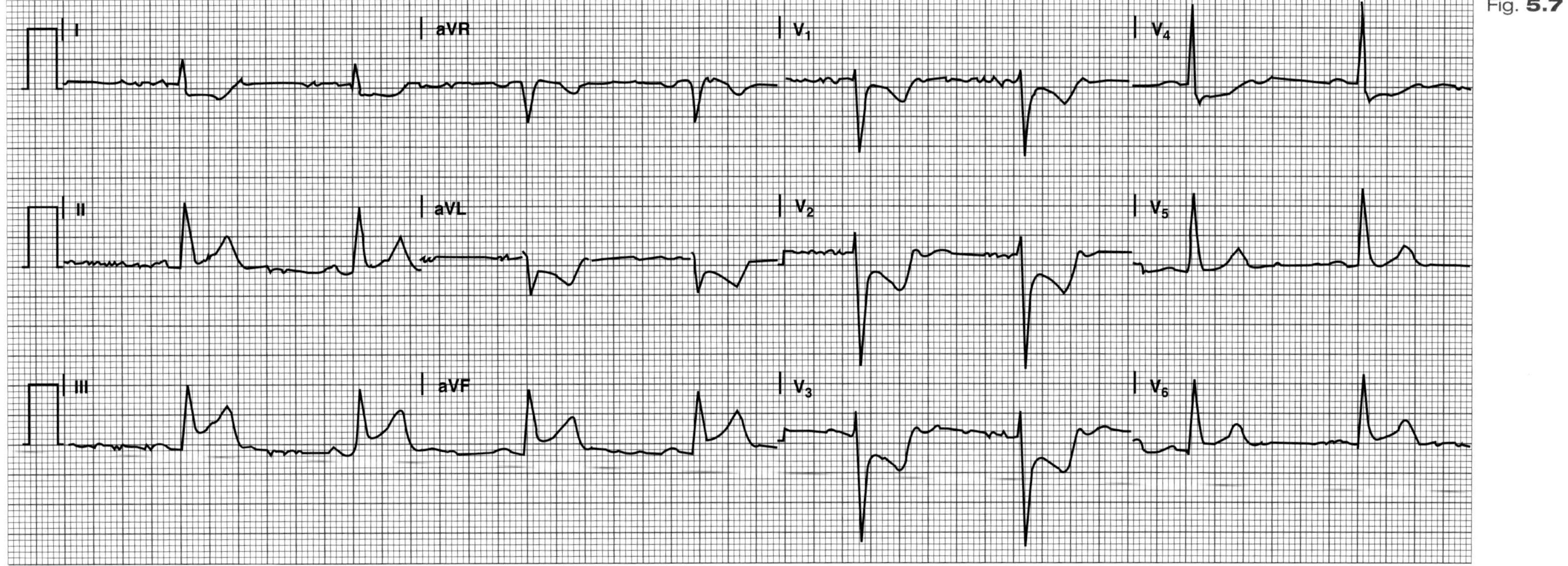

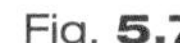
Fig. **5.7**

Rate and rhythm? ______________________ Pathologic Q waves? ______________________

STE? ______________________ ST depression? ______________________ T-wave changes? ______________________

Reciprocal changes? ______________________ Imposter present? ______________________ Axis? ______________________

Interpretation: ____

Inferior: II, III, aVF | **Septum: V_1, V_2** | **Anterior: V_3, V_4** | **Lateral: I, aVL, V_5, V_6**

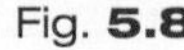

Fig. **5.8**

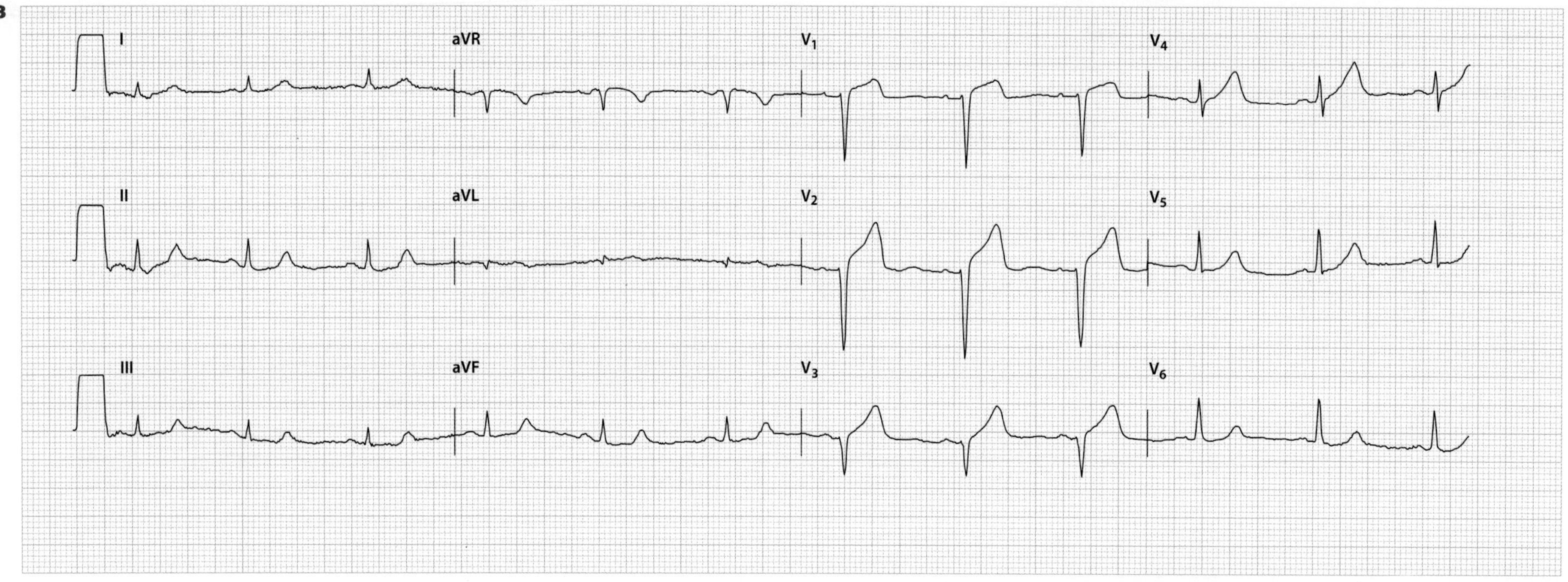

Rate and rhythm? ______________________ Pathologic Q waves? ______________________

STE? ______________________ ST depression? ______________________ T-wave changes? ______________________

Reciprocal changes? ______________________ Imposter present? ______________________ Axis? ______________________

Interpretation: ______________________

Inferior: II, III, aVF | Septum: V_1, V_2 | Anterior: V_3, V_4 | Lateral: I, aVL, V_5, V_6

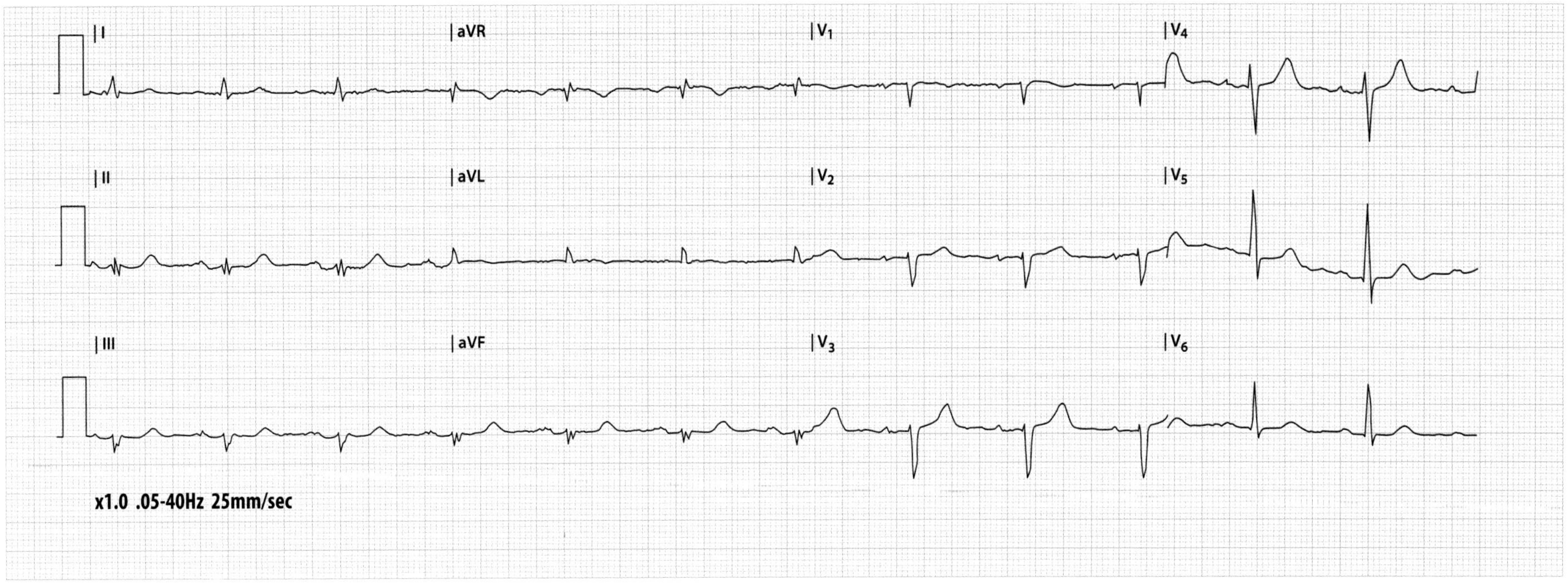

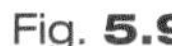

Fig. **5.9**

I | aVR | V1 | V4

II | aVL | V2 | V5

III | aVF | V3 | V6

x1.0 .05-40Hz 25mm/sec

Rate and rhythm? ______ Pathologic Q waves? ______

STE? ______ ST depression? ______ T-wave changes? ______

Reciprocal changes? ______ Imposter present? ______ Axis? ______

Interpretation: ______

Inferior: II, III, aVF | **Septum: V_1, V_2** | Anterior: V_3, V_4 | **Lateral: I, aVL, V_5, V_6**

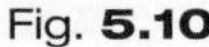

Fig. **5.10**

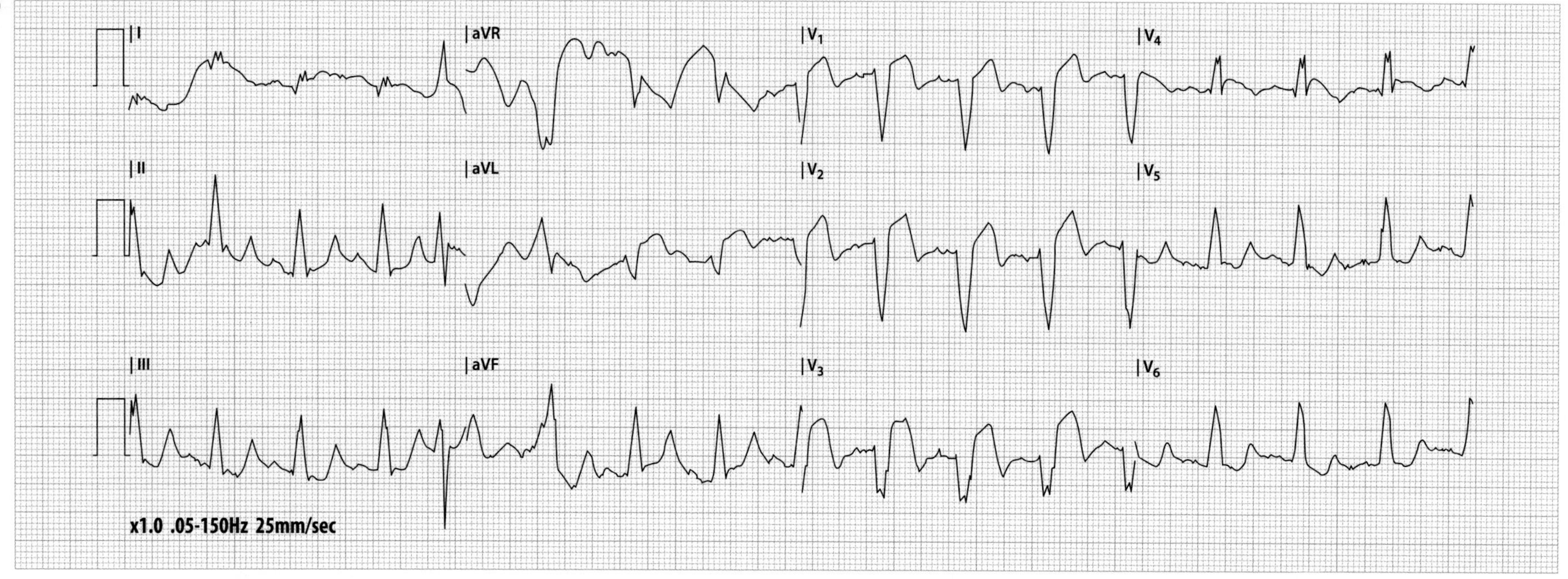

Rate and rhythm? ______ Pathologic Q waves? ______

STE? ______ ST depression? ______ T-wave changes? ______

Reciprocal changes? ______ Imposter present? ______ Axis? ______

Interpretation: ______

Inferior: II, III, aVF | **Septum: V_1, V_2** | Anterior: V_3, V_4 | **Lateral: I, aVL, V_5, V_6**

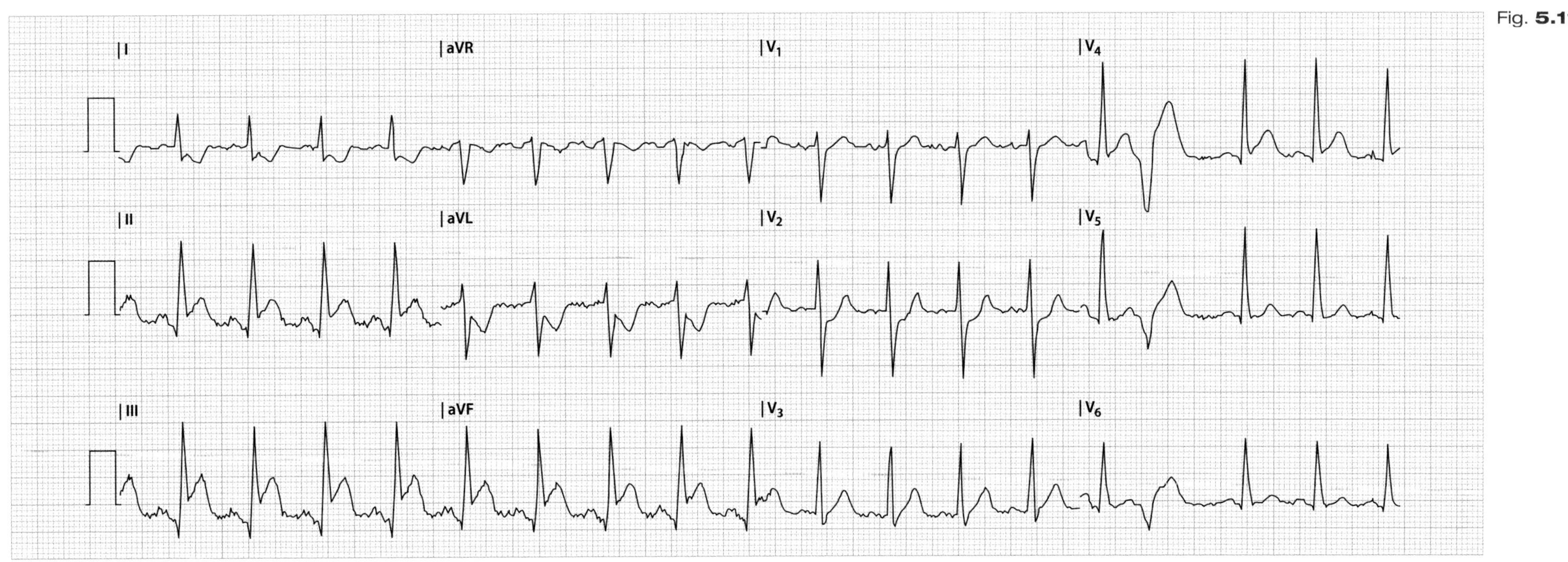

Fig. **5.11**

Rate and rhythm? ______ Pathologic Q waves? ______

STE? ______ ST depression? ______ T-wave changes? ______

Reciprocal changes? ______ Imposter present? ______ Axis? ______

Interpretation: ______

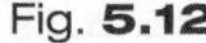

Fig. 5.12

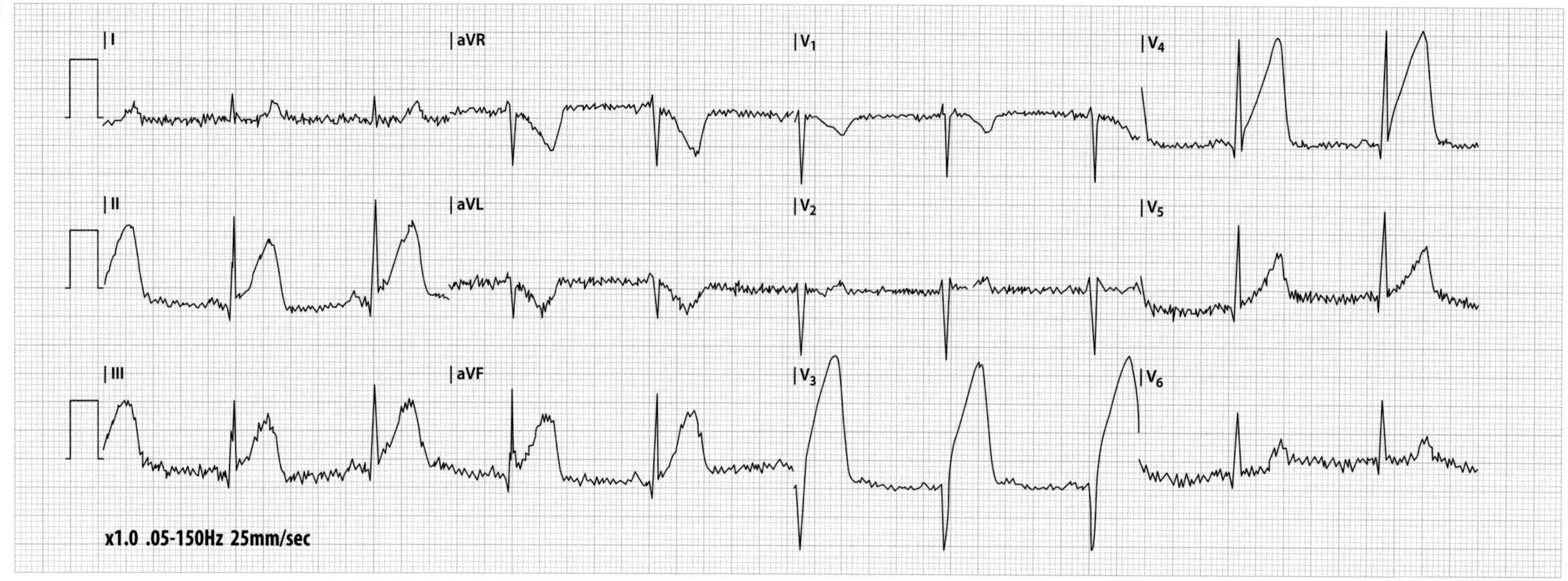

Rate and rhythm? ______________________ Pathologic Q waves? ______________________

STE? ______________________ ST depression? ______________________ T-wave changes? ______________________

Reciprocal changes? ______________________ Imposter present? ______________________ Axis? ______________________

Interpretation: ______________________

Inferior: II, III, aVF | **Septum: V_1, V_2** | **Anterior: V_3, V_4** | **Lateral: I, aVL, V_5, V_6**

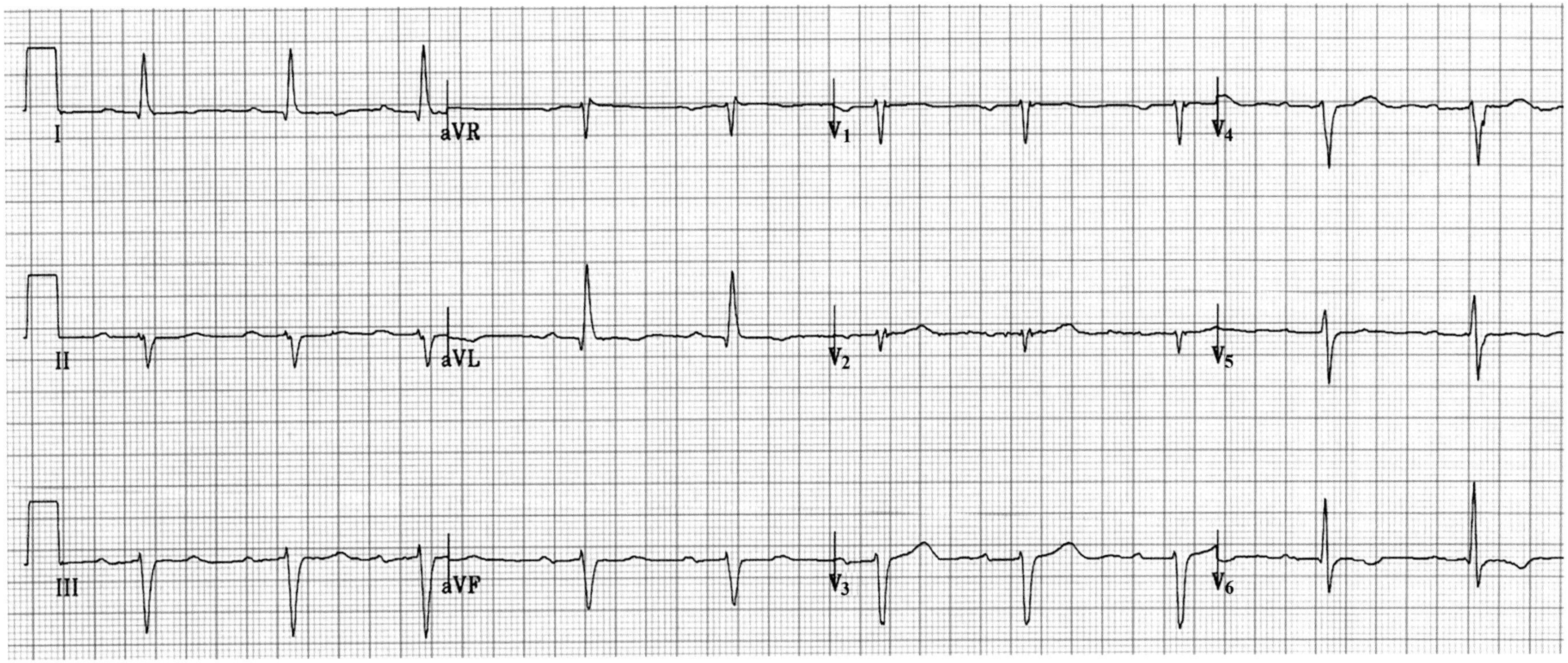

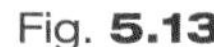

Fig. **5.13**

Rate and rhythm? __________ Pathologic Q waves? __________

STE? __________ ST depression? __________ T-wave changes? __________

Reciprocal changes? __________ Imposter present? __________ Axis? __________

Interpretation: __________

Inferior: II, III, aVF | **Septum: V_1, V_2** | **Anterior: V_3, V_4** | **Lateral: I, aVL, V_5, V_6**

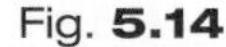

Fig. **5.14**

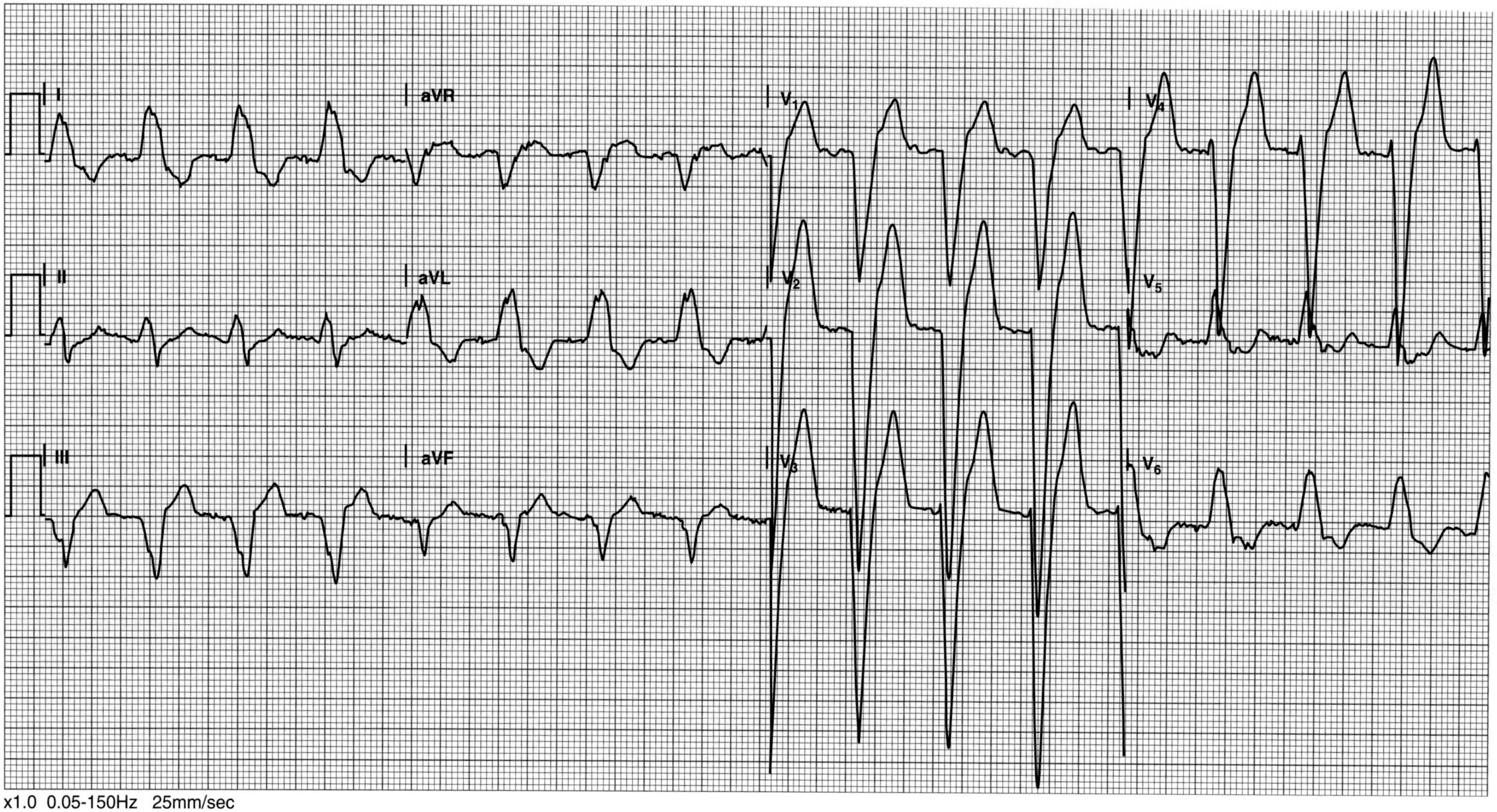

I aVR V_1 V_4

II aVL V_2 V_5

III aVF V_3 V_6

x1.0 0.05-150Hz 25mm/sec

Rate and rhythm? ______________________ Pathologic Q waves? ______________________

STE? ______________________ ST depression? ______________________ T-wave changes? ______________________

Reciprocal changes? ______________________ Imposter present? ______________________ Axis? ______________________

Interpretation: ____

Inferior: II, III, aVF | **Septum: V_1, V_2** | Anterior: V_3, V_4 | **Lateral: I, aVL, V_5, V_6**

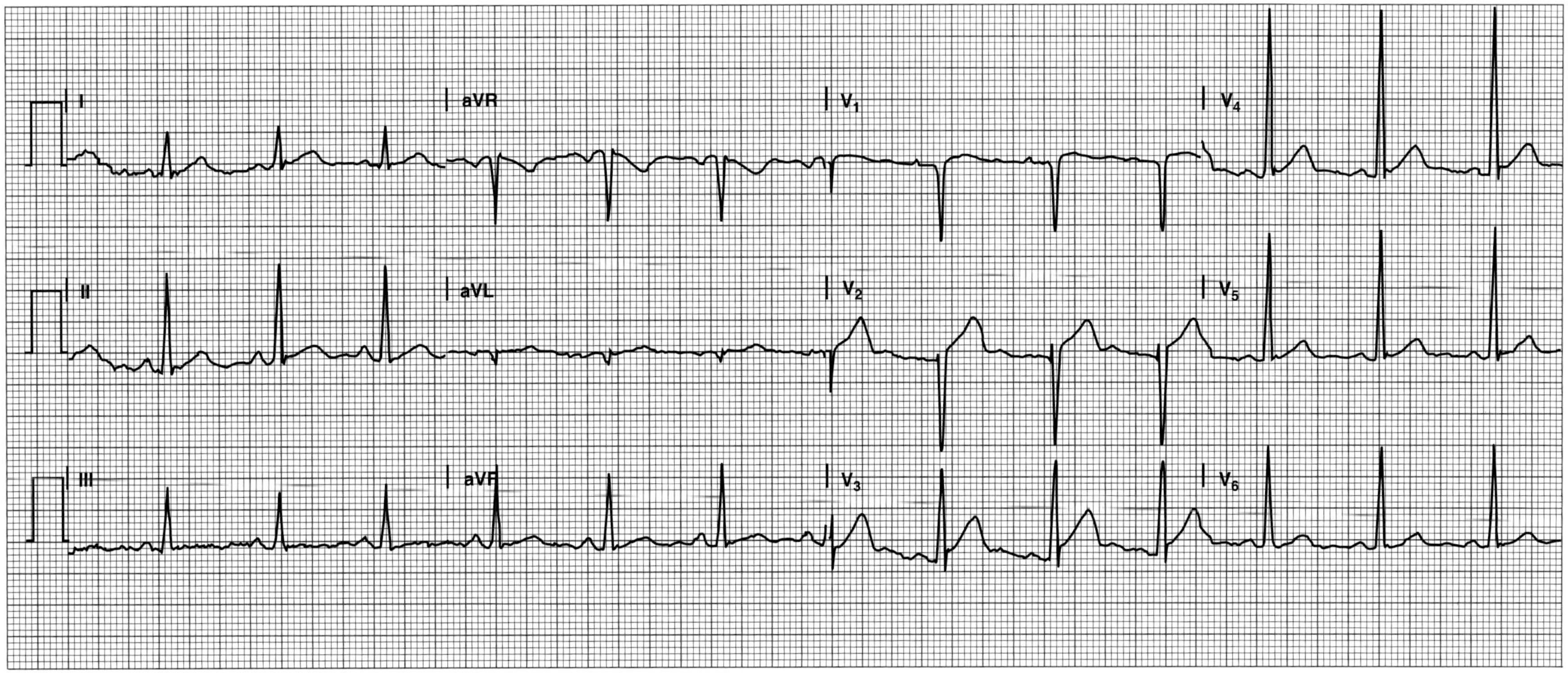

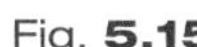

Fig. 5.15

x1.0 0.05-150Hz 25mm/sec

Rate and rhythm? ______ Pathologic Q waves? ______

STE? ______ ST depression? ______ T-wave changes? ______

Reciprocal changes? ______ Imposter present? ______ Axis? ______

Interpretation: ______

Fig. **5.16**

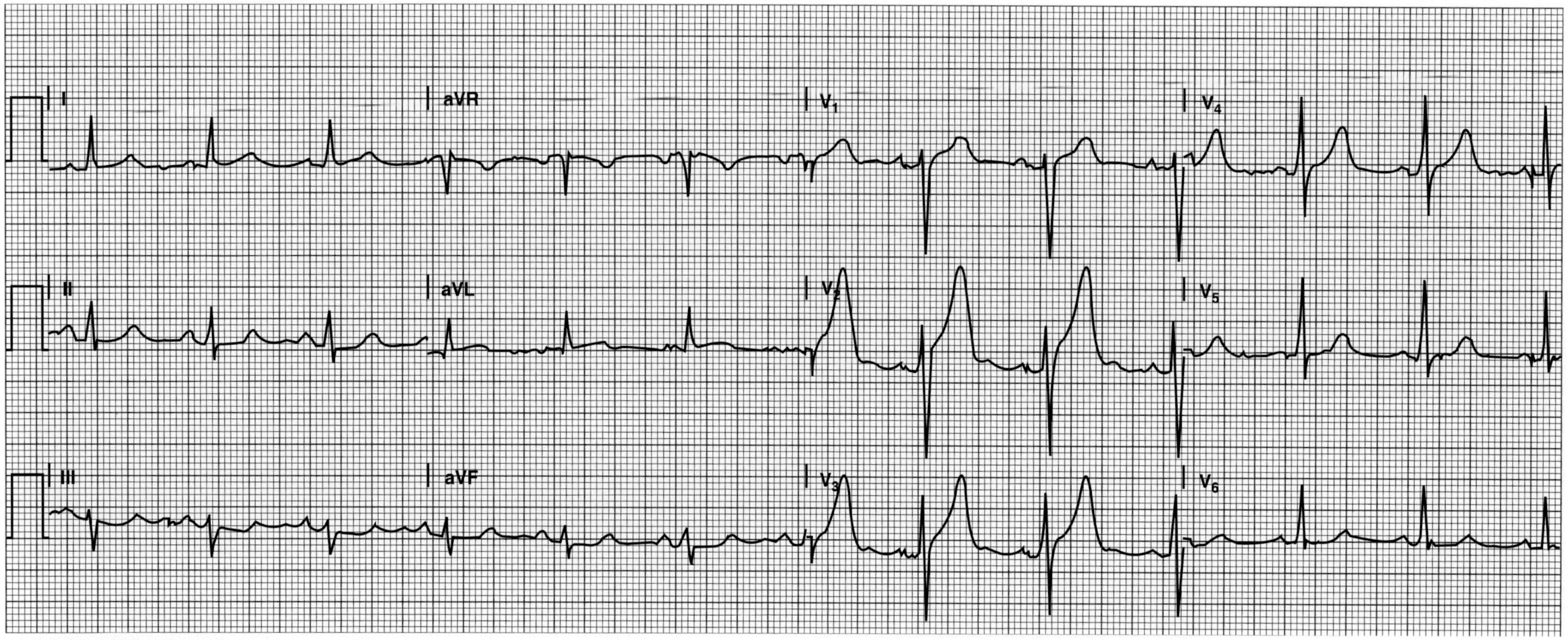

x1.0 0.05-150Hz 25mm/sec

Rate and rhythm? ______________________ Pathologic Q waves? ______________________

STE? ______________________ ST depression? ______________________ T-wave changes? ______________________

Reciprocal changes? ______________________ Imposter present? ______________________ Axis? ______________________

Interpretation: ______________________

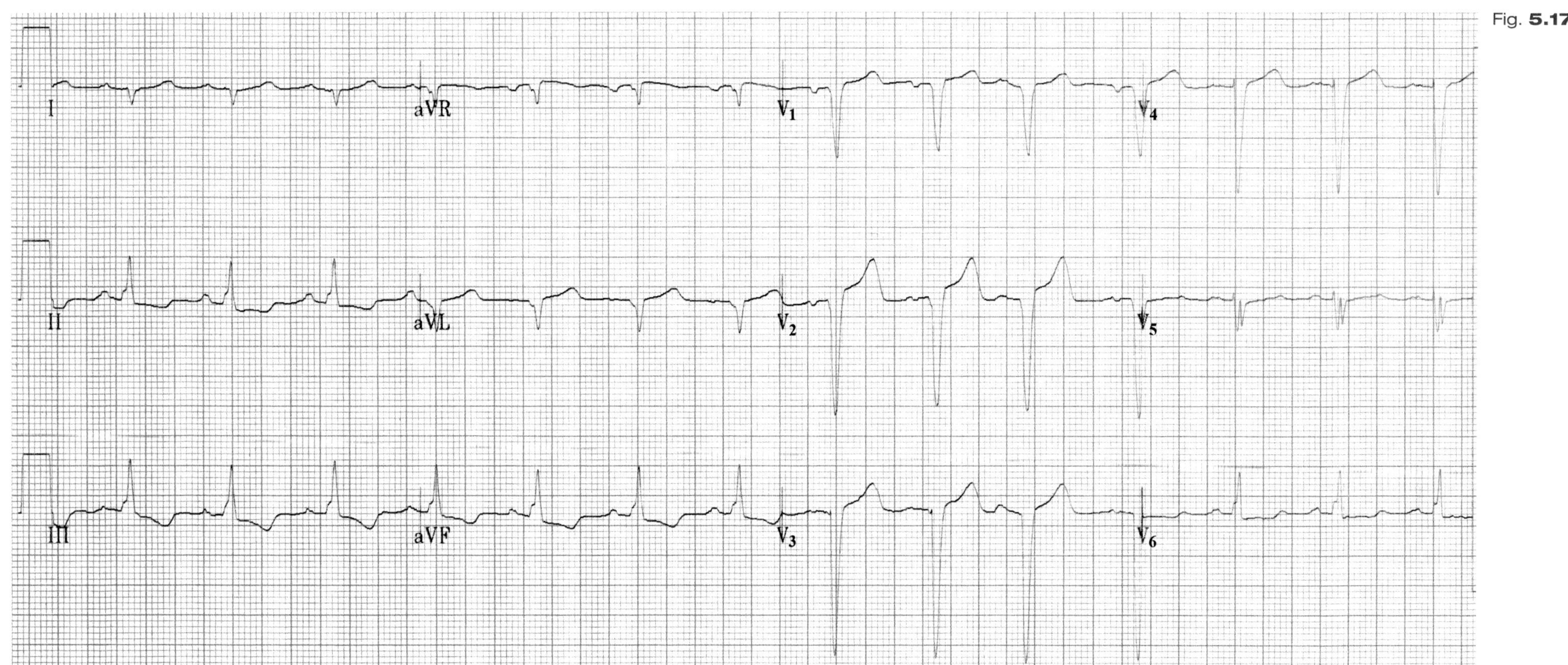

Fig. 5.17

Rate and rhythm? ____________________ Pathologic Q waves? ____________________

STE? ____________________ ST depression? ____________________ T-wave changes? ____________________

Reciprocal changes? ____________________ Imposter present? ____________________ Axis? ____________________

Interpretation: ____

Inferior: II, III, aVF | **Septum: V_1, V_2** | Anterior: V_3, V_4 | **Lateral: I, aVL, V_5, V_6**

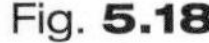

Fig. 5.18

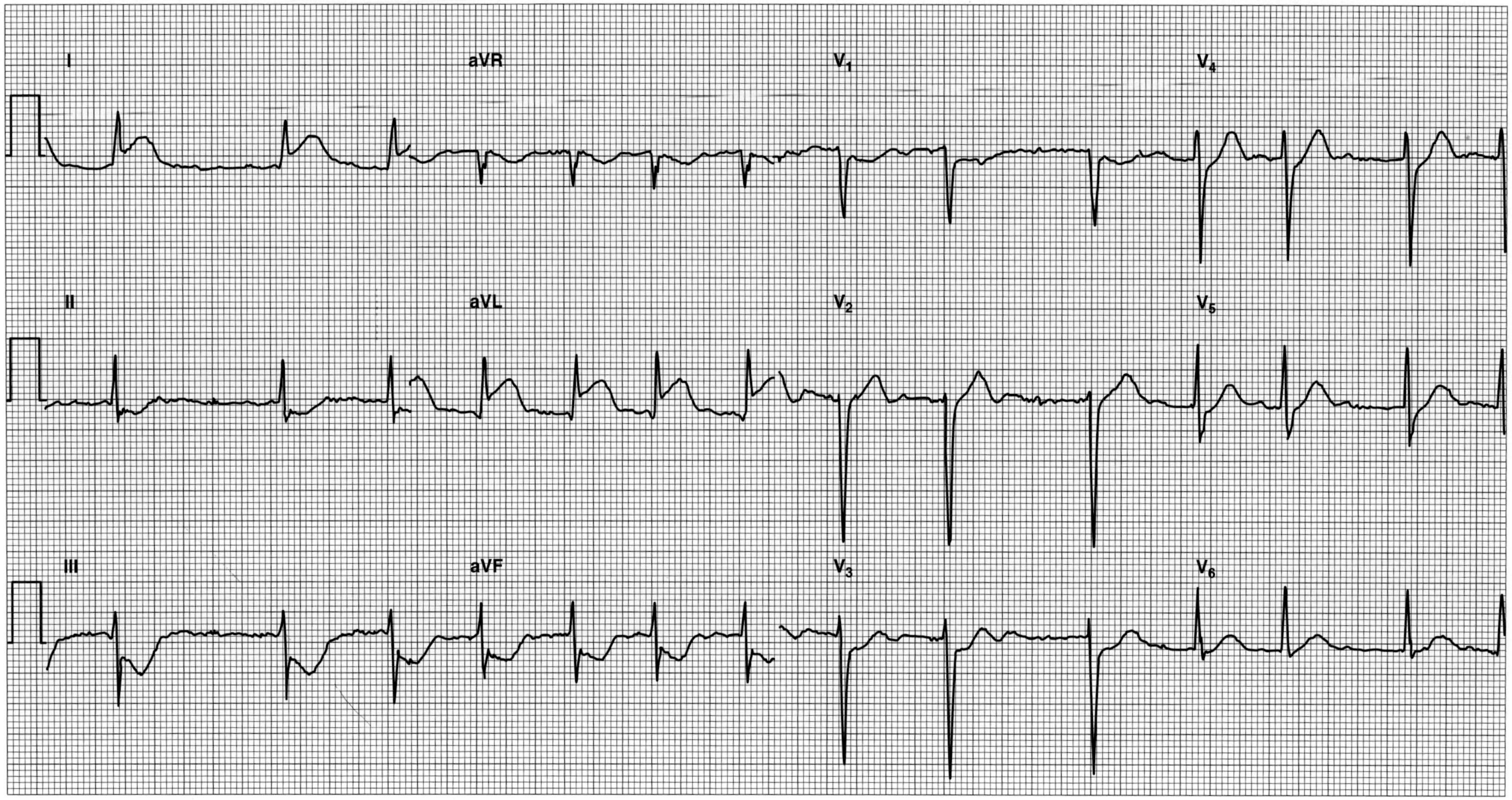

Rate and rhythm? ______________________ Pathologic Q waves? ______________________

STE? ______________________ ST depression? ______________________ T-wave changes? ______________________

Reciprocal changes? ______________________ Imposter present? ______________________ Axis? ______________________

Interpretation: ______________________

Inferior: II, III, aVF | **Septum: V_1, V_2** | **Anterior: V_3, V_4** | **Lateral: I, aVL, V_5, V_6**

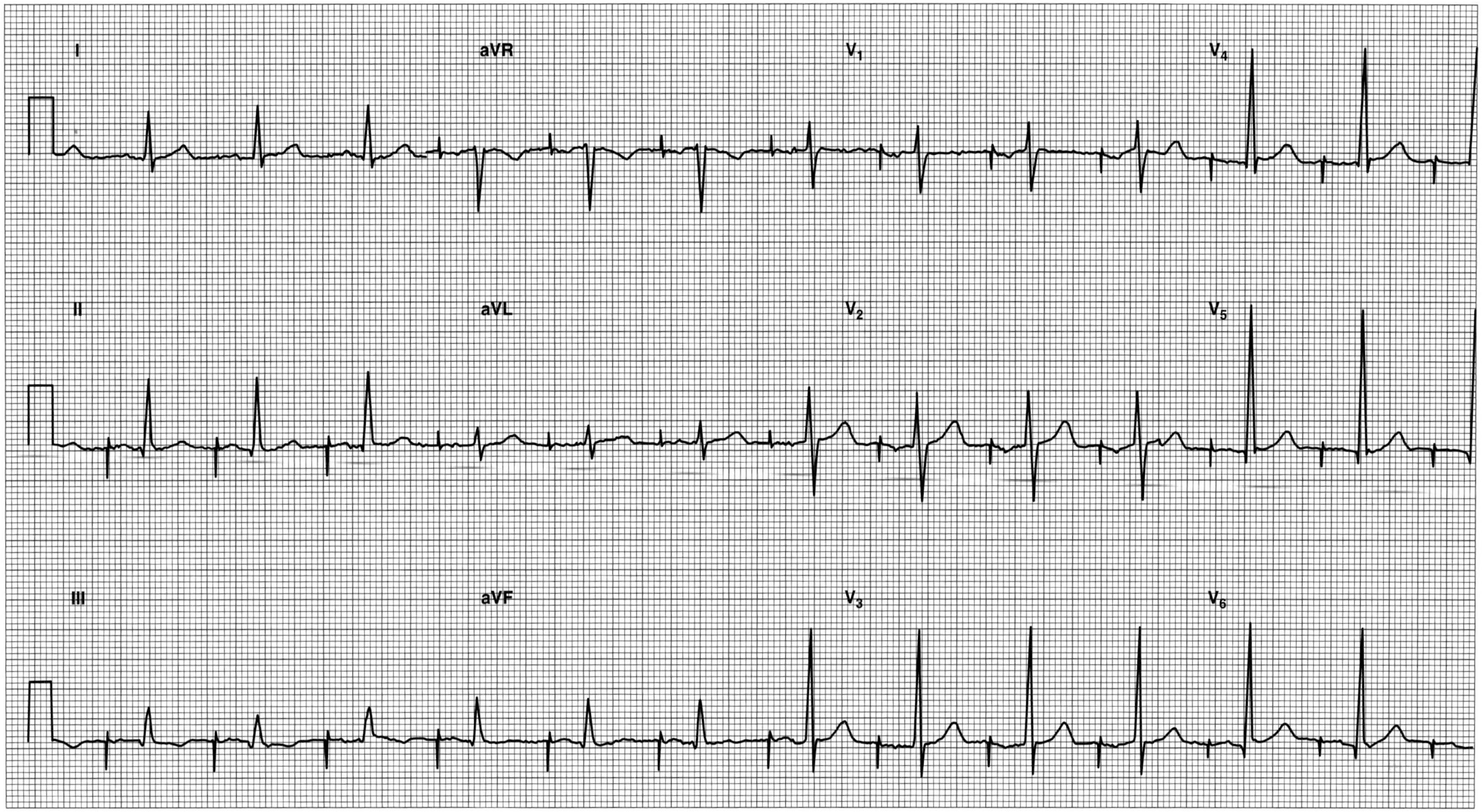

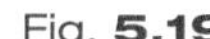

Fig. 5.19

Rate and rhythm? ______________________ Pathologic Q waves? ______________________

STE? ______________________ ST depression? ______________________ T-wave changes? ______________________

Reciprocal changes? ______________________ Imposter present? ______________________ Axis? ______________________

Interpretation: ______________________

Inferior: II, III, aVF | **Septum: V_1, V_2** | Anterior: V_3, V_4 | **Lateral: I, aVL, V_5, V_6**

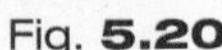
Fig. 5.20

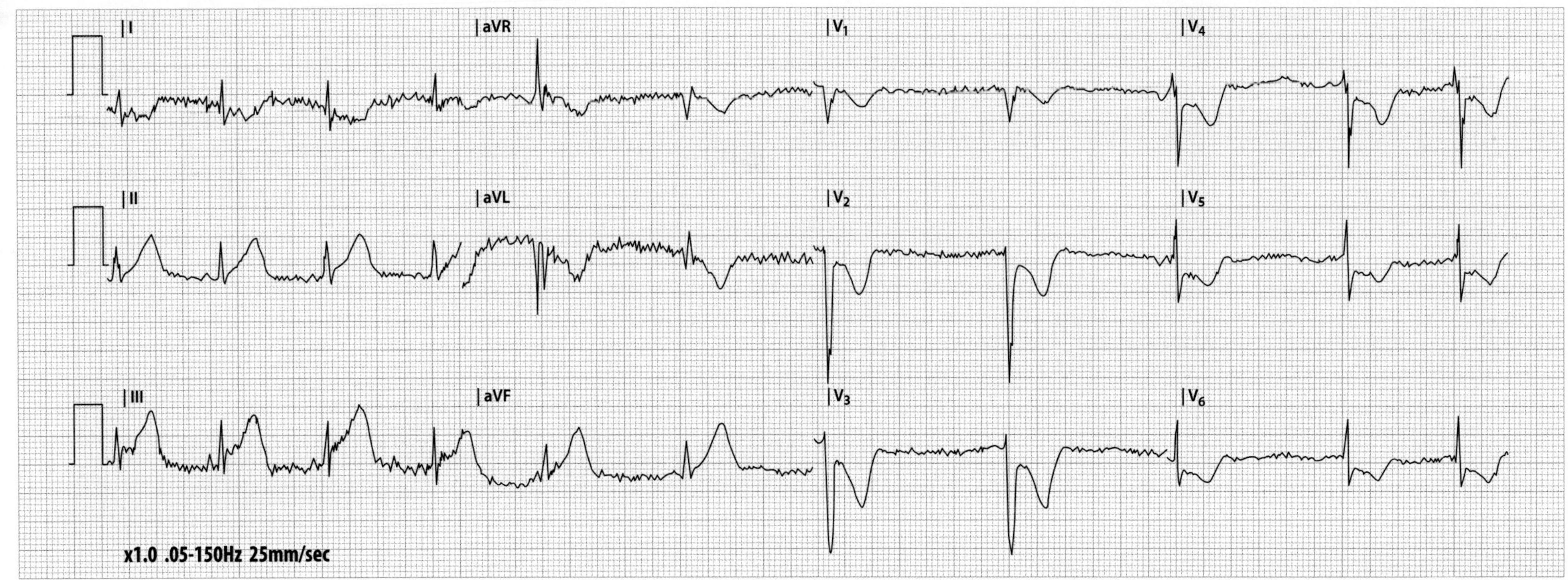

Rate and rhythm? ______ Pathologic Q waves? ______

STE? ______ ST depression? ______ T-wave changes? ______

Reciprocal changes? ______ Imposter present? ______ Axis? ______

Interpretation: ______

Inferior: II, III, aVF | **Septum: V_1, V_2** | **Anterior: V_3, V_4** | **Lateral: I, aVL, V_5, V_6**

Fig. **5.21**

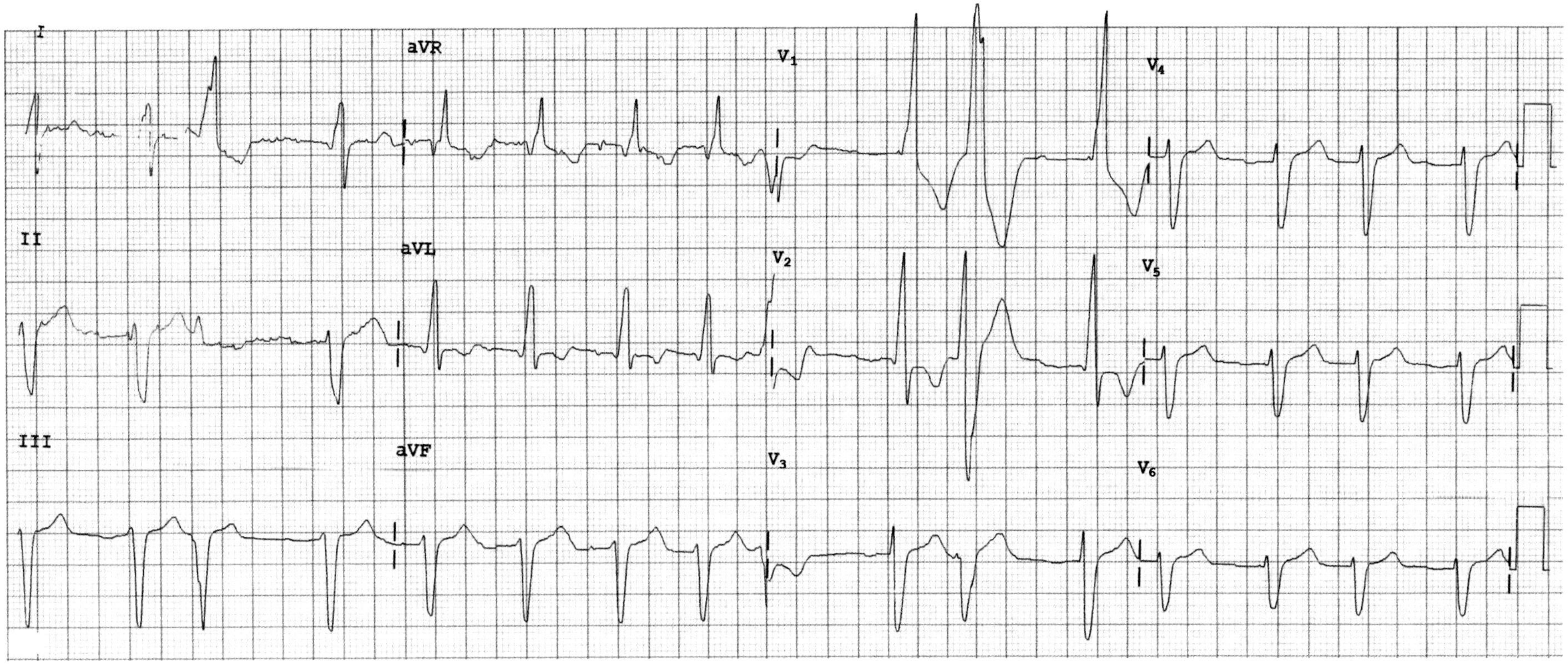

Rate and rhythm? ______________________ Pathologic Q waves? ______________________

STE? ______________________ ST depression? ______________________ T-wave changes? ______________________

Reciprocal changes? ______________________ Imposter present? ______________________ Axis? ______________________

Interpretation: ____

Inferior: II, III, aVF | **Septum: V_1, V_2** | Anterior: V_3, V_4 | **Lateral: I, aVL, V_5, V_6**

Fig. **5.22**

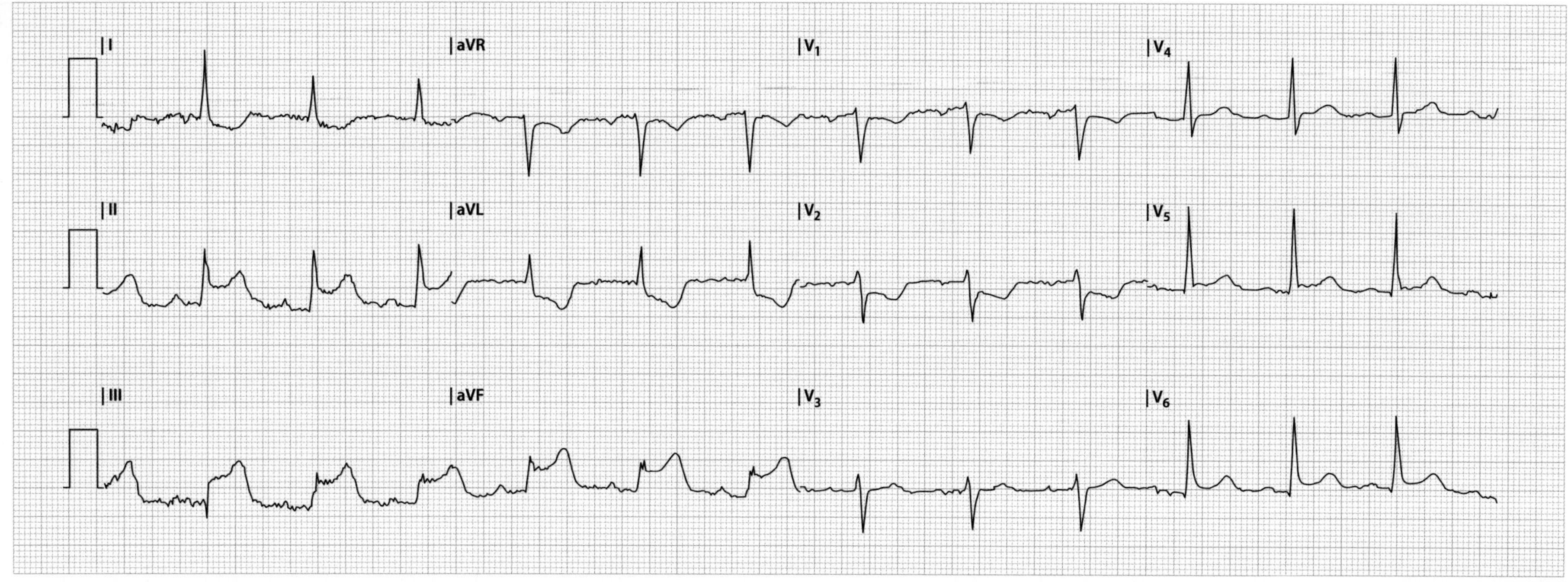

Rate and rhythm? ____________ Pathologic Q waves? ____________

STE? ____________ ST depression? ____________ T-wave changes? ____________

Reciprocal changes? ____________ Imposter present? ____________ Axis? ____________

Interpretation: ____________

Inferior: II, III, aVF | **Septum: V_1, V_2** | **Anterior: V_3, V_4** | **Lateral: I, aVL, V_5, V_6**

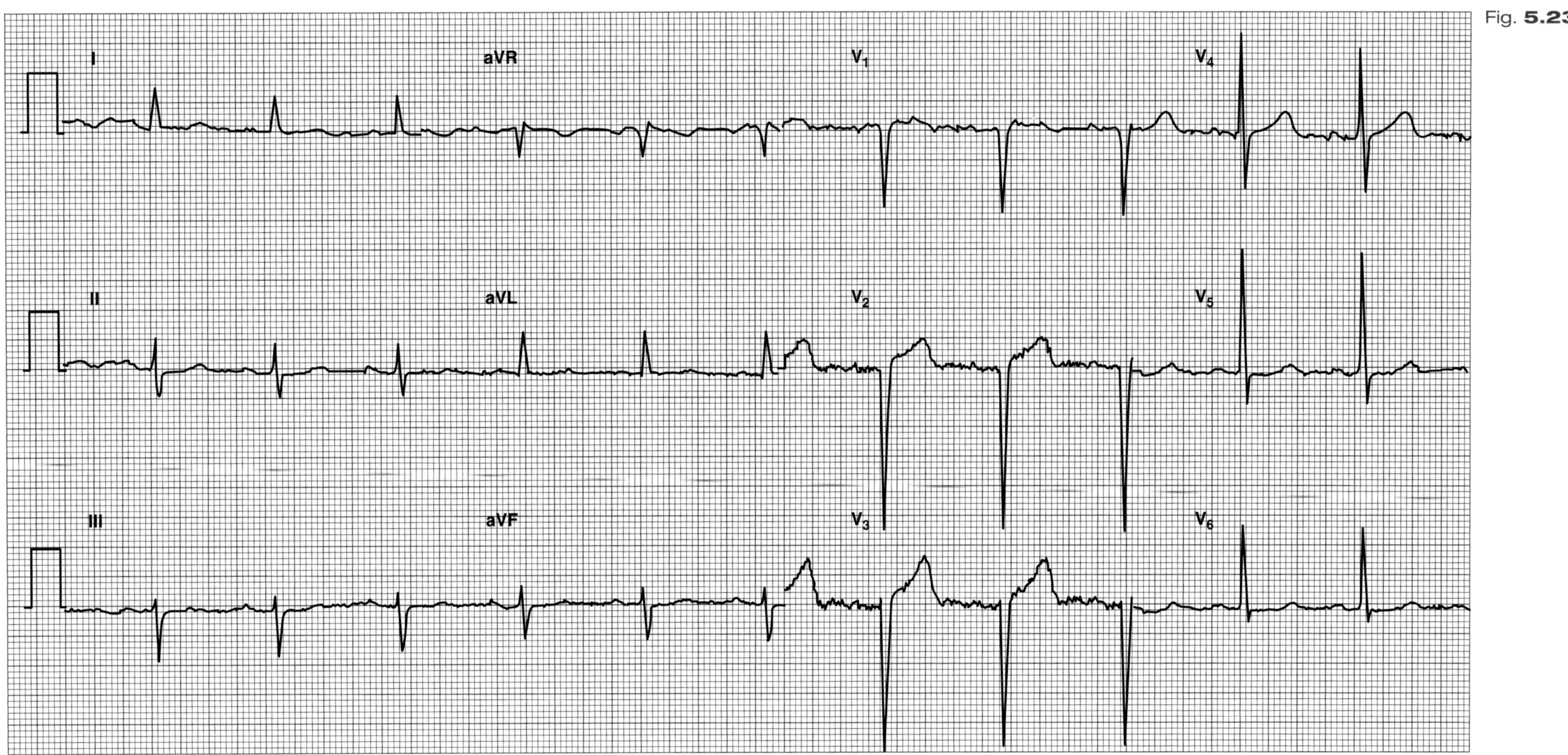

Fig. 5.23

Rate and rhythm? ______ Pathologic Q waves? ______

STE? ______ ST depression? ______ T-wave changes? ______

Reciprocal changes? ______ Imposter present? ______ Axis? ______

Interpretation: ______

Inferior: II, III, aVF | **Septum: V_1, V_2** | **Anterior: V_3, V_4** | **Lateral: I, aVL, V_5, V_6**

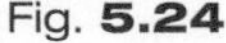
Fig. **5.24**

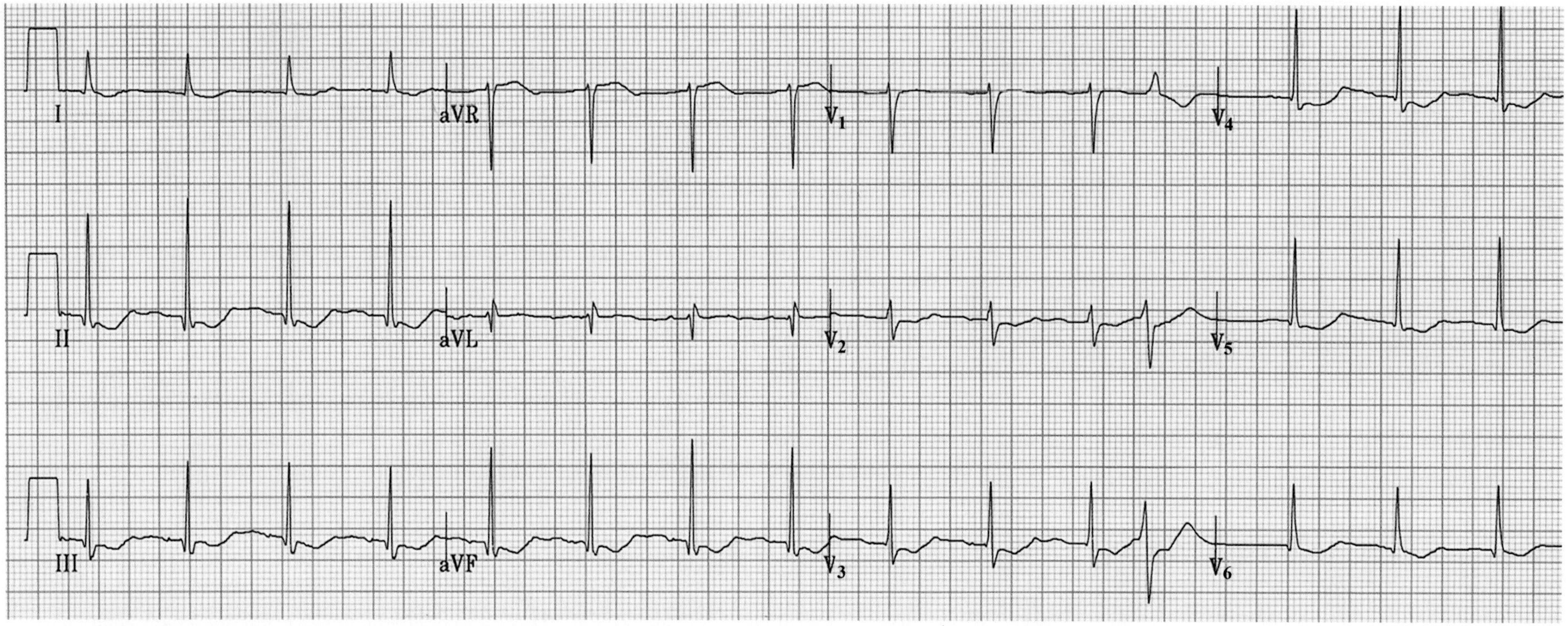

Rate and rhythm? ______________________ Pathologic Q waves? ______________________

STE? ______________________ ST depression? ______________________ T-wave changes? ______________________

Reciprocal changes? ______________________ Imposter present? ______________________ Axis? ______________________

Interpretation: ______________________

Inferior: II, III, aVF | **Septum: V_1, V_2** | **Anterior: V_3, V_4** | **Lateral: I, aVL, V_5, V_6**

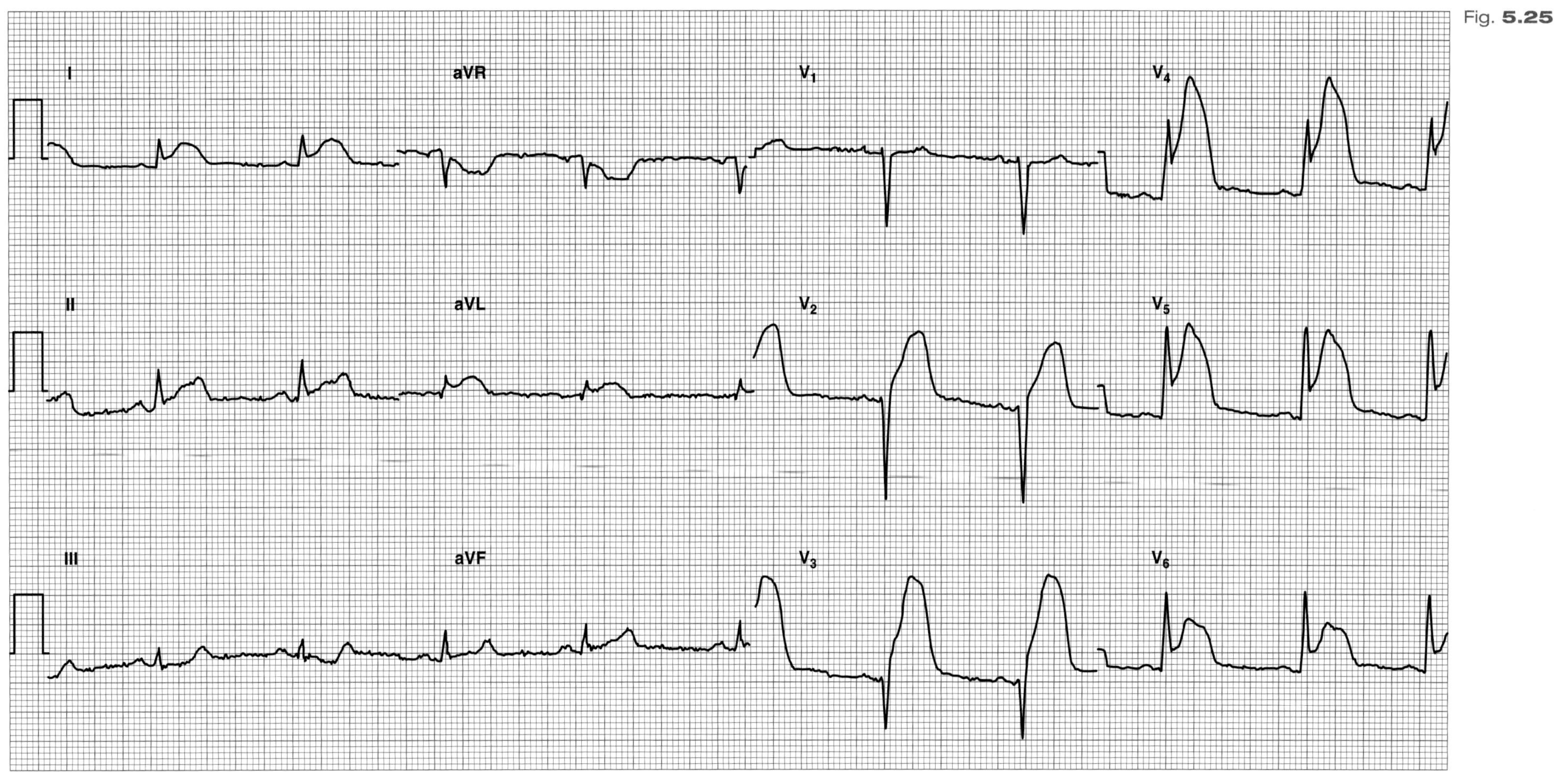

Fig. 5.25

Rate and rhythm? ______ Pathologic Q waves? ______

STE? ______ ST depression? ______ T-wave changes? ______

Reciprocal changes? ______ Imposter present? ______ Axis? ______

Interpretation: ______

Inferior: II, III, aVF | **Septum: V_1, V_2** | **Anterior: V_3, V_4** | **Lateral: I, aVL, V_5, V_6**

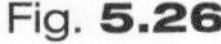

Fig. **5.26**

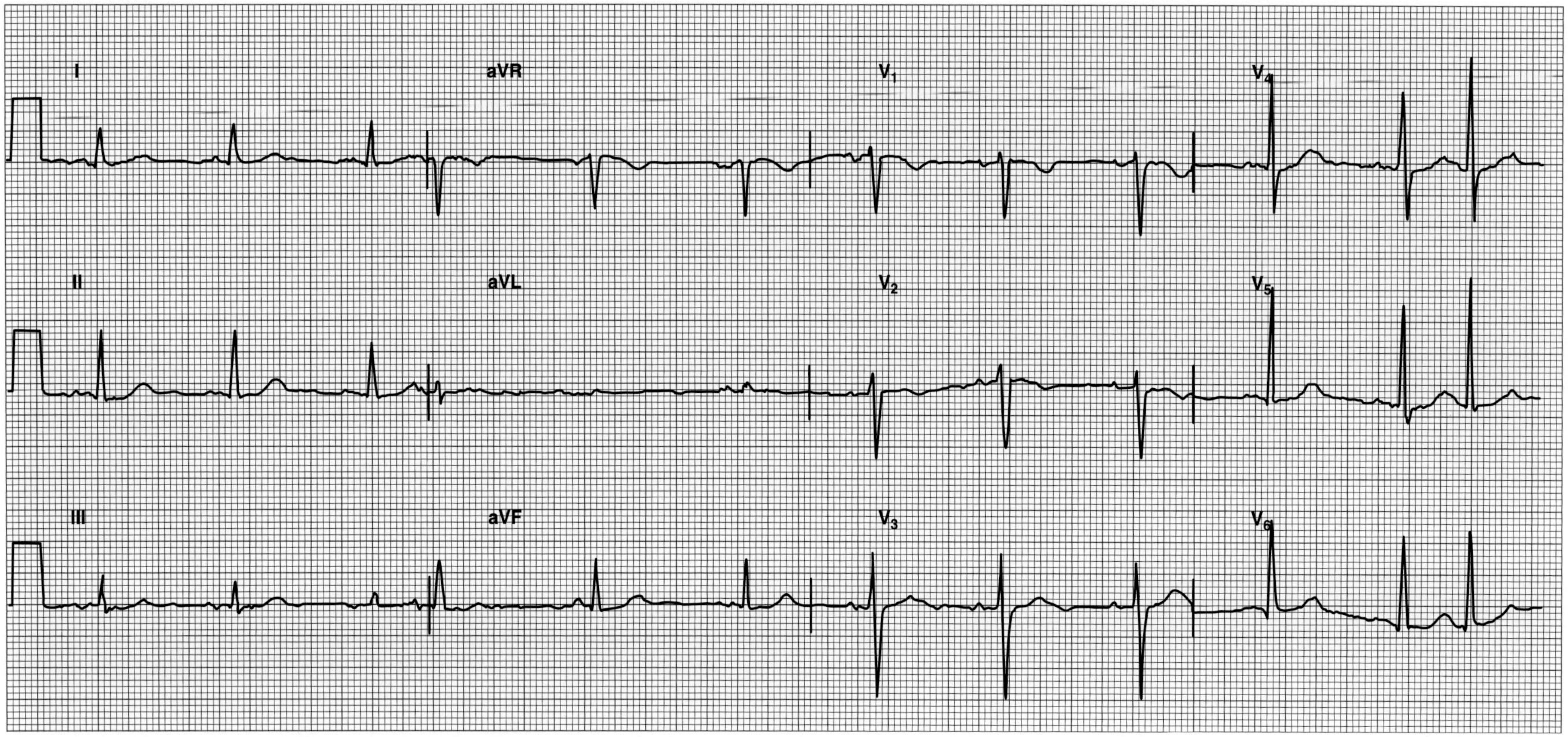

Rate and rhythm? ______ Pathologic Q waves? ______

STE? ______ ST depression? ______ T-wave changes? ______

Reciprocal changes? ______ Imposter present? ______ Axis? ______

Interpretation: ______

Inferior: II, III, aVF | **Septum: V_1, V_2** | **Anterior: V_3, V_4** | **Lateral: I, aVL, V_5, V_6**

Fig. **5.27**

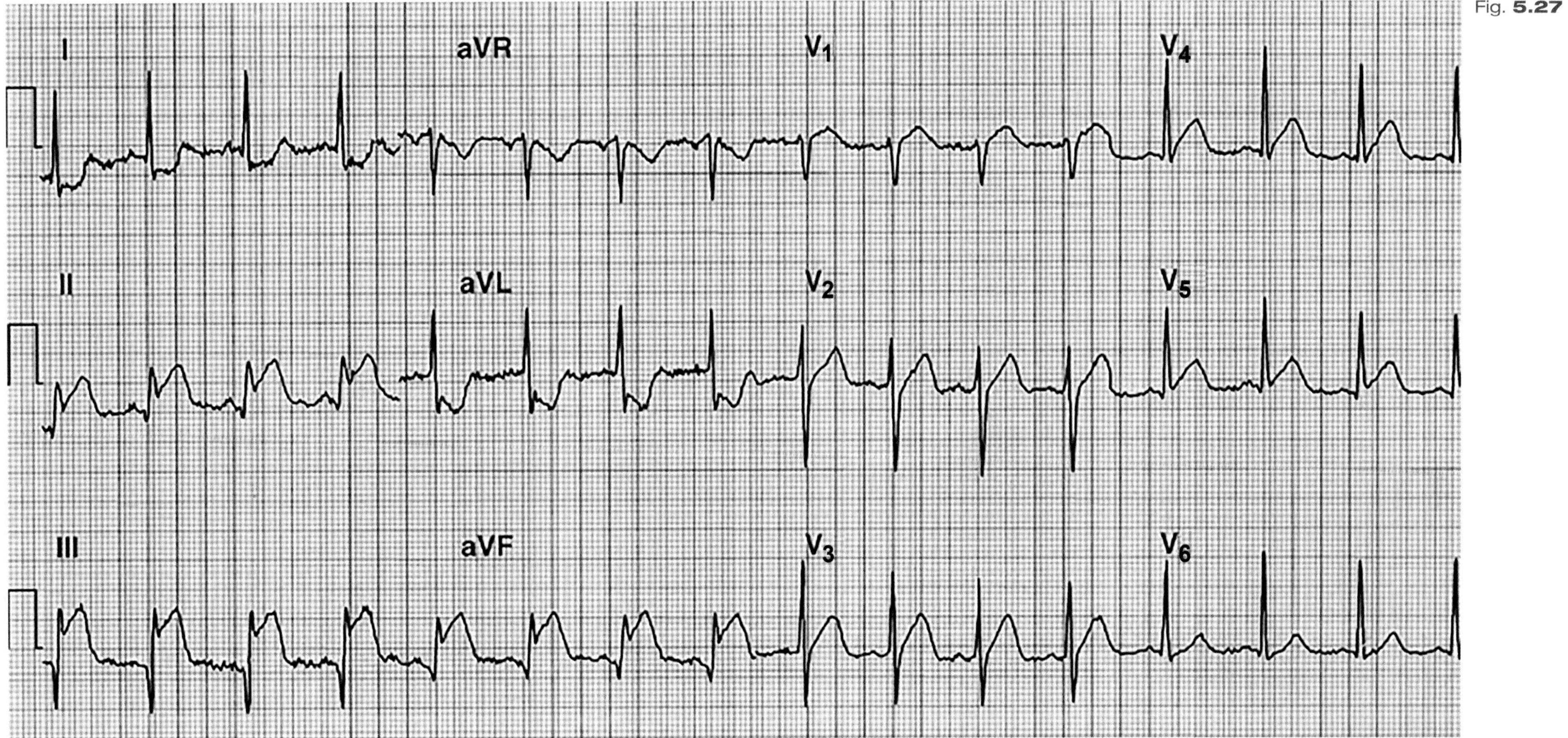

Rate and rhythm? ______ Pathologic Q waves? ______

STE? ______ ST depression? ______ T-wave changes? ______

Reciprocal changes? ______ Imposter present? ______ Axis? ______

Interpretation: ______

Inferior: II, III, aVF | **Septum: V_1, V_2** | **Anterior: V_3, V_4** | **Lateral: I, aVL, V_5, V_6**

Fig. **5.28**

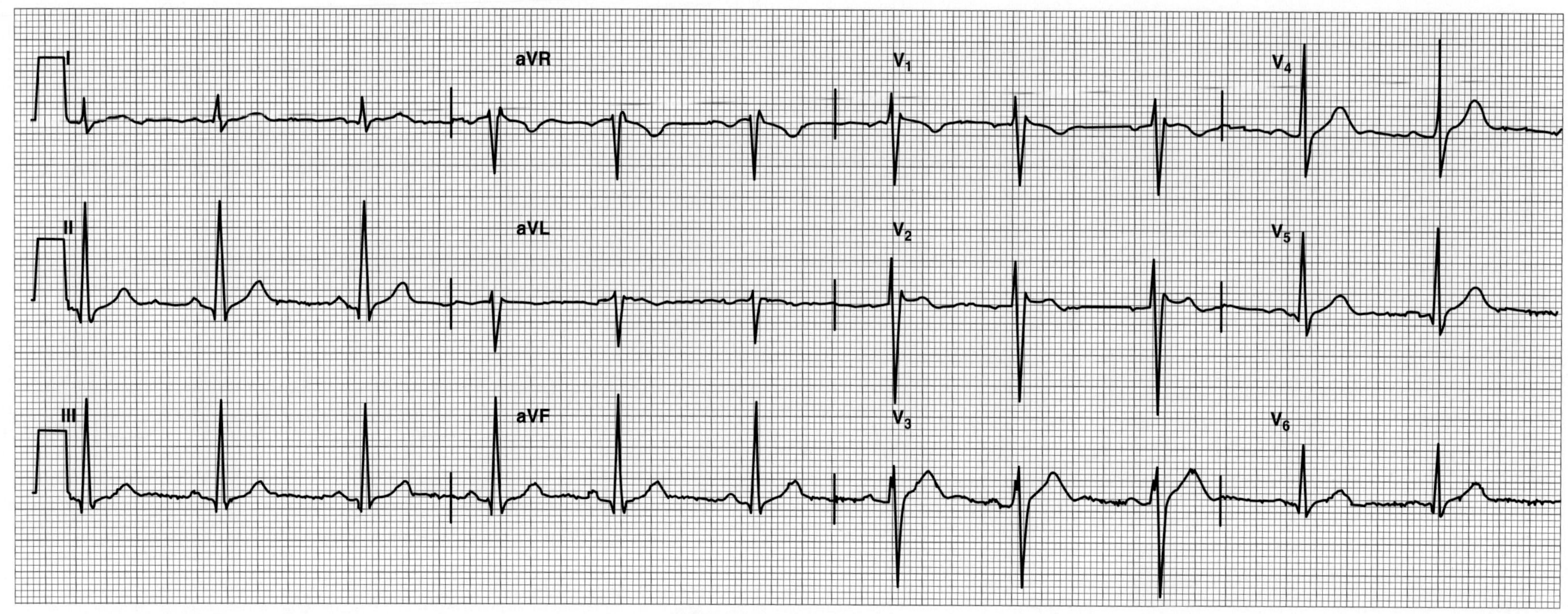

Rate and rhythm? ______ Pathologic Q waves? ______

STE? ______ ST depression? ______ T-wave changes? ______

Reciprocal changes? ______ Imposter present? ______ Axis? ______

Interpretation: ______

Inferior: II, III, aVF | Septum: V_1, V_2 | Anterior: V_3, V_4 | Lateral: I, aVL, V_5, V_6

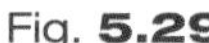
Fig. 5.29

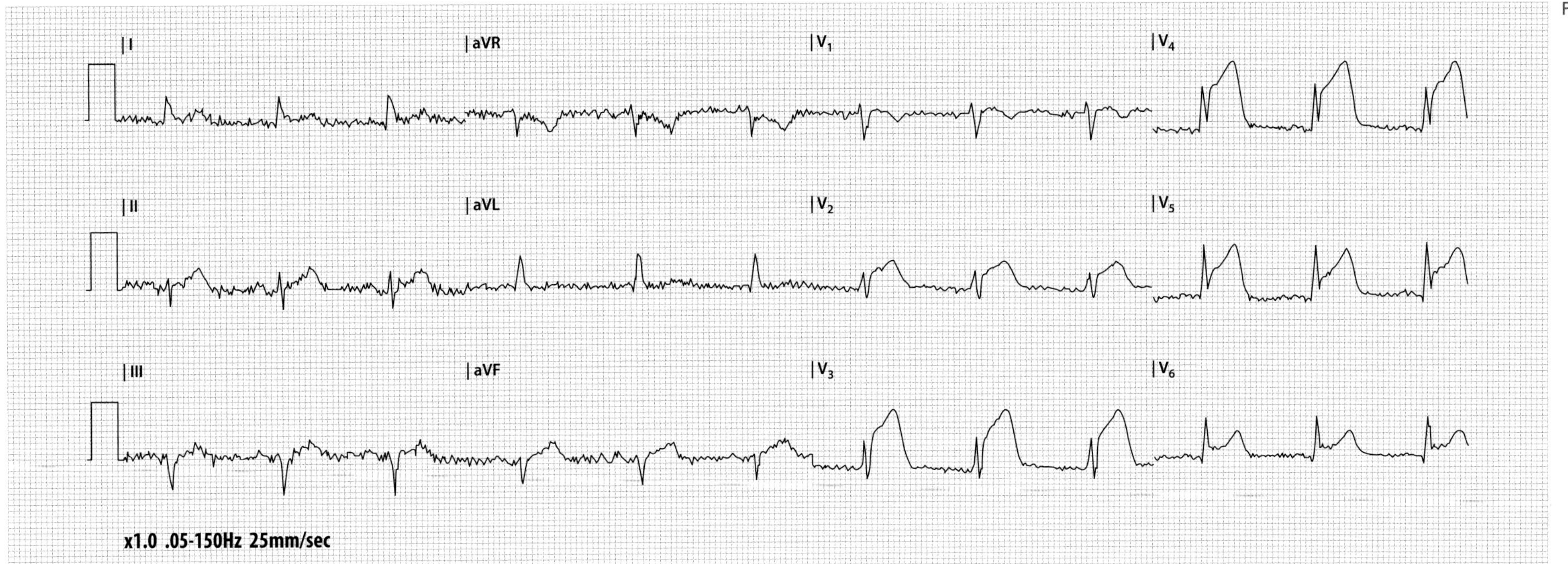

Rate and rhythm? ______ Pathologic Q waves? ______

STE? ______ ST depression? ______ T-wave changes? ______

Reciprocal changes? ______ Imposter present? ______ Axis? ______

Interpretation: ______

Inferior: II, III, aVF | **Septum:** V_1, V_2 | Anterior: V_3, V_4 | **Lateral:** I, aVL, V_5, V_6

Fig. **5.30**

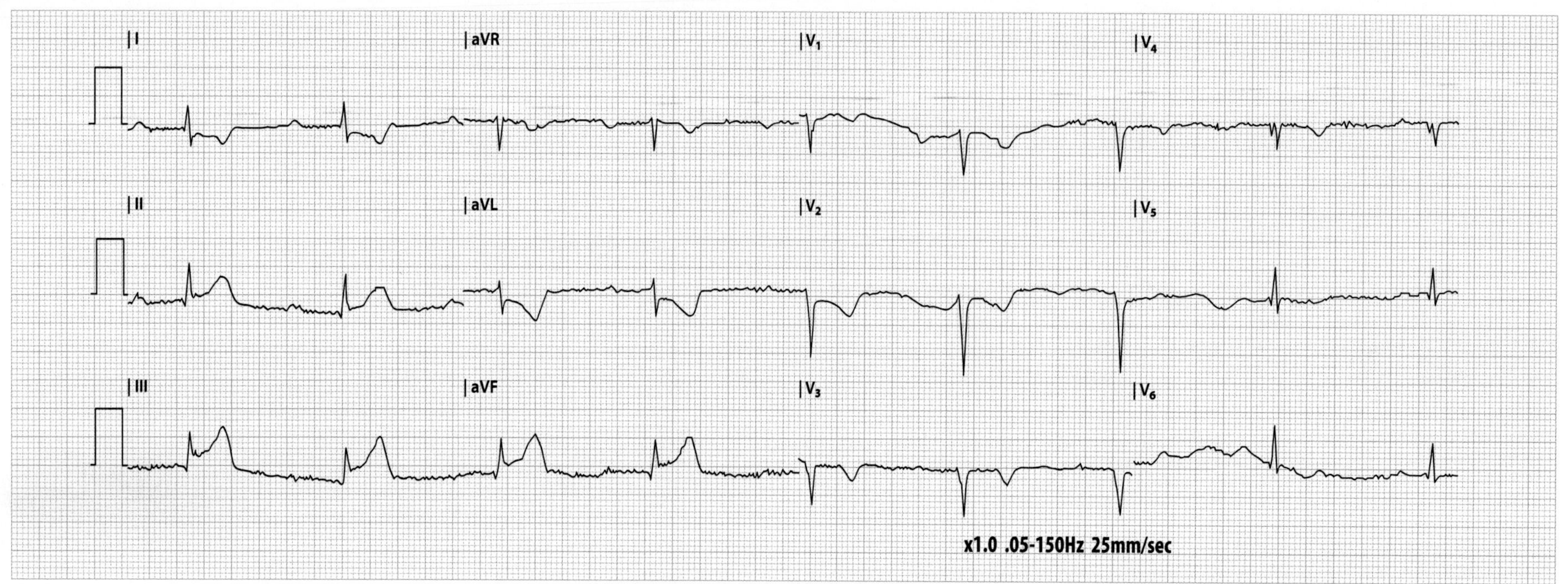

Rate and rhythm? ______ Pathologic Q waves? ______

STE? ______ ST depression? ______ T-wave changes? ______

Reciprocal changes? ______ Imposter present? ______ Axis? ______

Interpretation: ______

Inferior: II, III, aVF | **Septum: V_1, V_2** | **Anterior: V_3, V_4** | **Lateral: I, aVL, V_5, V_6**

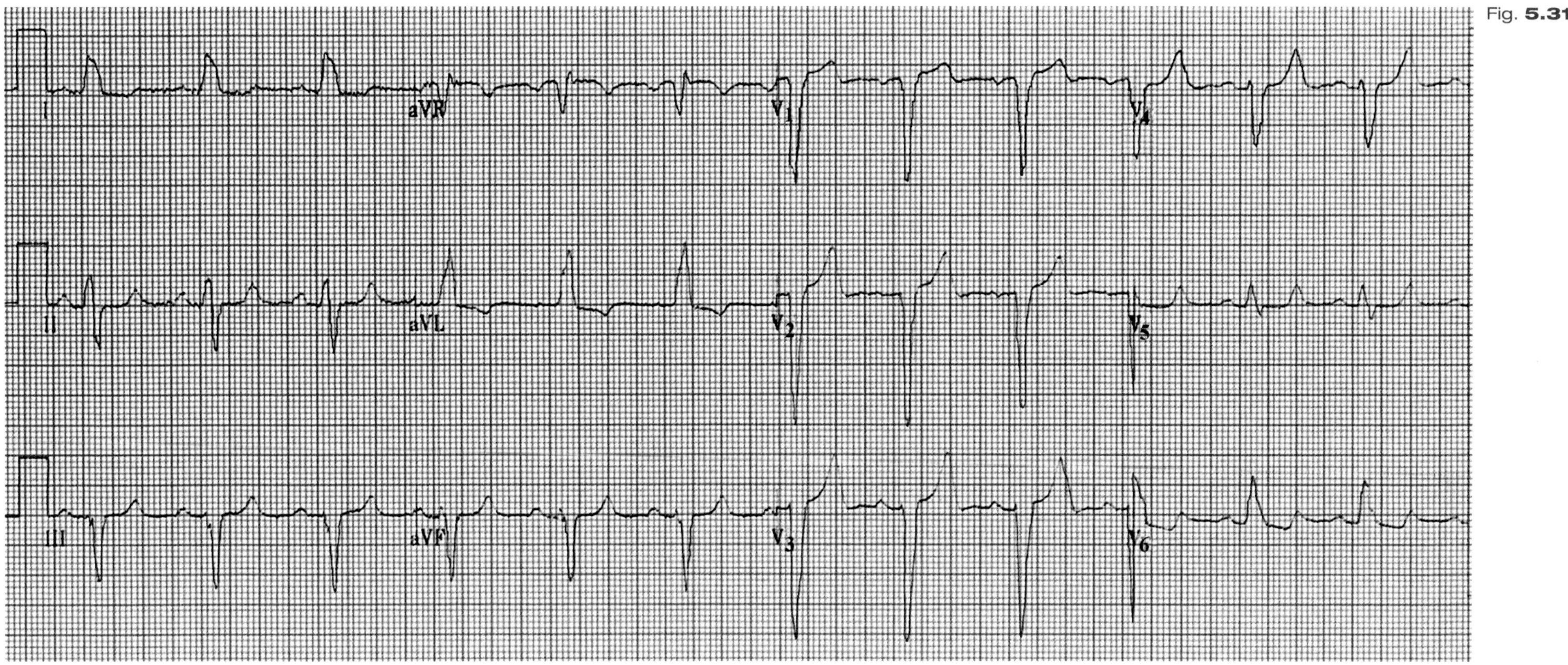

Fig. 5.31

Rate and rhythm? ______ Pathologic Q waves? ______

STE? ______ ST depression? ______ T-wave changes? ______

Reciprocal changes? ______ Imposter present? ______ Axis? ______

Interpretation: ______

Inferior: II, III, aVF | **Septum: V_1, V_2** | **Anterior: V_3, V_4** | **Lateral: I, aVL, V_5, V_6**

Fig. **5.32**

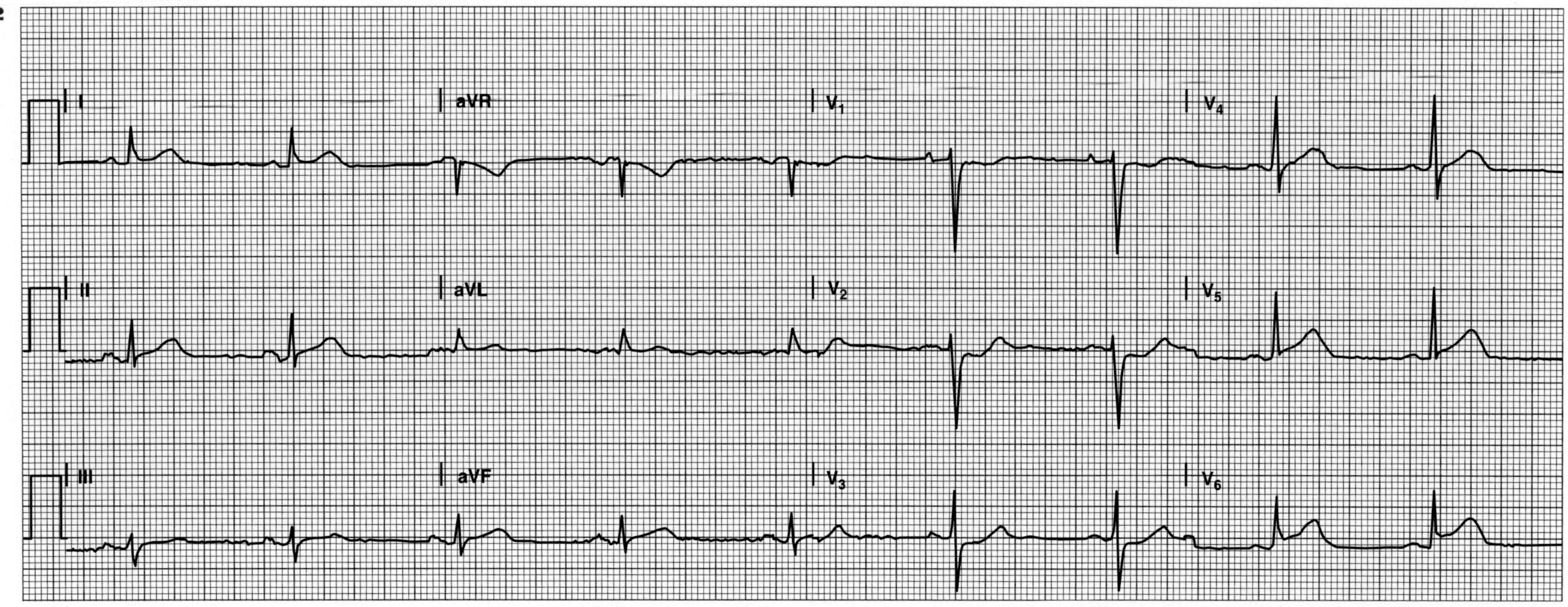

Rate and rhythm? ______ Pathologic Q waves? ______

STE? ______ ST depression? ______ T-wave changes? ______

Reciprocal changes? ______ Imposter present? ______ Axis? ______

Interpretation: ______

Inferior: II, III, aVF | **Septum: V_1, V_2** | **Anterior: V_3, V_4** | **Lateral: I, aVL, V_5, V_6**

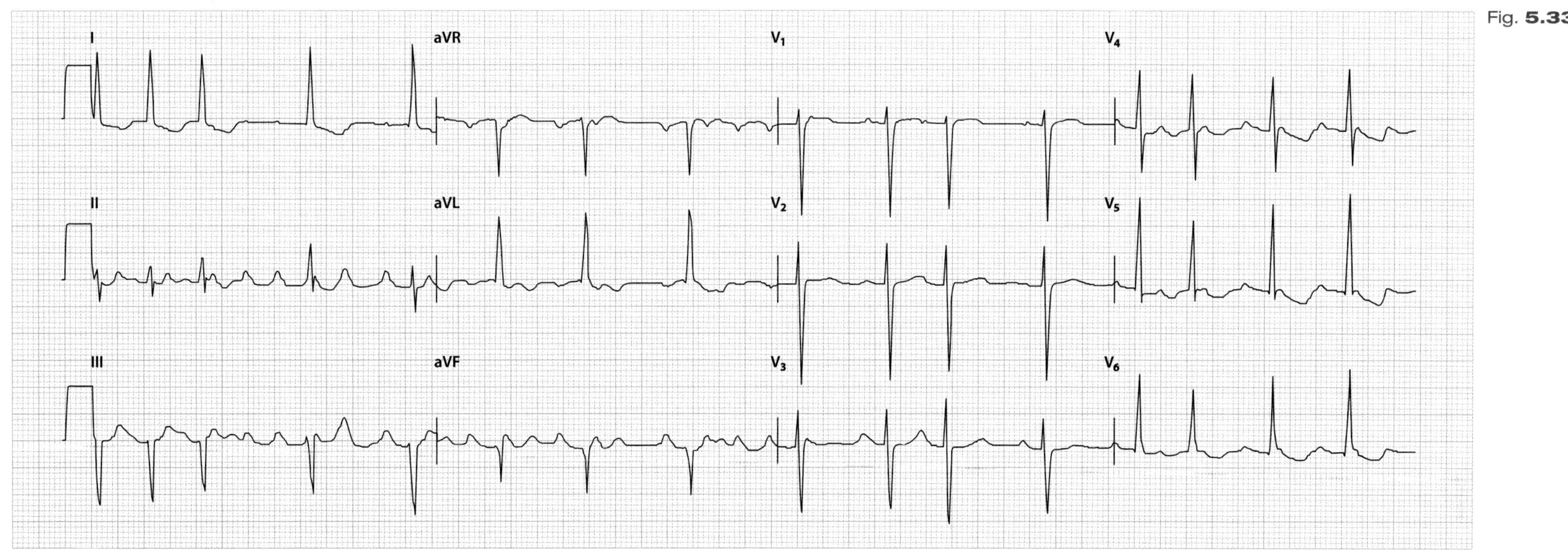

Fig. **5.33**

Rate and rhythm? ______________________ Pathologic Q waves? ______________________

STE? ______________________ ST depression? ______________________ T-wave changes? ______________________

Reciprocal changes? ______________________ Imposter present? ______________________ Axis? ______________________

Interpretation: ____

Inferior: II, III, aVF | **Septum: V_1, V_2** | Anterior: V_3, V_4 | **Lateral: I, aVL, V_5, V_6**

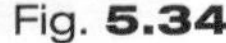

Fig. **5.34**

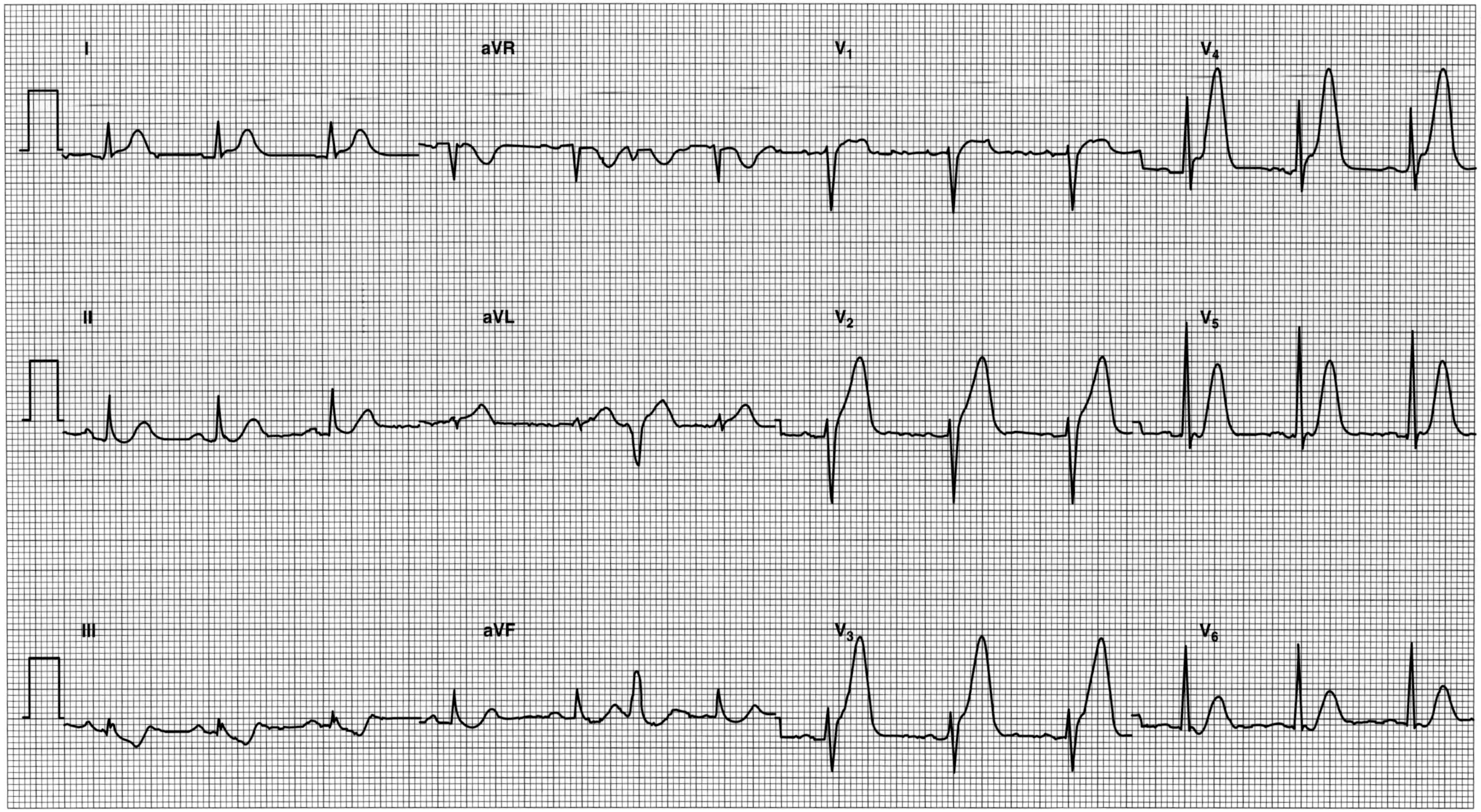

Rate and rhythm? __________ Pathologic Q waves? __________

STE? __________ ST depression? __________ T-wave changes? __________

Reciprocal changes? __________ Imposter present? __________ Axis? __________

Interpretation: __________

Inferior: II, III, aVF | **Septum: V_1, V_2** | **Anterior: V_3, V_4** | **Lateral: I, aVL, V_5, V_6**

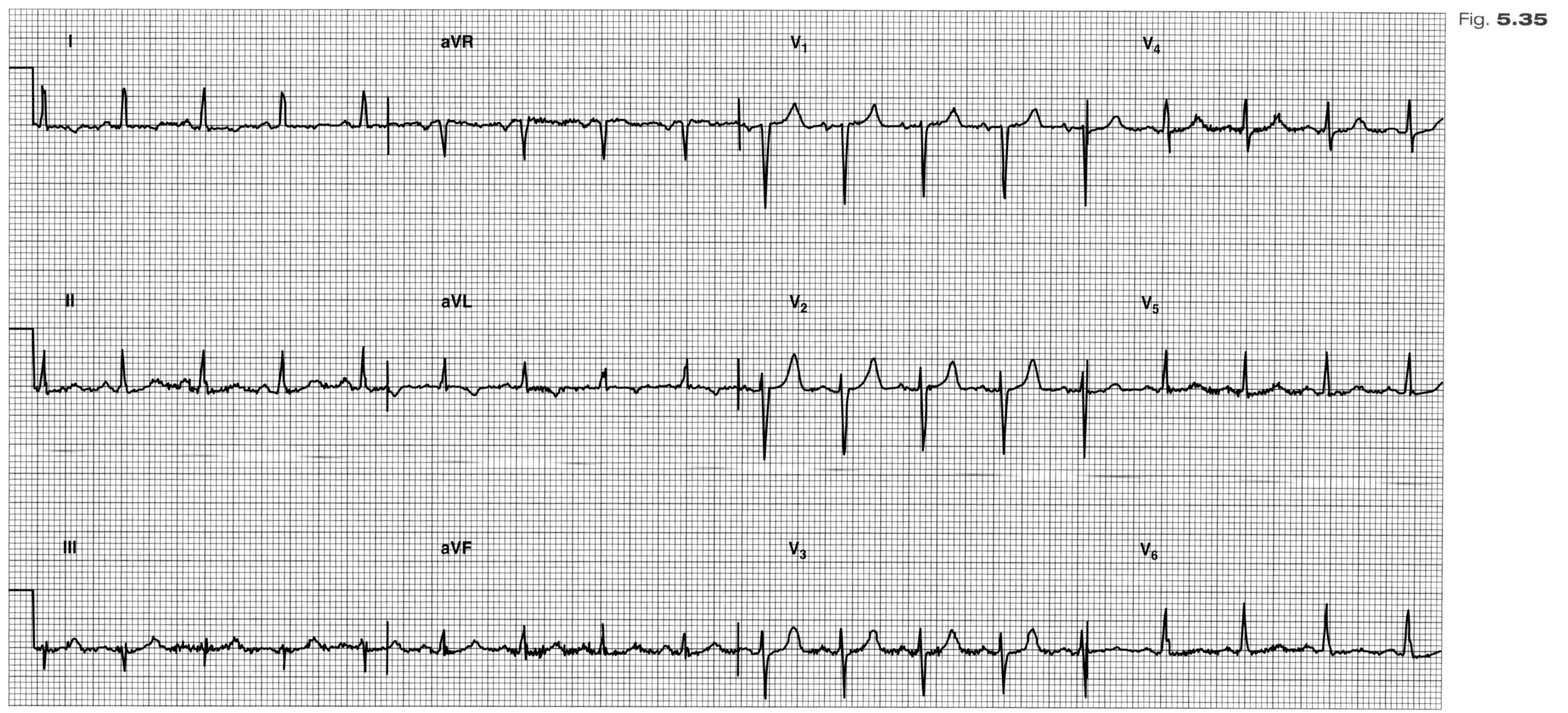

Fig. 5.35

Rate and rhythm? ______________________ Pathologic Q waves? ______________________

STE? ______________________ ST depression? ______________________ T-wave changes?______________________

Reciprocal changes? ______________________ Imposter present? ______________________ Axis? ______________________

Interpretation:______________________

Inferior: II, III, aVF | **Septum: V_1, V_2** | Anterior: V_3, V_4 | **Lateral: I, aVL, V_5, V_6**

Fig. **5.36**

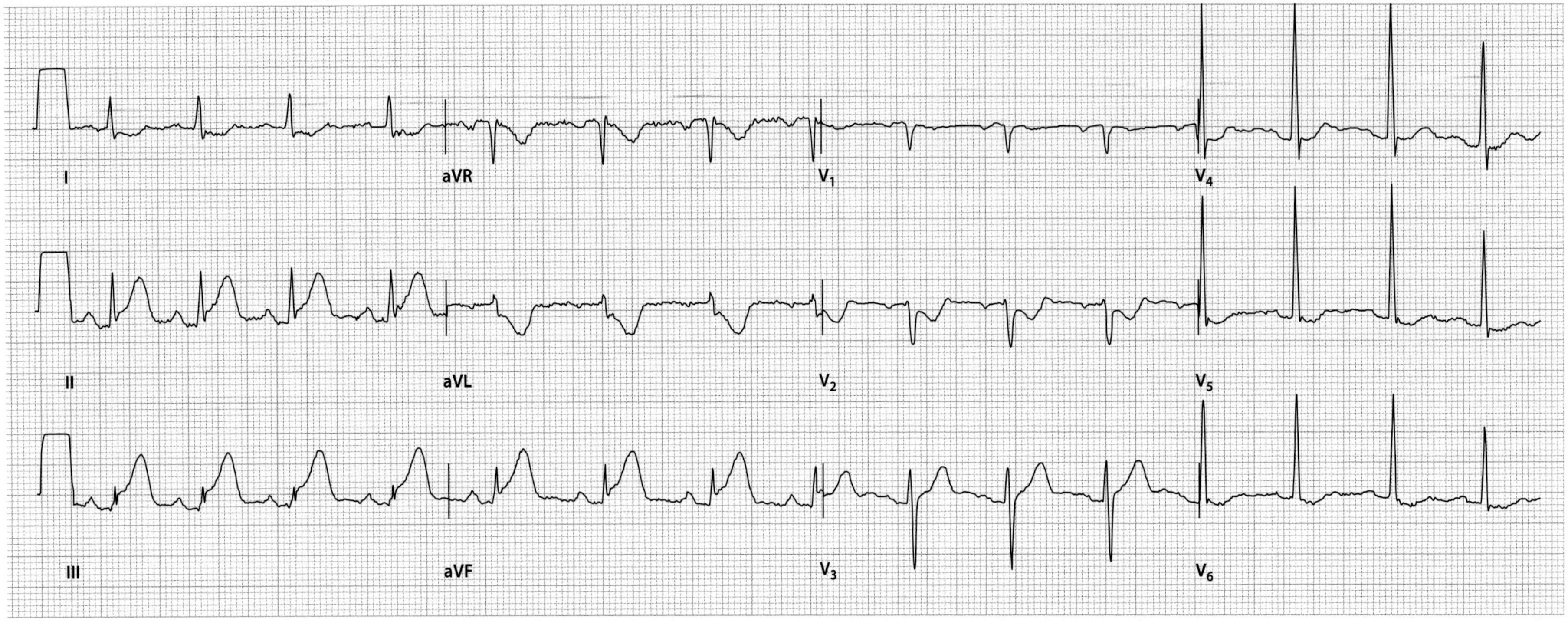

Rate and rhythm? ______________________ Pathologic Q waves? ______________________

STE? ______________________ ST depression? ______________________ T-wave changes? ______________________

Reciprocal changes? ______________________ Imposter present? ______________________ Axis? ______________________

Interpretation: ______________________

Inferior: II, III, aVF | **Septum: V_1, V_2** | **Anterior: V_3, V_4** | **Lateral: I, aVL, V_5, V_6**

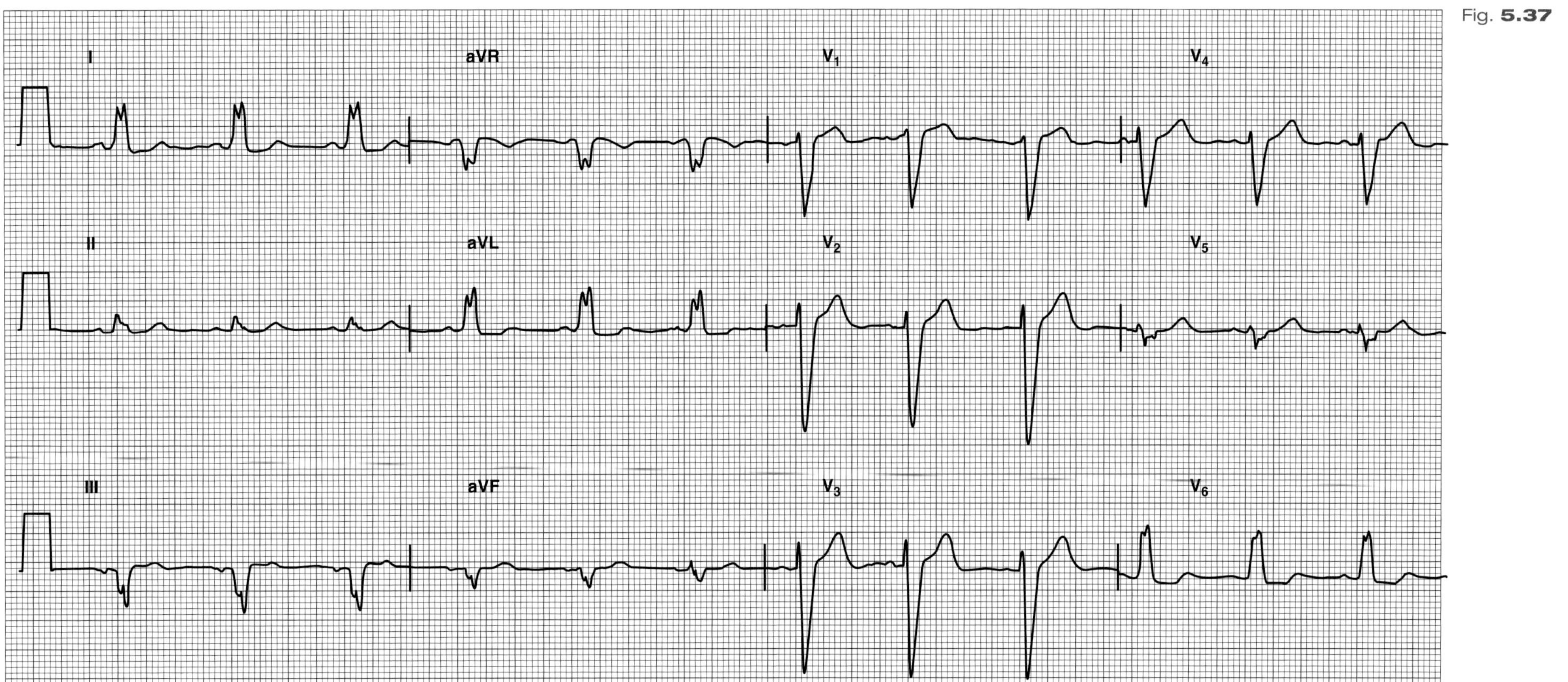

Fig. 5.37

Rate and rhythm? ______ Pathologic Q waves? ______

STE? ______ ST depression? ______ T-wave changes? ______

Reciprocal changes? ______ Imposter present? ______ Axis? ______

Interpretation: ______

Inferior: II, III, aVF | **Septum: V_1, V_2** | Anterior: V_3, V_4 | **Lateral: I, aVL, V_5, V_6**

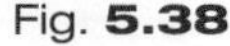

Fig. **5.38**

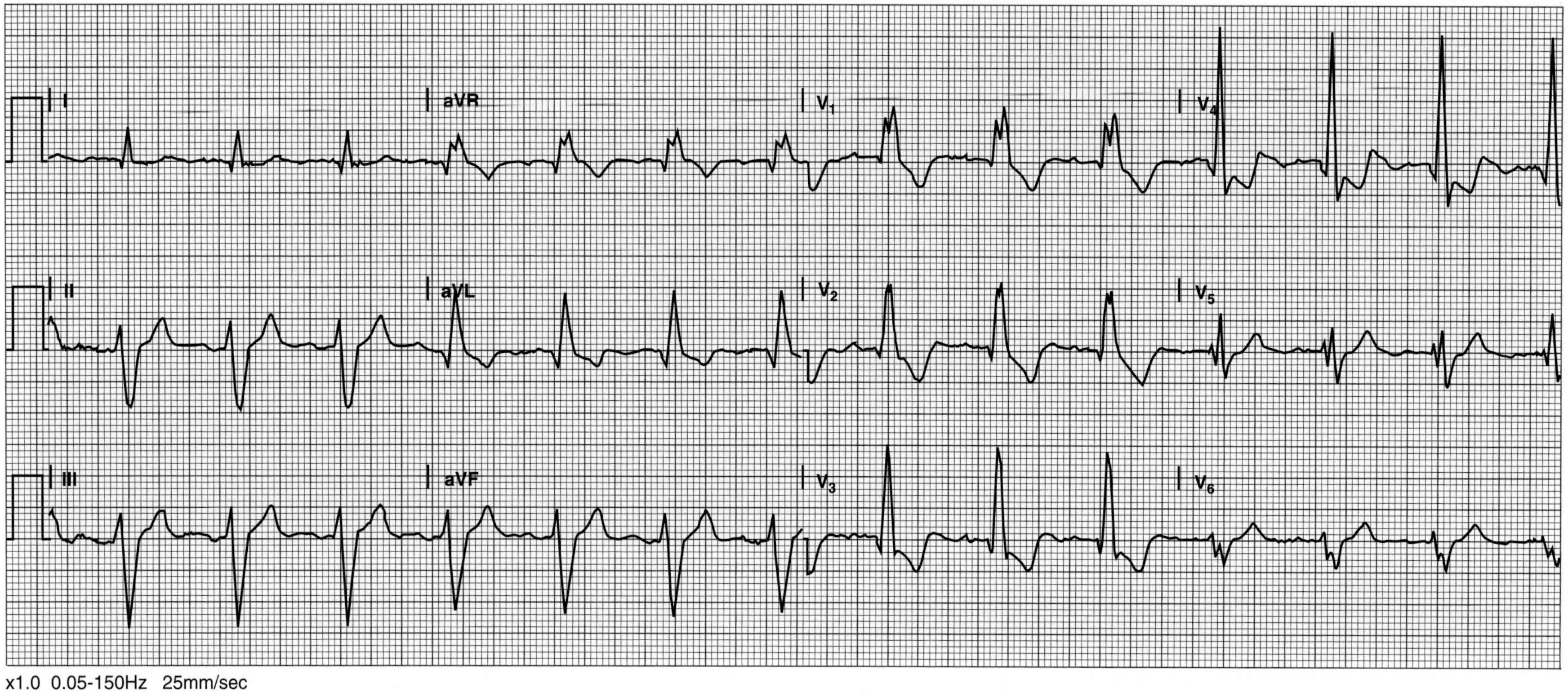

x1.0 0.05-150Hz 25mm/sec

Rate and rhythm? ______________________ Pathologic Q waves? ______________________

STE? ______________________ ST depression? ______________________ T-wave changes?______________________

Reciprocal changes? ______________________ Imposter present? ______________________ Axis? ______________________

Interpretation:____

Inferior: II, III, aVF | **Septum: V_1, V_2** | Anterior: V_3, V_4 | **Lateral: I, aVL, V_5, V_6**

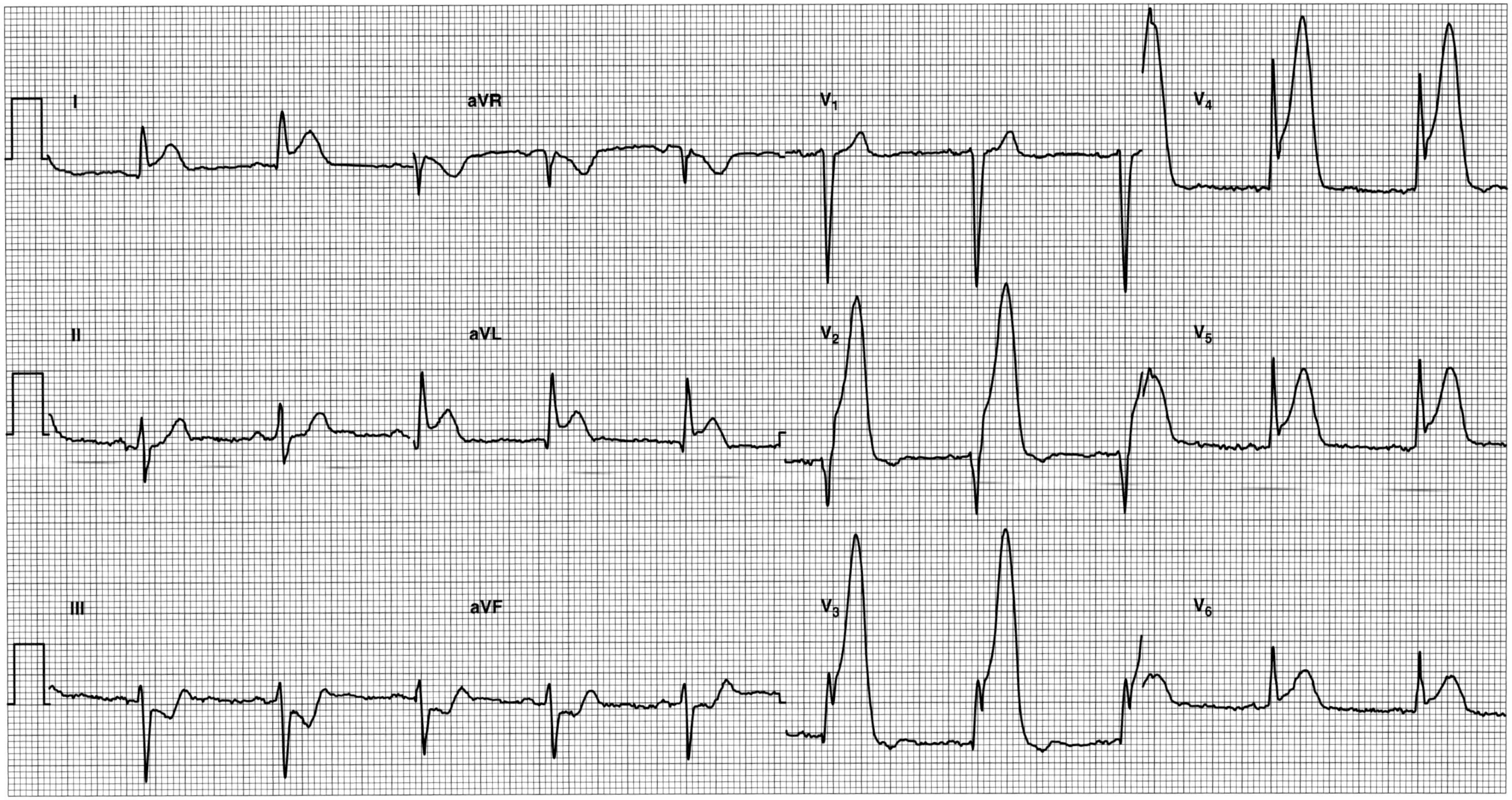

Fig. **5.39**

Rate and rhythm? ____________________ Pathologic Q waves? ____________________

STE? ____________________ ST depression? ____________________ T-wave changes? ____________________

Reciprocal changes? ____________________ Imposter present? ____________________ Axis? ____________________

Interpretation: ____

Inferior: II, III, aVF | **Septum: V_1, V_2** | **Anterior: V_3, V_4** | **Lateral: I, aVL, V_5, V_6**

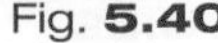

Fig. 5.40

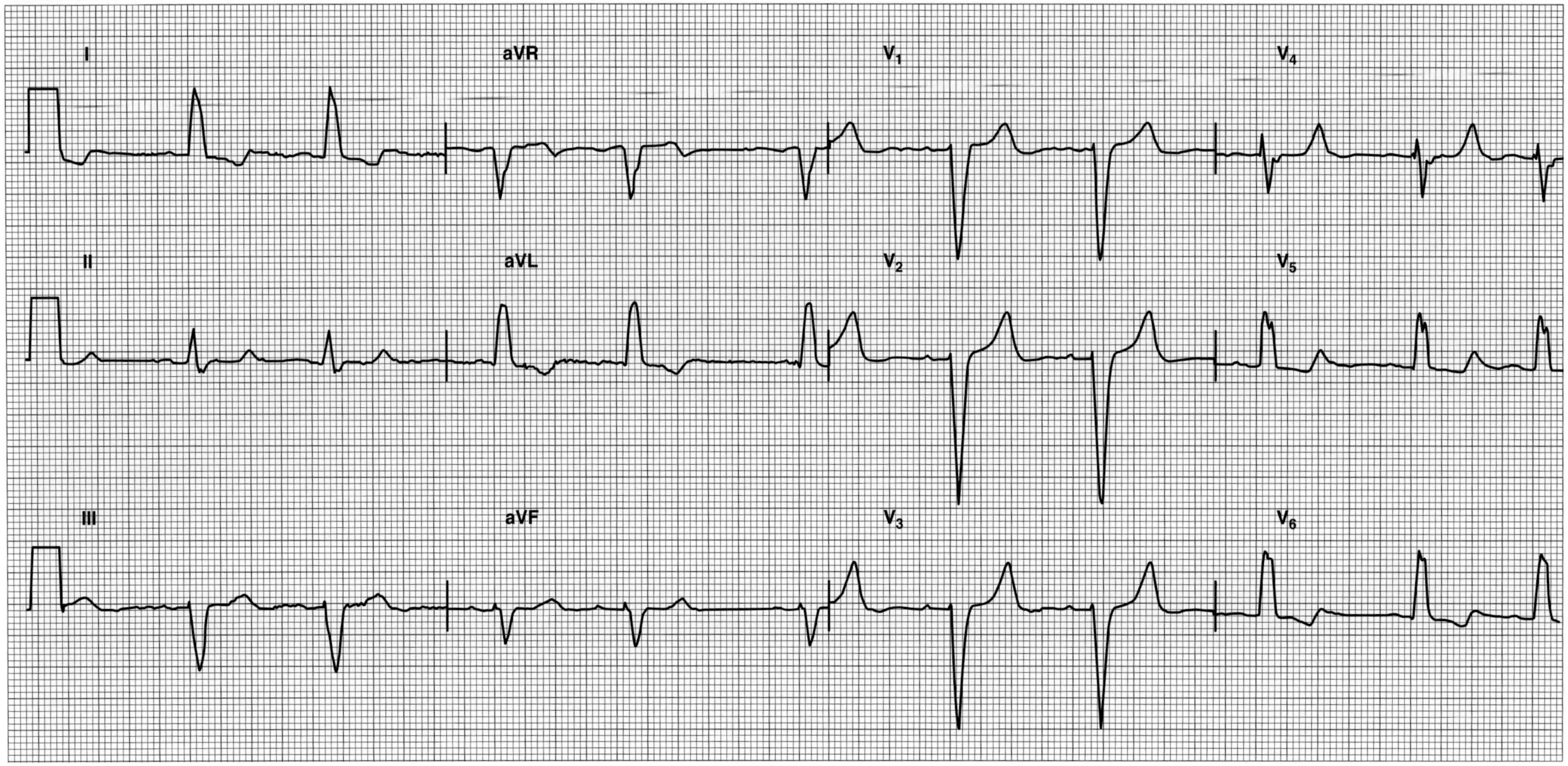

I aVR V_1 V_4

II aVL V_2 V_5

III aVF V_3 V_6

Rate and rhythm? ______________________ Pathologic Q waves? ______________________

STE? ______________________ ST depression? ______________________ T-wave changes? ______________________

Reciprocal changes? ______________________ Imposter present? ______________________ Axis? ______________________

Interpretation: ____

Inferior: II, III, aVF | **Septum: V_1, V_2** | **Anterior: V_3, V_4** | **Lateral: I, aVL, V_5, V_6**

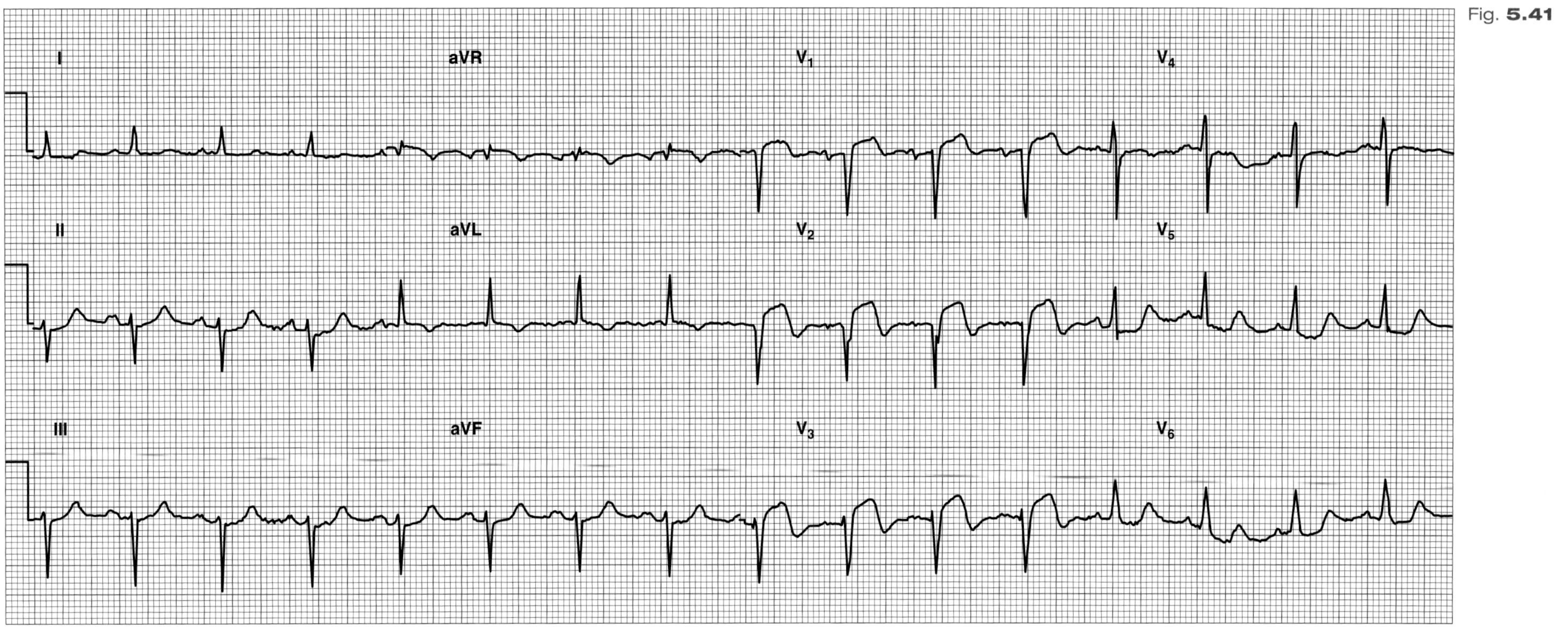

Fig. **5.41**

Rate and rhythm? ____________________ Pathologic Q waves? ____________________

STE? ____________________ ST depression? ____________________ T-wave changes?____________________

Reciprocal changes? ____________________ Imposter present? ____________________ Axis? ____________________

Interpretation:____________________

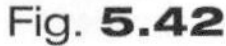

Fig. 5.42

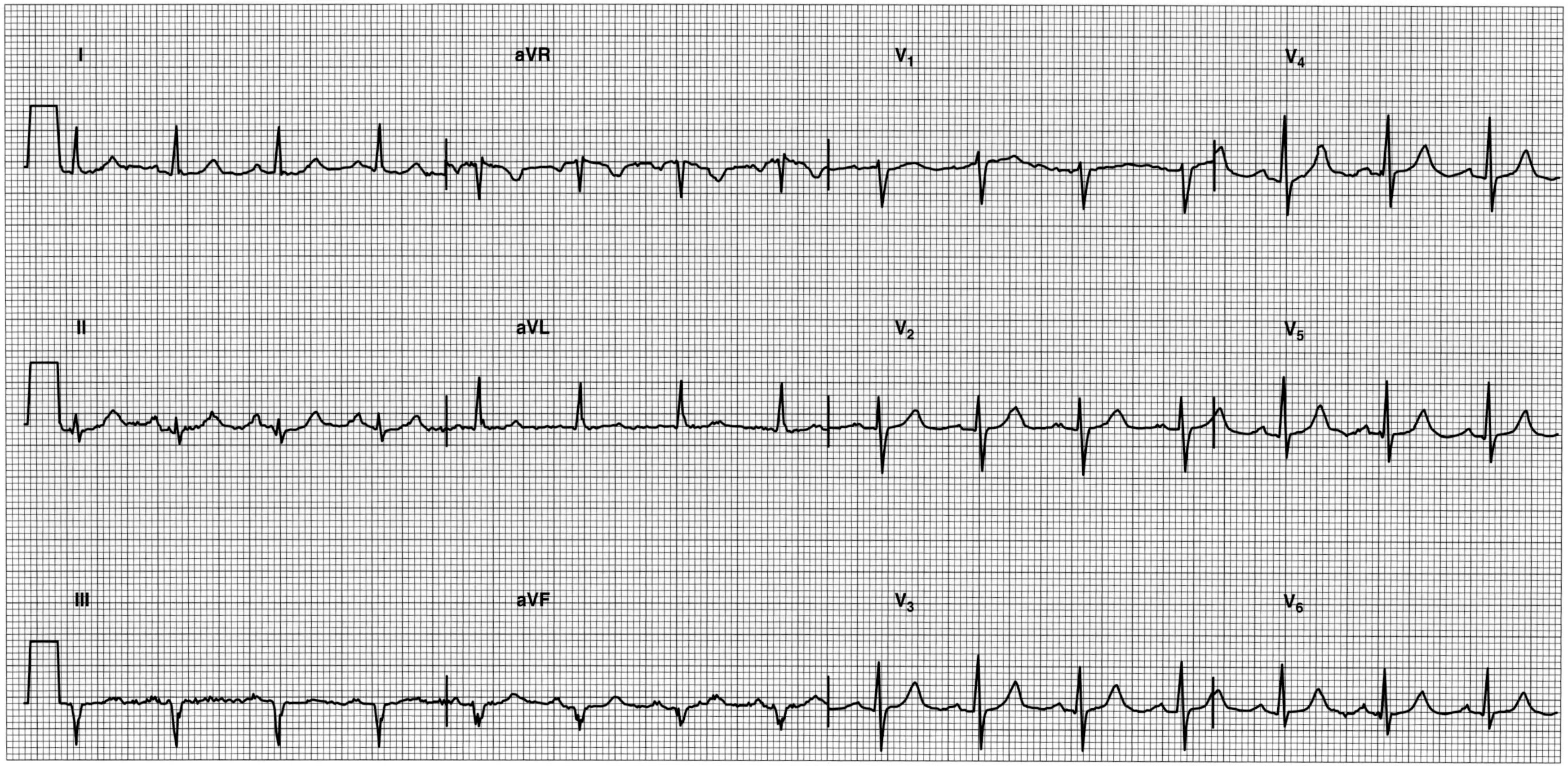

Rate and rhythm? ______________________ Pathologic Q waves? ______________________

STE? ______________________ ST depression? ______________________ T-wave changes? ______________________

Reciprocal changes? ______________________ Imposter present? ______________________ Axis? ______________________

Interpretation: ____

Inferior: II, III, aVF | **Septum: V_1, V_2** | **Anterior: V_3, V_4** | **Lateral: I, aVL, V_5, V_6**

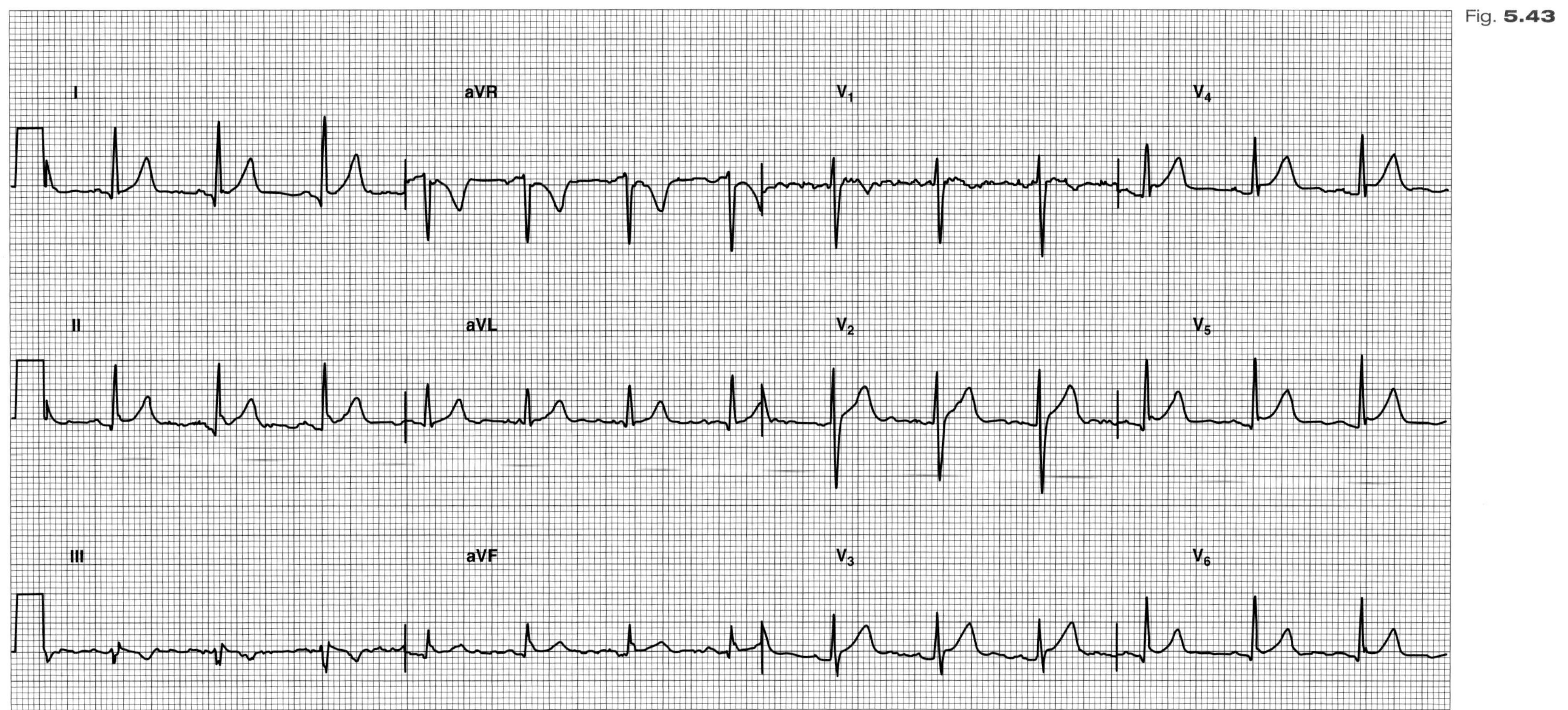

Fig. **5.43**

Rate and rhythm? ______ Pathologic Q waves? ______

STE? ______ ST depression? ______ T-wave changes? ______

Reciprocal changes? ______ Imposter present? ______ Axis? ______

Interpretation: ______

Inferior: II, III, aVF | **Septum: V_1, V_2** | Anterior: V_3, V_4 | **Lateral: I, aVL, V_5, V_6**

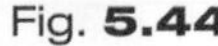

Fig. **5.44**

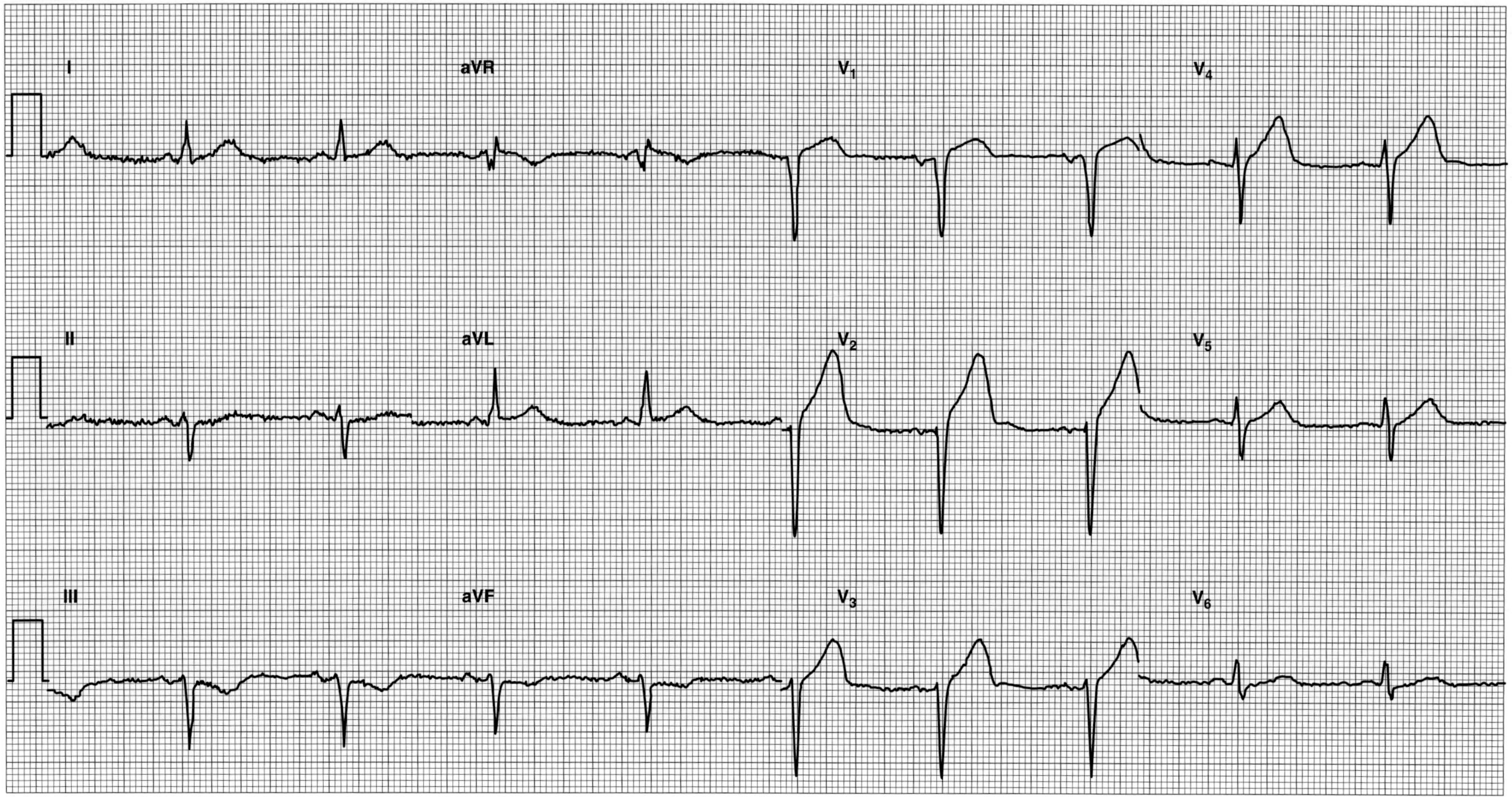

Rate and rhythm? __________ Pathologic Q waves? __________

STE? __________ ST depression? __________ T-wave changes? __________

Reciprocal changes? __________ Imposter present? __________ Axis? __________

Interpretation: __________

Inferior: II, III, aVF | **Septum: V_1, V_2** | **Anterior: V_3, V_4** | **Lateral: I, aVL, V_5, V_6**

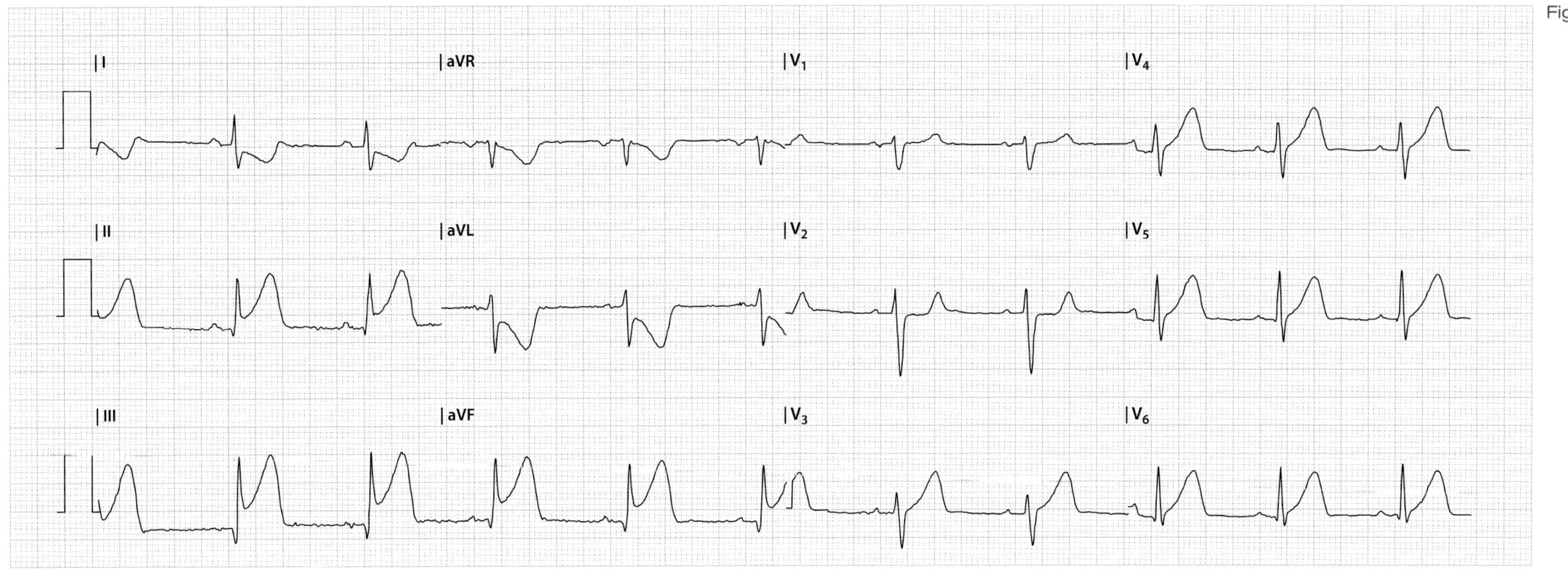

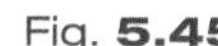
Fig. 5.45

Rate and rhythm? ______________________ Pathologic Q waves? ______________________

STE? ______________________ ST depression? ______________________ T-wave changes? ______________________

Reciprocal changes? ______________________ Imposter present? ______________________ Axis? ______________________

Interpretation: ____

Inferior: II, III, aVF | **Septum: V_1, V_2** | **Anterior: V_3, V_4** | **Lateral: I, aVL, V_5, V_6**

Fig. **5.46**

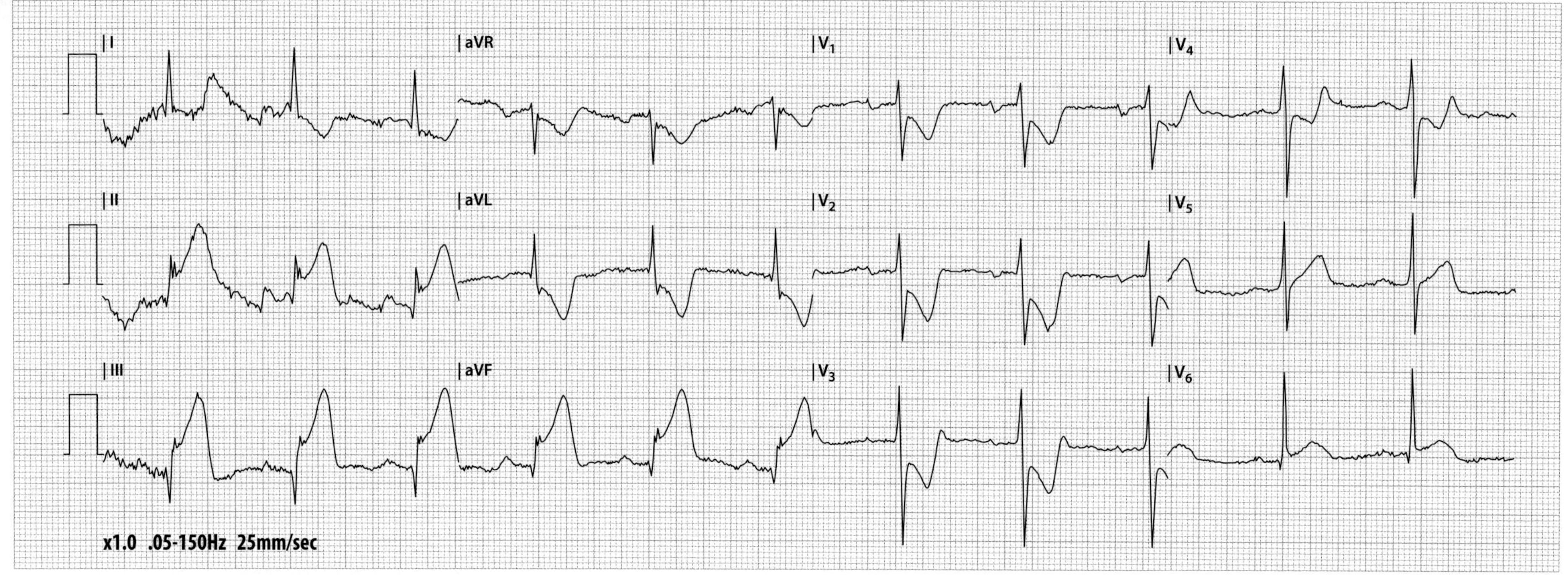

Rate and rhythm? ______ Pathologic Q waves? ______

STE? ______ ST depression? ______ T-wave changes? ______

Reciprocal changes? ______ Imposter present? ______ Axis? ______

Interpretation: ______

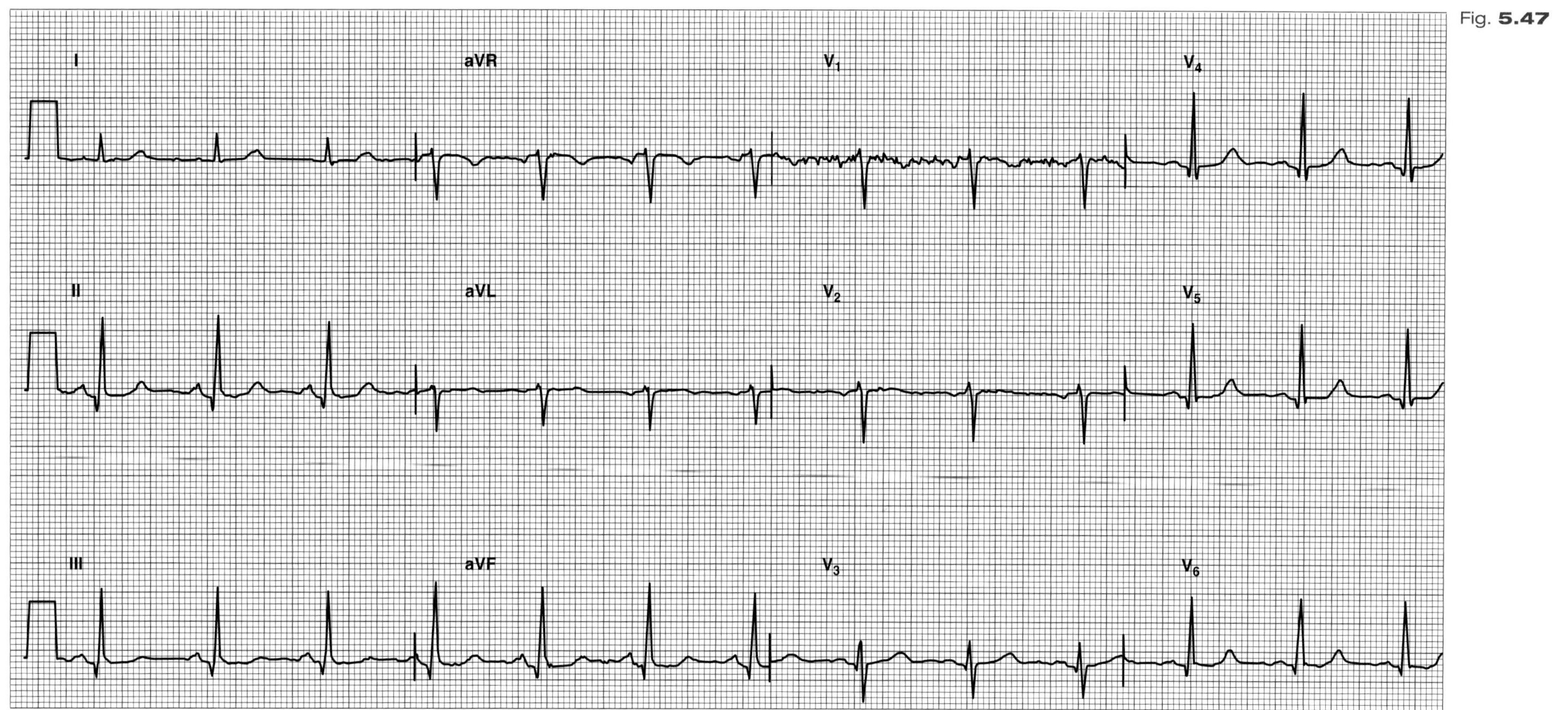

Fig. 5.47

Rate and rhythm? ____________________ Pathologic Q waves? ____________________

STE? ____________________ ST depression? ____________________ T-wave changes? ____________________

Reciprocal changes? ____________________ Imposter present? ____________________ Axis? ____________________

Interpretation: ____________________

Inferior: II, III, aVF | Septum: V_1, V_2 | Anterior: V_3, V_4 | Lateral: I, aVL, V_5, V_6

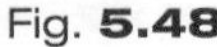

Fig. **5.48**

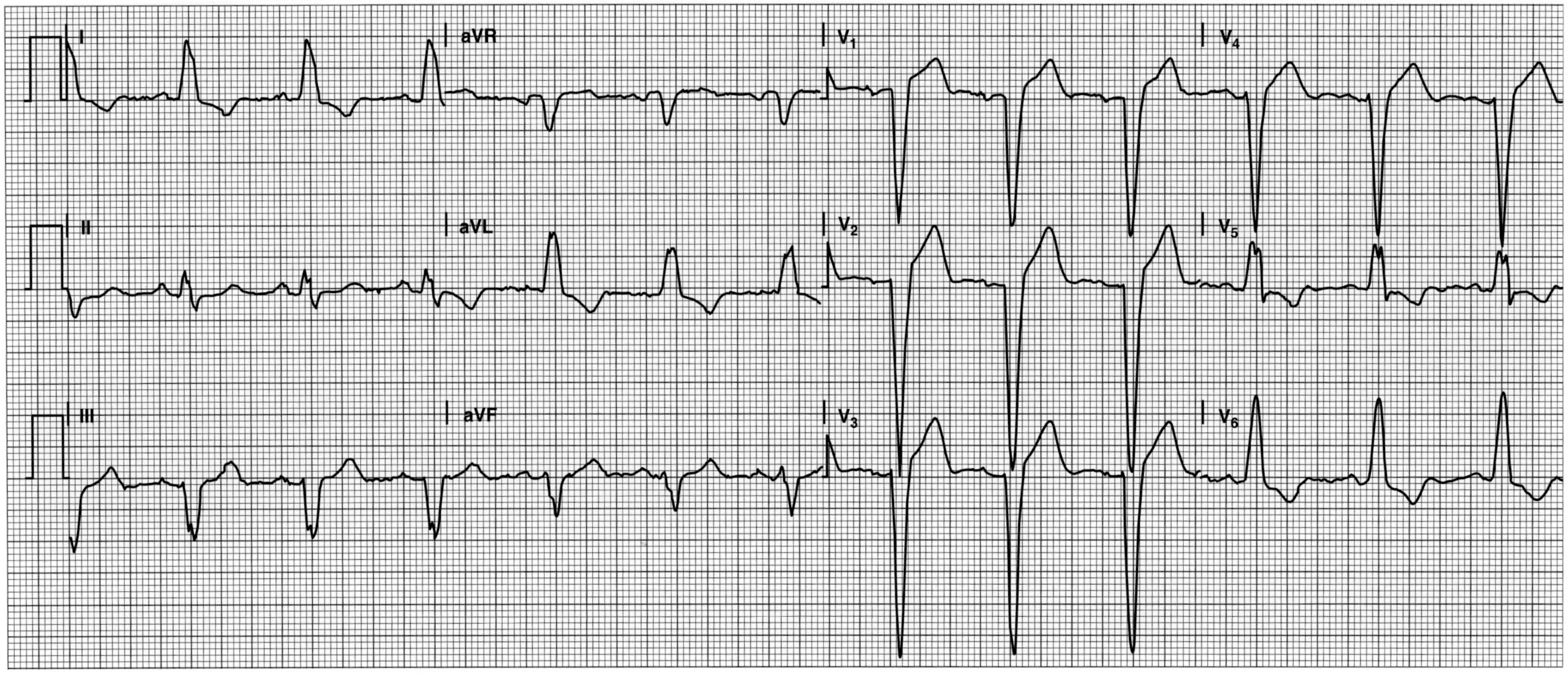

Rate and rhythm? ______________________ Pathologic Q waves? ______________________

STE? ______________________ ST depression? ______________________ T-wave changes? ______________________

Reciprocal changes? ______________________ Imposter present? ______________________ Axis? ______________________

Interpretation: ______________________

Inferior: II, III, aVF | **Septum: V_1, V_2** | Anterior: V_3, V_4 | **Lateral: I, aVL, V_5, V_6**

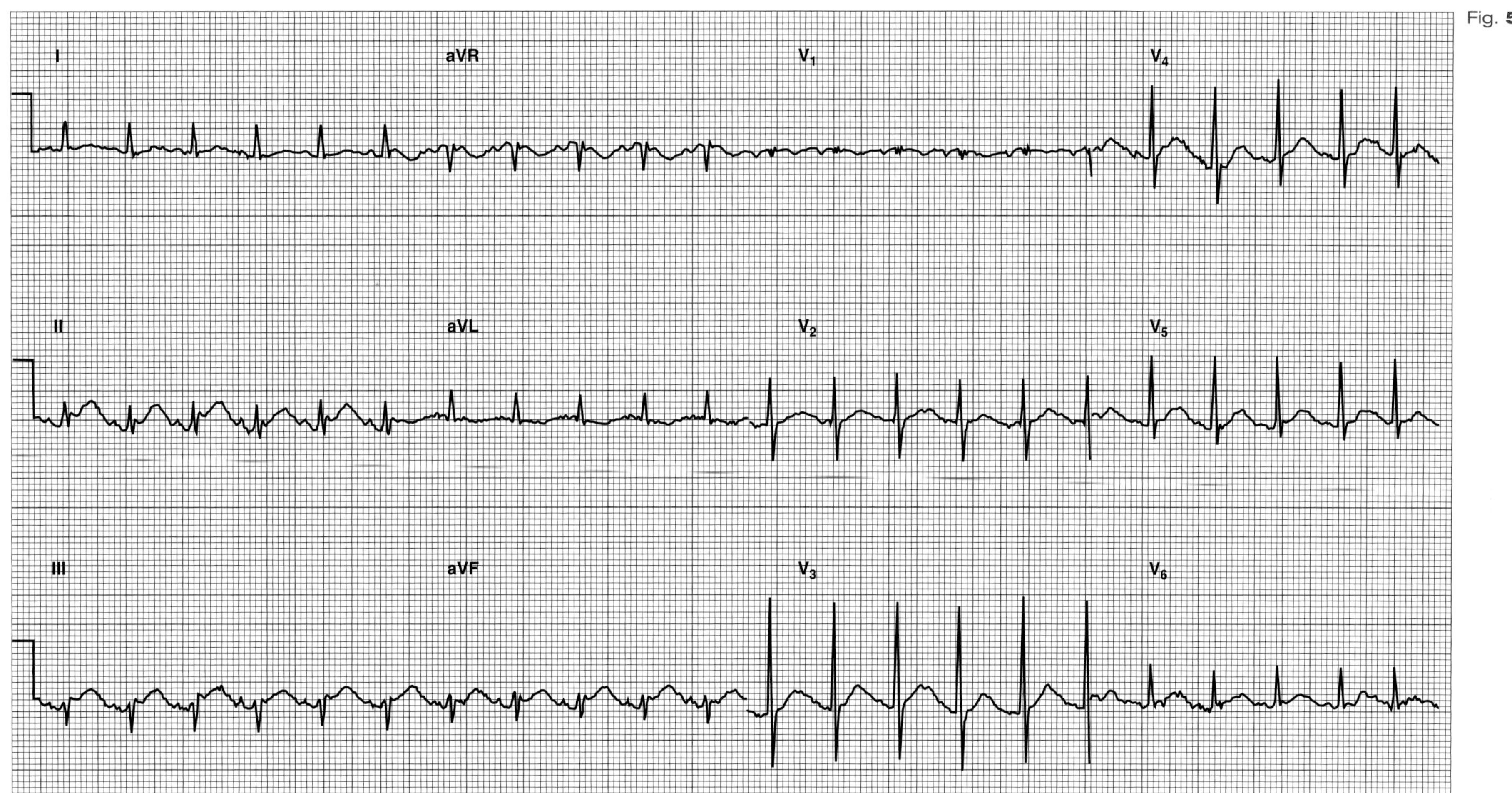

Fig. 5.49

Rate and rhythm? ____________________ Pathologic Q waves? ____________________

STE? ____________________ ST depression? ____________________ T-wave changes?____________________

Reciprocal changes? ____________________ Imposter present? ____________________ Axis? ____________________

Interpretation:____________________

Inferior: II, III, aVF | **Septum: V_1, V_2** | **Anterior: V_3, V_4** | **Lateral: I, aVL, V_5, V_6**

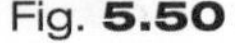

Fig. **5.50**

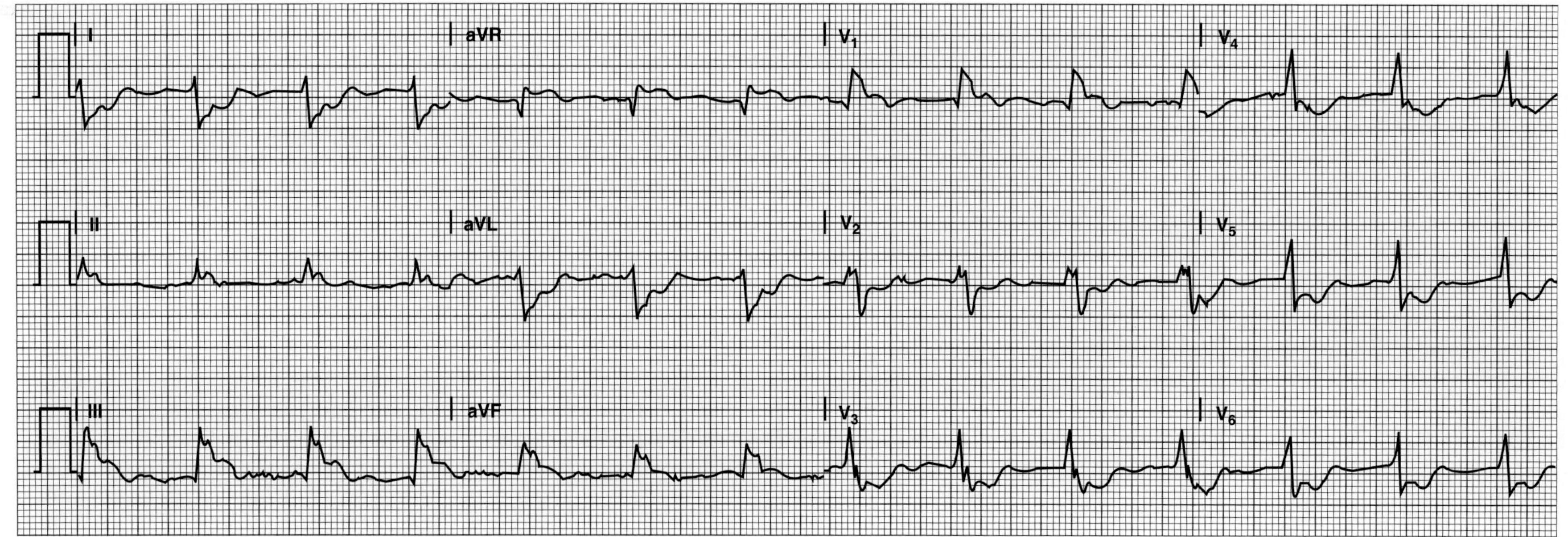

Rate and rhythm? ______________ Pathologic Q waves? ______________

STE? ______________ ST depression? ______________ T-wave changes? ______________

Reciprocal changes? ______________ Imposter present? ______________ Axis? ______________

Interpretation: ______________

Inferior: II, III, aVF | **Septum: V_1, V_2** | **Anterior: V_3, V_4** | **Lateral: I, aVL, V_5, V_6**

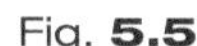

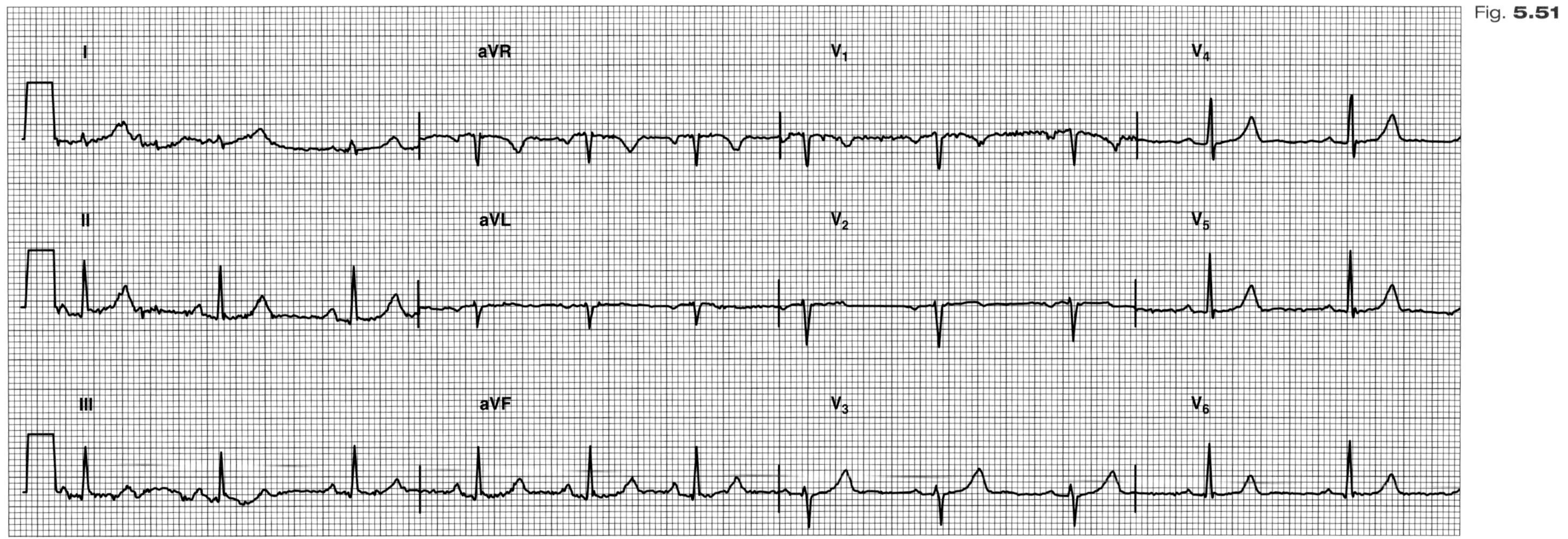

Fig. **5.51**

Rate and rhythm? ______ Pathologic Q waves? ______

STE? ______ ST depression? ______ T-wave changes? ______

Reciprocal changes? ______ Imposter present? ______ Axis? ______

Interpretation: ______

Inferior: II, III, aVF | **Septum: V_1, V_2** | Anterior: V_3, V_4 | **Lateral: I, aVL, V_5, V_6**

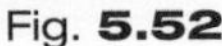

Fig. **5.52**

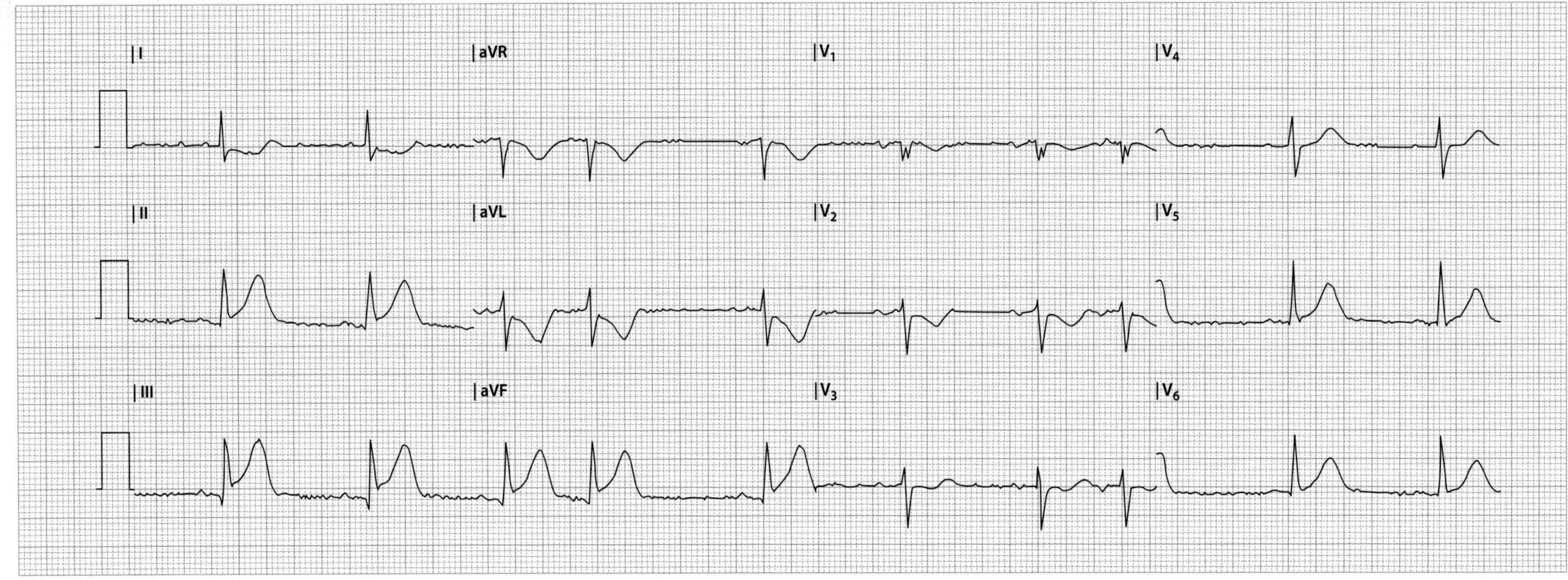

Rate and rhythm? ______ Pathologic Q waves? ______

STE? ______ ST depression? ______ T-wave changes?______

Reciprocal changes? ______ Imposter present? ______ Axis? ______

Interpretation:______

Inferior: II, III, aVF | **Septum: V_1, V_2** | **Anterior: V_3, V_4** | **Lateral: I, aVL, V_5, V_6**

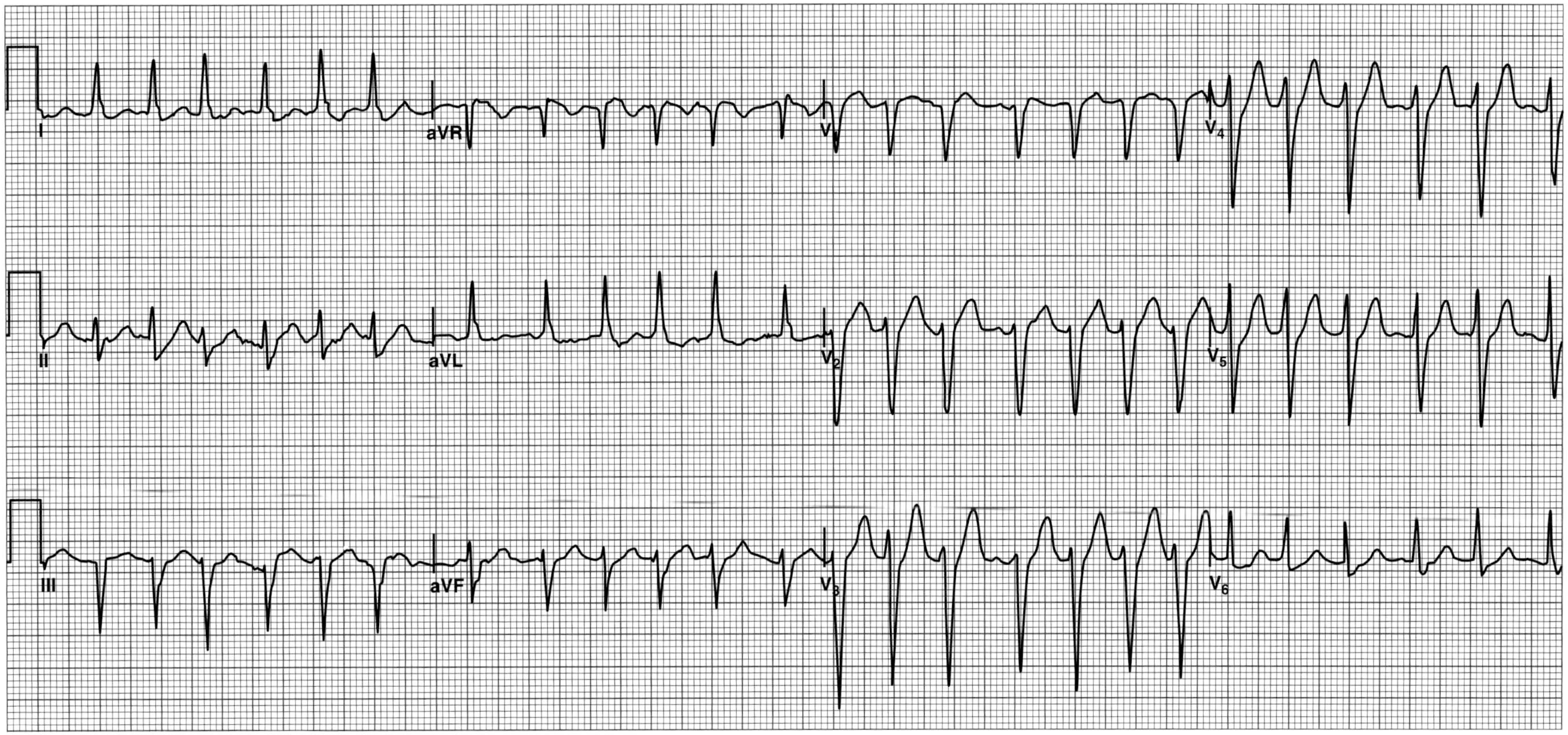

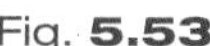

Fig. 5.53

Rate and rhythm? ______ Pathologic Q waves? ______

STE? ______ ST depression? ______ T-wave changes?______

Reciprocal changes? ______ Imposter present? ______ Axis? ______

Interpretation:______

Inferior: II, III, aVF | **Septum: V_1, V_2** | **Anterior: V_3, V_4** | **Lateral: I, aVL, V_5, V_6**

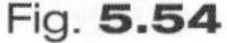

Fig. **5.54**

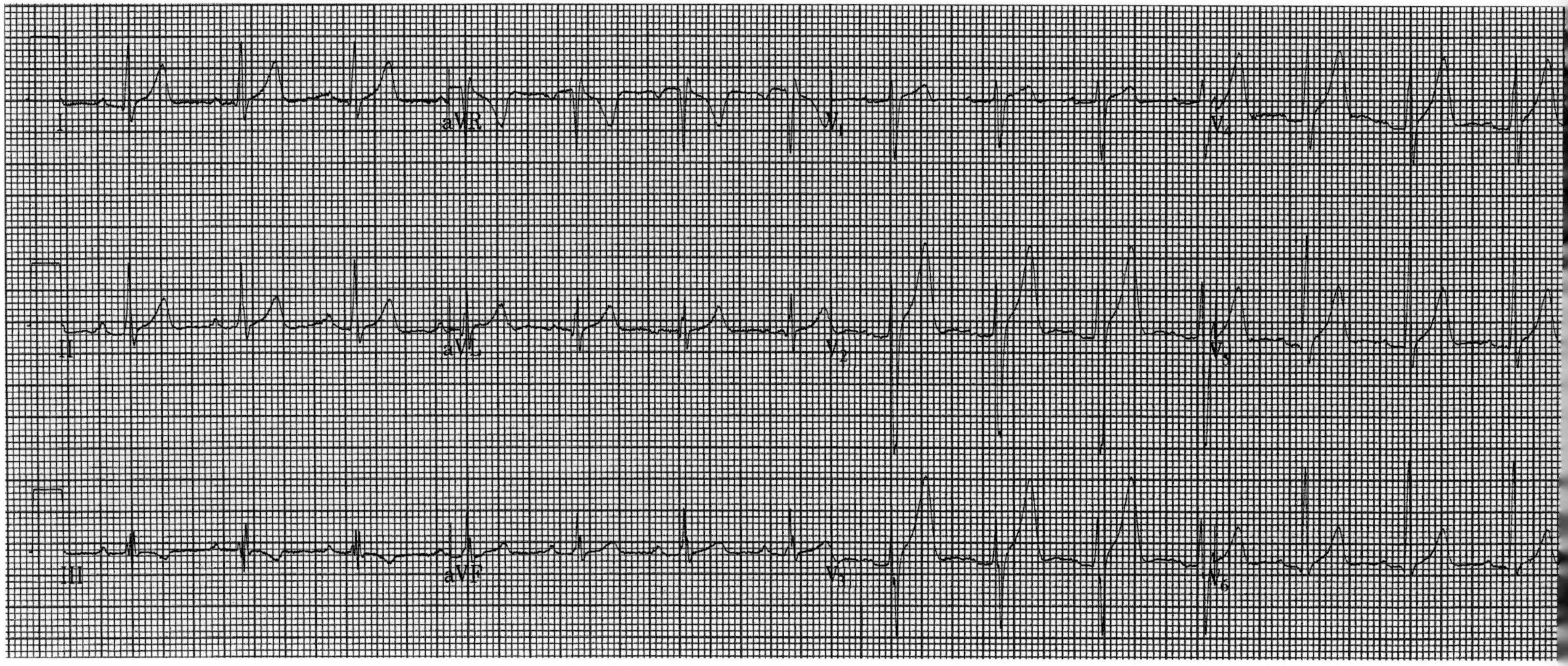

Rate and rhythm? ______________________ Pathologic Q waves? ______________________

STE? ______________________ ST depression? ______________________ T-wave changes?______________________

Reciprocal changes? ______________________ Imposter present? ______________________ Axis? ______________________

Interpretation:____

Inferior: II, III, aVF | **Septum: V_1, V_2** | **Anterior: V_3, V_4** | **Lateral: I, aVL, V_5, V_6**

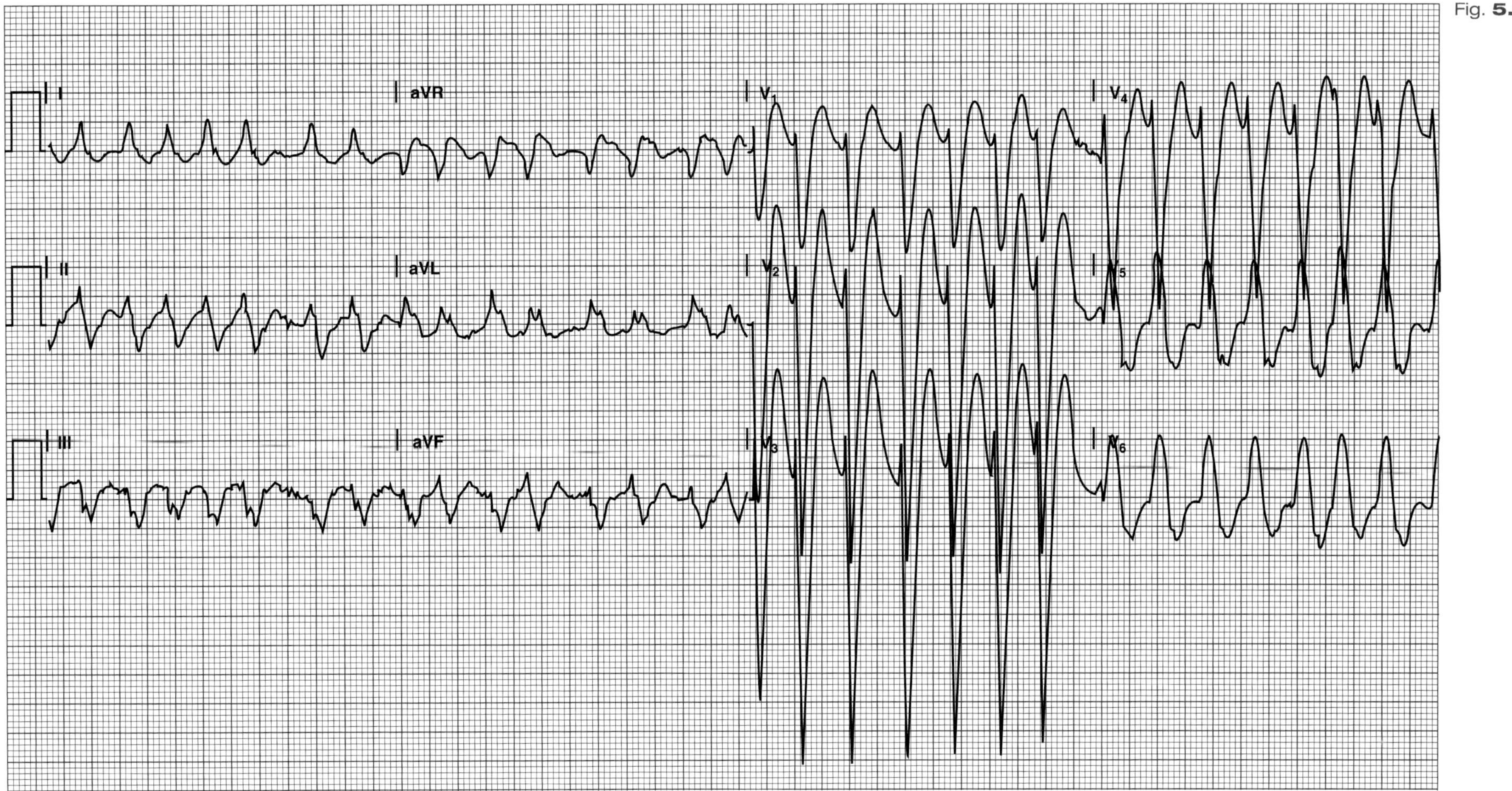

Fig. 5.55

Rate and rhythm? ______ Pathologic Q waves? ______

STE? ______ ST depression? ______ T-wave changes? ______

Reciprocal changes? ______ Imposter present? ______ Axis? ______

Interpretation: ______

Inferior: II, III, aVF | **Septum: V_1, V_2** | **Anterior: V_3, V_4** | **Lateral: I, aVL, V_5, V_6**

Fig. **5.56**

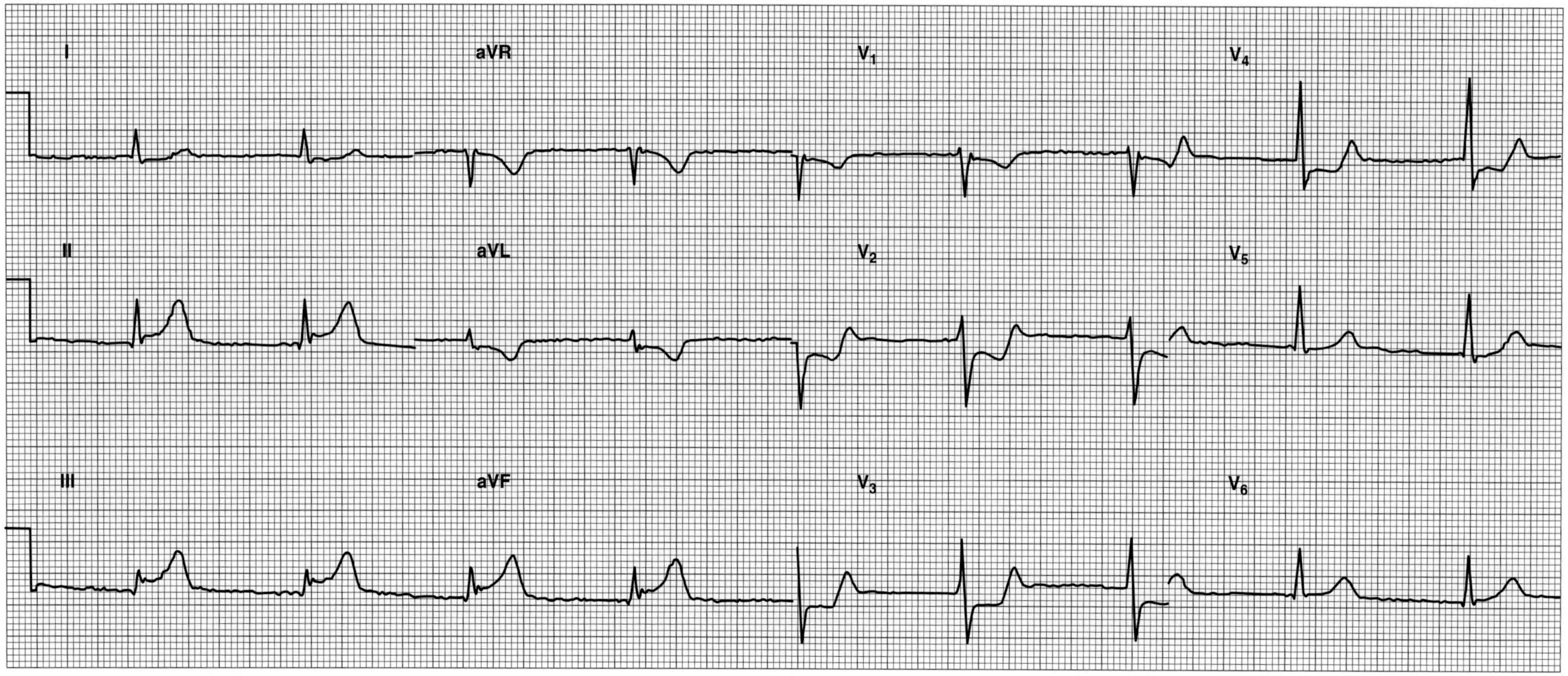

Rate and rhythm? ______________________ Pathologic Q waves? ______________________

STE? ______________________ ST depression? ______________________ T-wave changes? ______________________

Reciprocal changes? ______________________ Imposter present? ______________________ Axis? ______________________

Interpretation: ____

Inferior: II, III, aVF | **Septum: V_1, V_2** | **Anterior: V_3, V_4** | **Lateral: I, aVL, V_5, V_6**

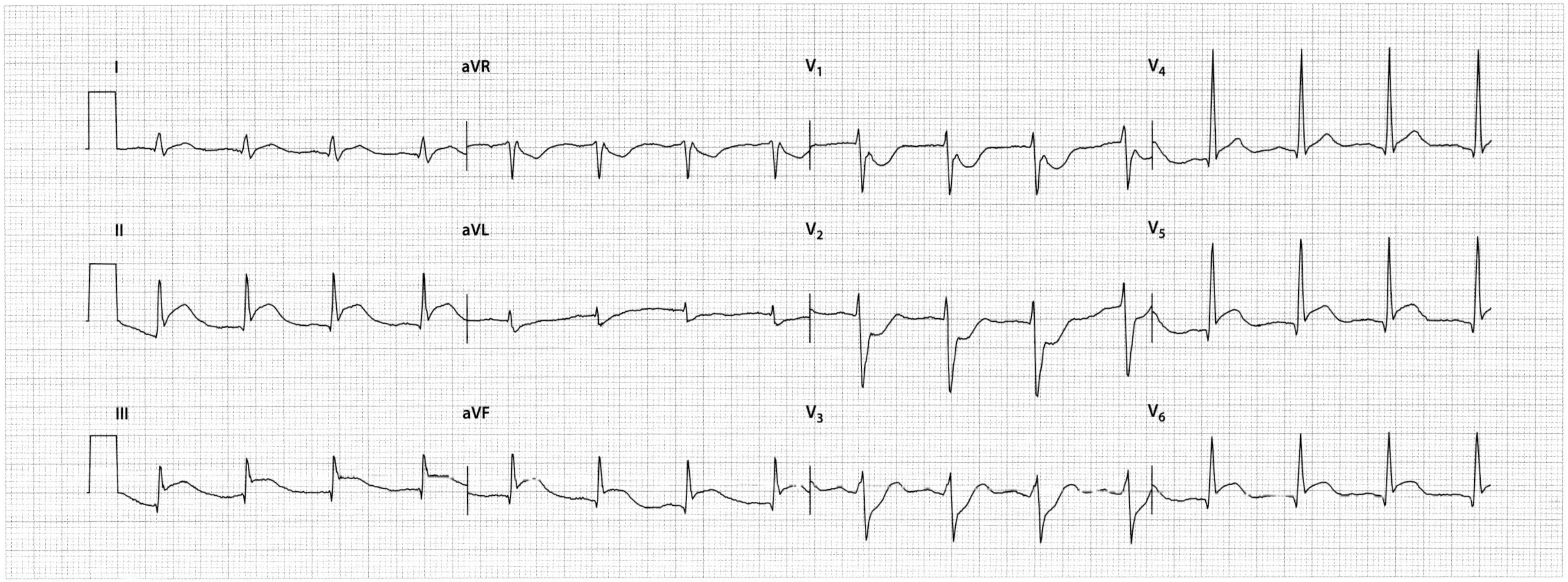

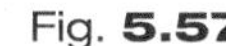

Fig. 5.57

Rate and rhythm? ______________________ Pathologic Q waves? ______________________

STE? ______________________ ST depression? ______________________ T-wave changes? ______________________

Reciprocal changes? ______________________ Imposter present? ______________________ Axis? ______________________

Interpretation: ____

Inferior: II, III, aVF | **Septum: V_1, V_2** | **Anterior: V_3, V_4** | **Lateral: I, aVL, V_5, V_6**

Fig. **5.58**

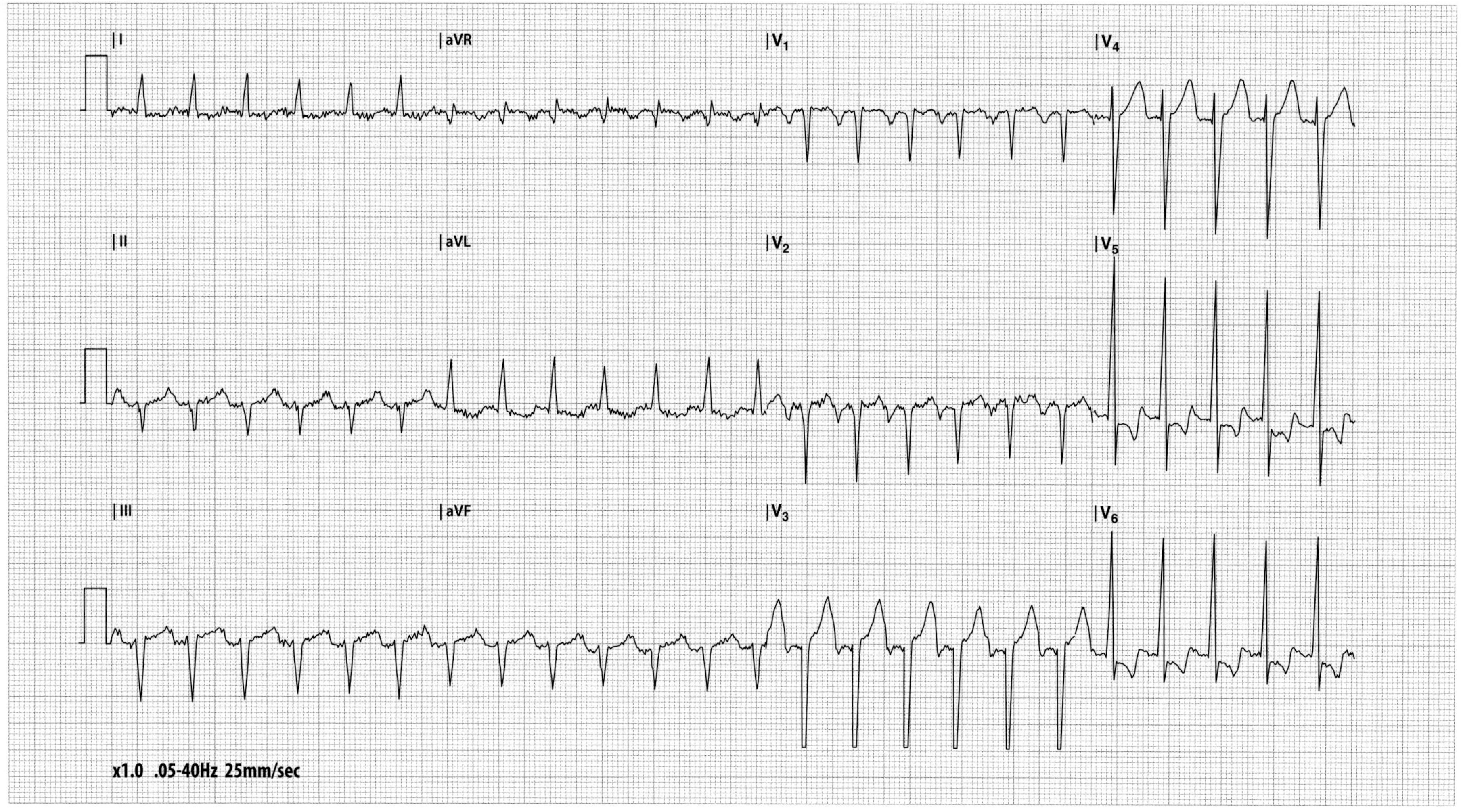

Rate and rhythm? ______ Pathologic Q waves? ______

STE? ______ ST depression? ______ T-wave changes? ______

Reciprocal changes? ______ Imposter present? ______ Axis? ______

Interpretation: ______

Inferior: II, III, aVF | **Septum: V_1, V_2** | **Anterior: V_3, V_4** | **Lateral: I, aVL, V_5, V_6**

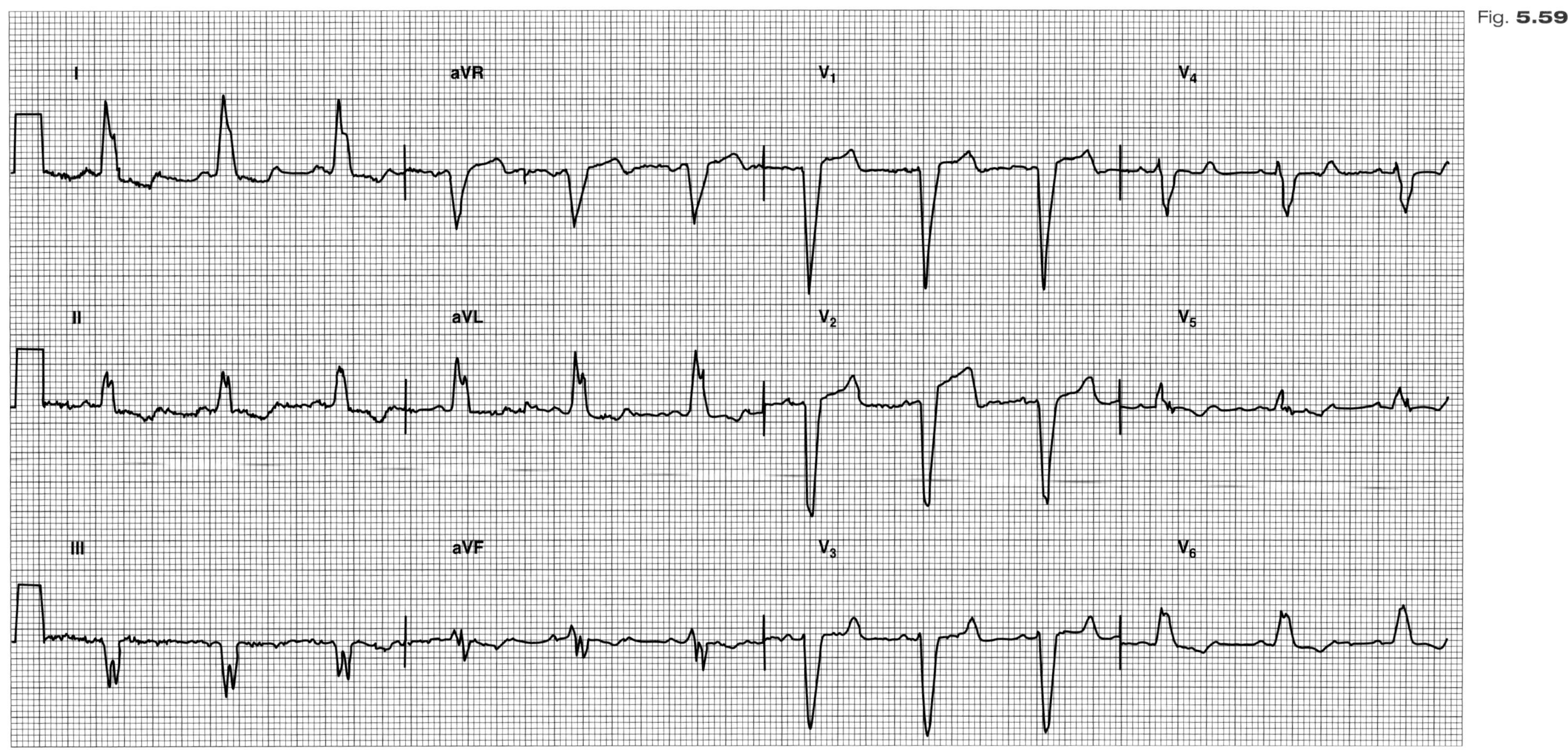

Fig. **5.59**

Rate and rhythm? ______ Pathologic Q waves? ______

STE? ______ ST depression? ______ T-wave changes? ______

Reciprocal changes? ______ Imposter present? ______ Axis? ______

Interpretation: ______

Inferior: II, III, aVF | **Septum: V_1, V_2** | Anterior: V_3, V_4 | **Lateral: I, aVL, V_5, V_6**

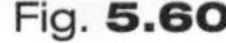

Fig. **5.60**

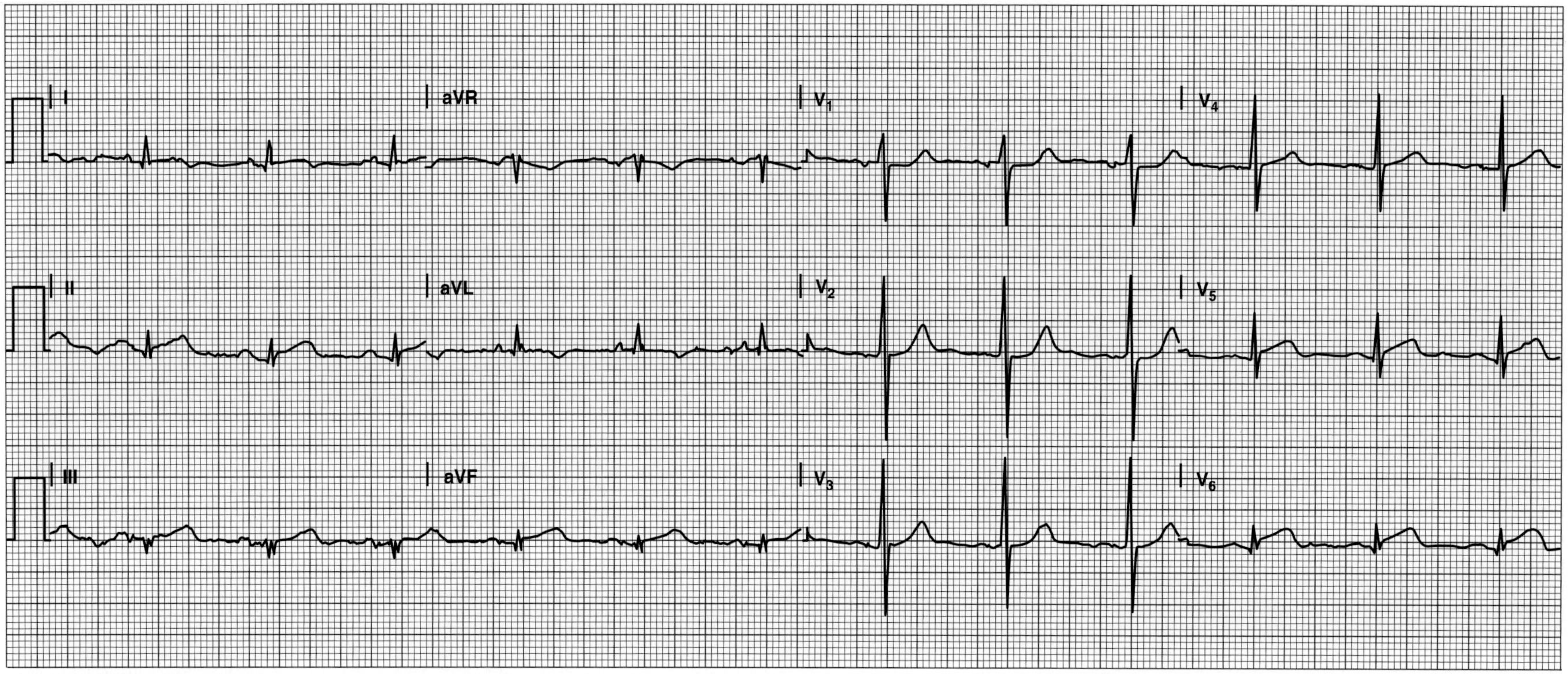

x1.0 0.05-150Hz 25mm/sec

Rate and rhythm? ______________________________ Pathologic Q waves? ______________________________

STE? ______________________ ST depression? ______________________ T-wave changes? ______________________

Reciprocal changes? ______________________ Imposter present? ______________________ Axis? ______________________

Interpretation: ____

Inferior: II, III, aVF | **Septum: V_1, V_2** | **Anterior: V_3, V_4** | **Lateral: I, aVL, V_5, V_6**

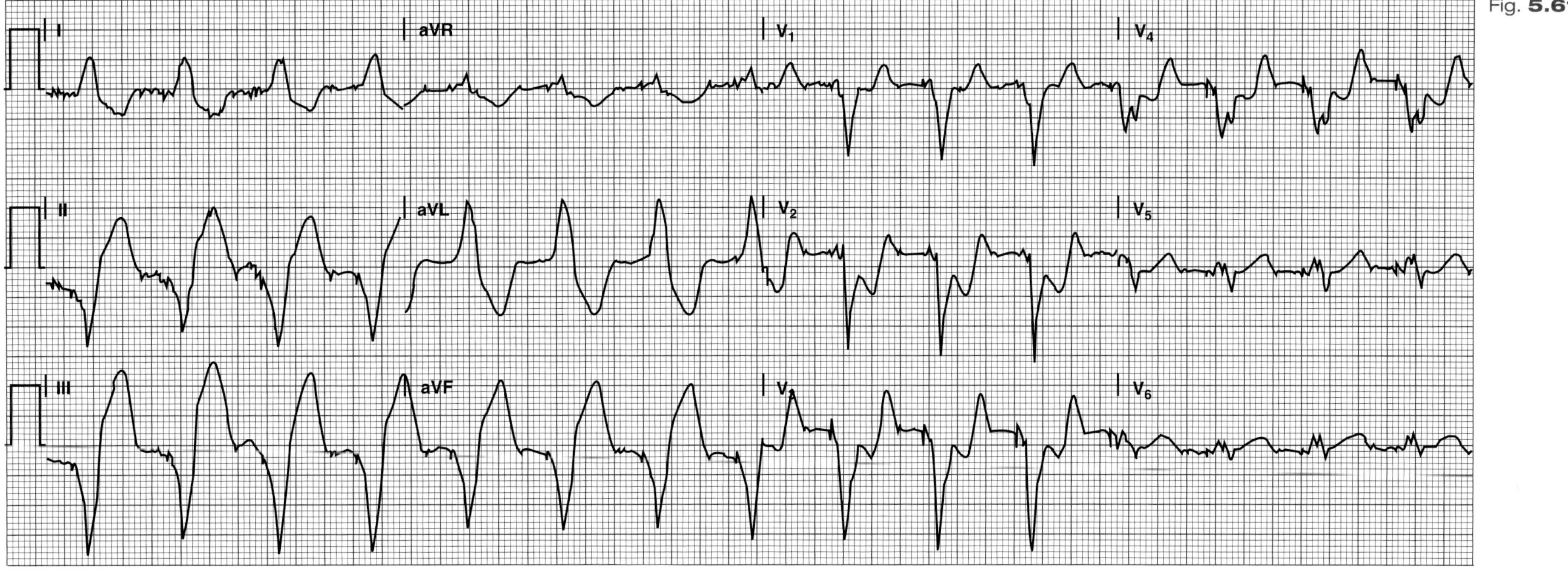

Fig. **5.61**

Rate and rhythm? ______ Pathologic Q waves? ______

STE? ______ ST depression? ______ T-wave changes? ______

Reciprocal changes? ______ Imposter present? ______ Axis? ______

Interpretation: ______

Inferior: II, III, aVF | **Septum: V_1, V_2** | **Anterior: V_3, V_4** | **Lateral: I, aVL, V_5, V_6**

Fig. **5.62**

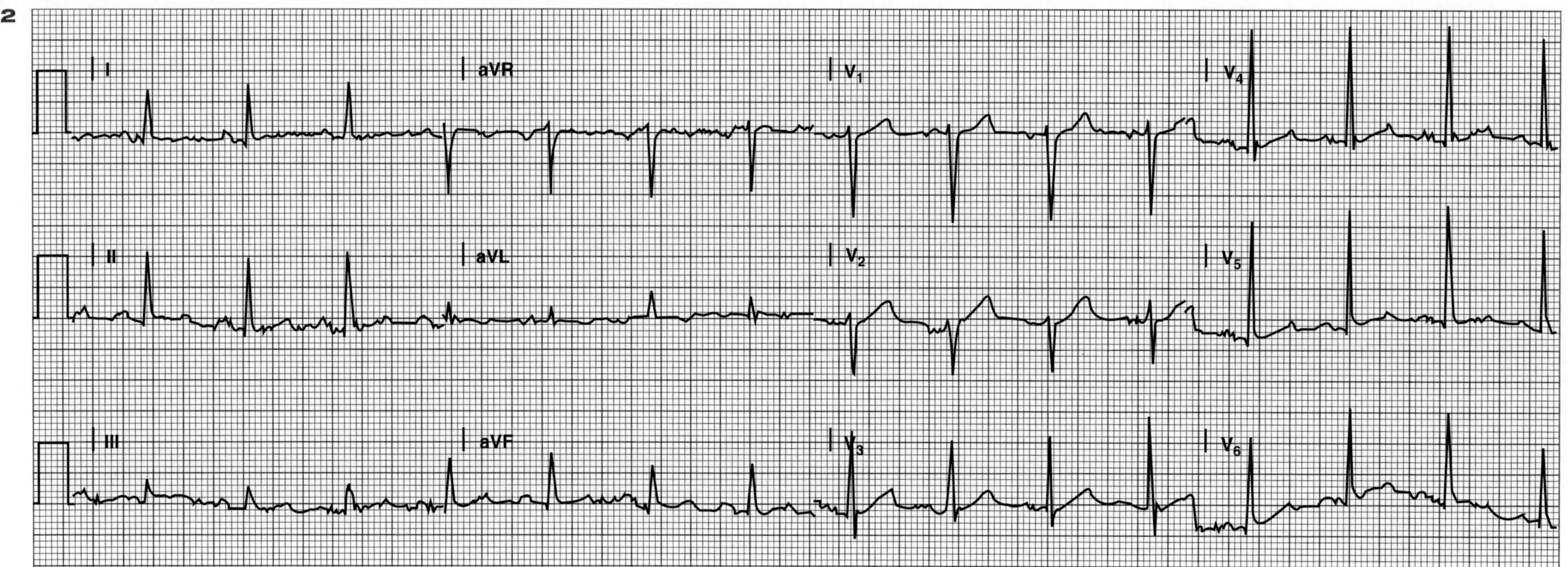

Rate and rhythm? ______________________ Pathologic Q waves? ______________________

STE? ______________________ ST depression? ______________________ T-wave changes?______________________

Reciprocal changes? ______________________ Imposter present? ______________________ Axis? ______________________

Interpretation:____

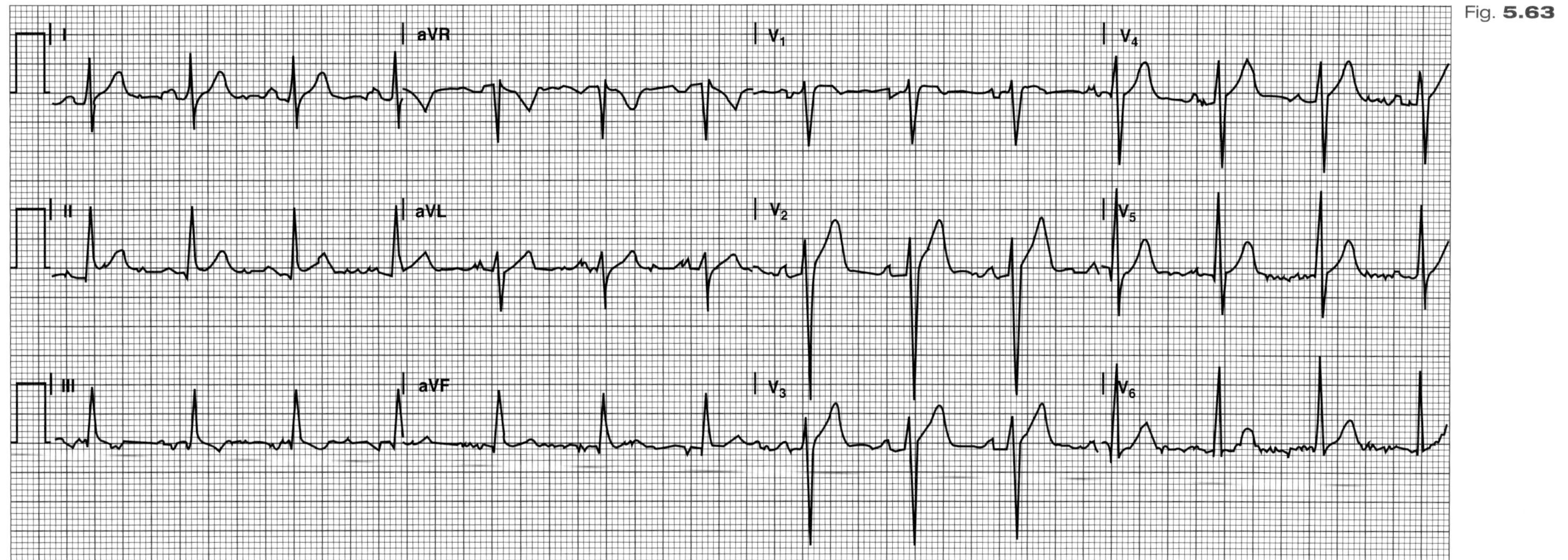

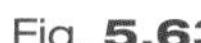
Fig. 5.63

Rate and rhythm? ______________________ Pathologic Q waves? ______________________

STE? ______________________ ST depression? ______________________ T-wave changes? ______________________

Reciprocal changes? ______________________ Imposter present? ______________________ Axis? ______________________

Interpretation: ____

Inferior: II, III, aVF | **Septum: V_1, V_2** | **Anterior: V_3, V_4** | **Lateral: I, aVL, V_5, V_6**

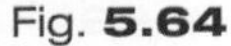

Fig. **5.64**

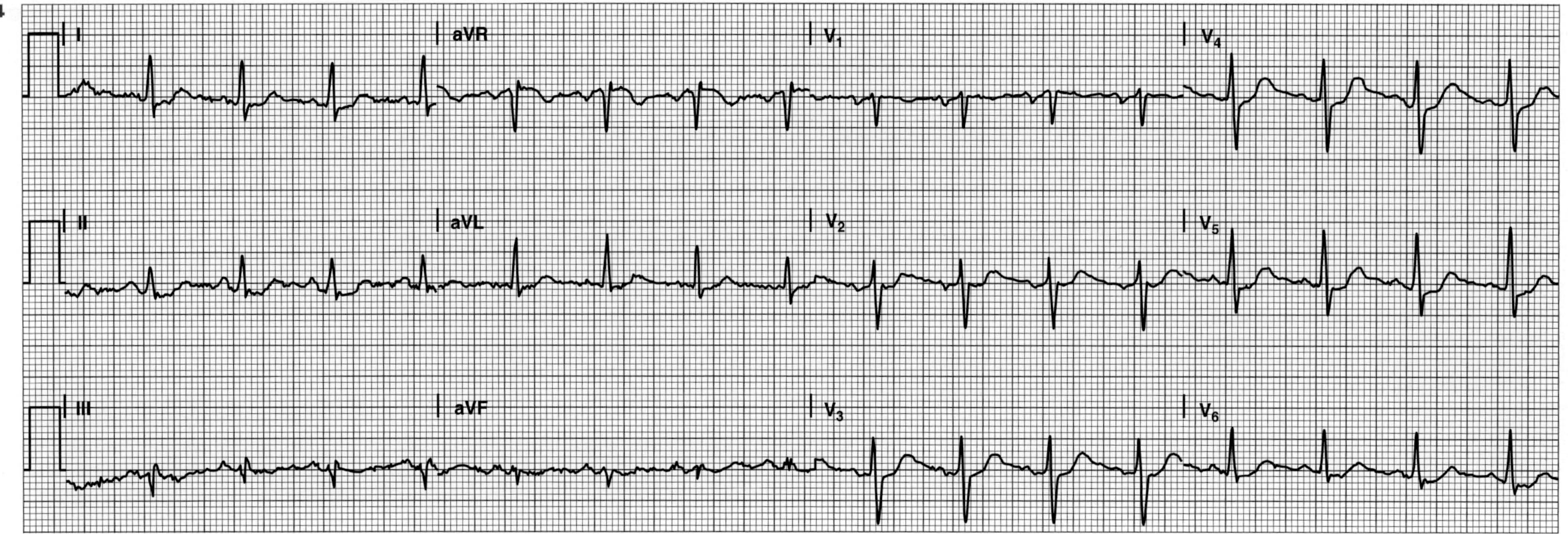

Rate and rhythm? ______________________ Pathologic Q waves? ______________________

STE? ______________________ ST depression? ______________________ T-wave changes? ______________________

Reciprocal changes? ______________________ Imposter present? ______________________ Axis? ______________________

Interpretation: ______________________

Inferior: II, III, aVF | **Septum: V_1, V_2** | **Anterior: V_3, V_4** | **Lateral: I, aVL, V_5, V_6**

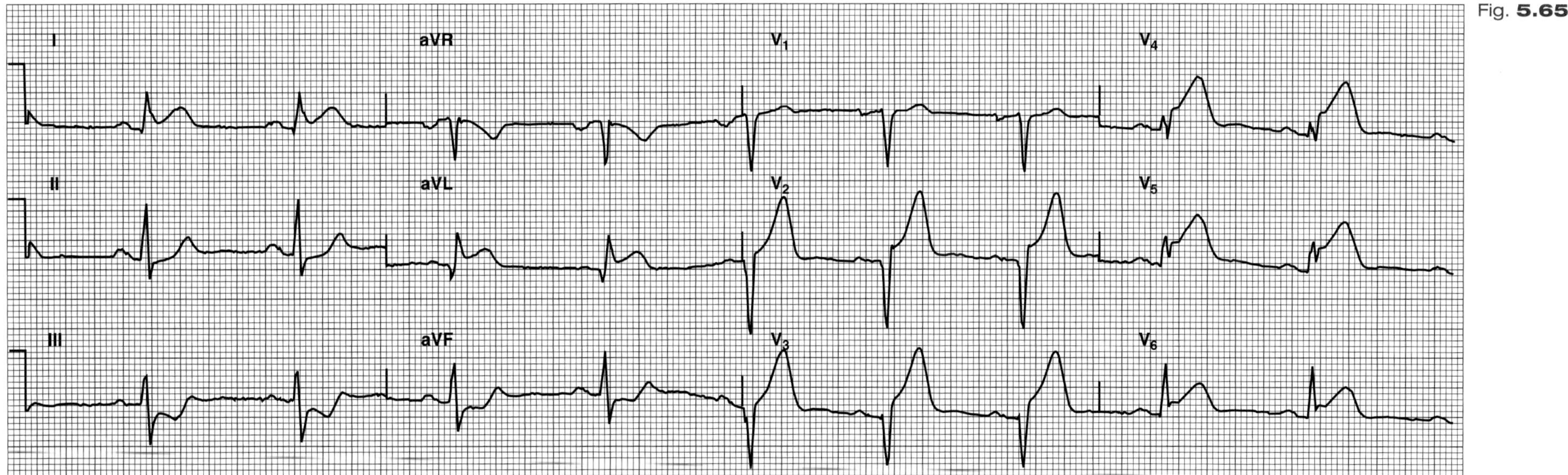

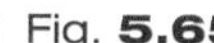
Fig. 5.65

Rate and rhythm? ______________________ Pathologic Q waves? ______________________

STE? ______________________ ST depression? ______________________ T-wave changes? ______________________

Reciprocal changes? ______________________ Imposter present? ______________________ Axis? ______________________

Interpretation: ____

Inferior: II, III, aVF | **Septum: V_1, V_2** | **Anterior: V_3, V_4** | **Lateral: I, aVL, V_5, V_6**

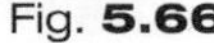

Fig. 5.66

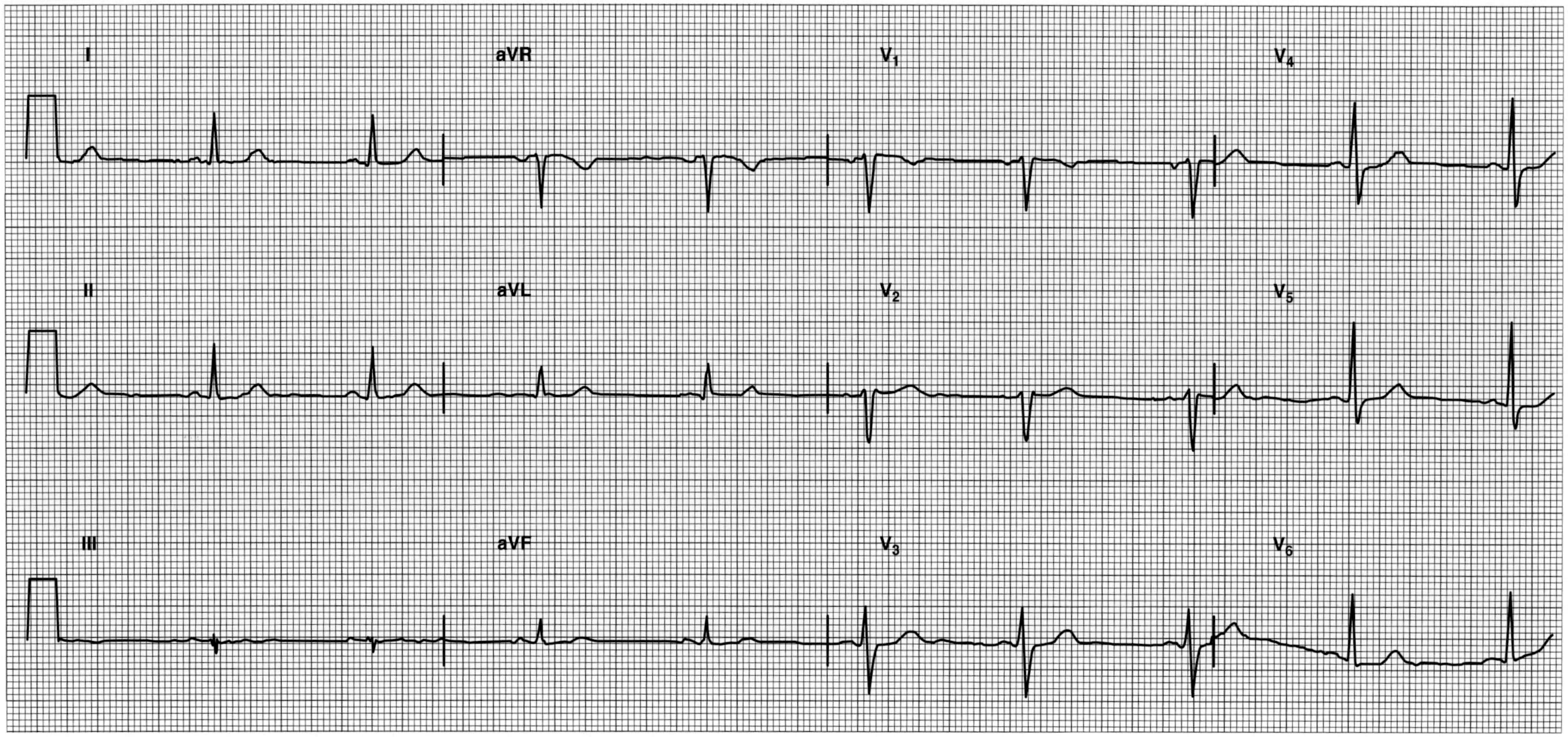

Rate and rhythm? ______ Pathologic Q waves? ______

STE? ______ ST depression? ______ T-wave changes? ______

Reciprocal changes? ______ Imposter present? ______ Axis? ______

Interpretation: ______

Inferior: II, III, aVF | **Septum: V_1, V_2** | **Anterior: V_3, V_4** | **Lateral: I, aVL, V_5, V_6**

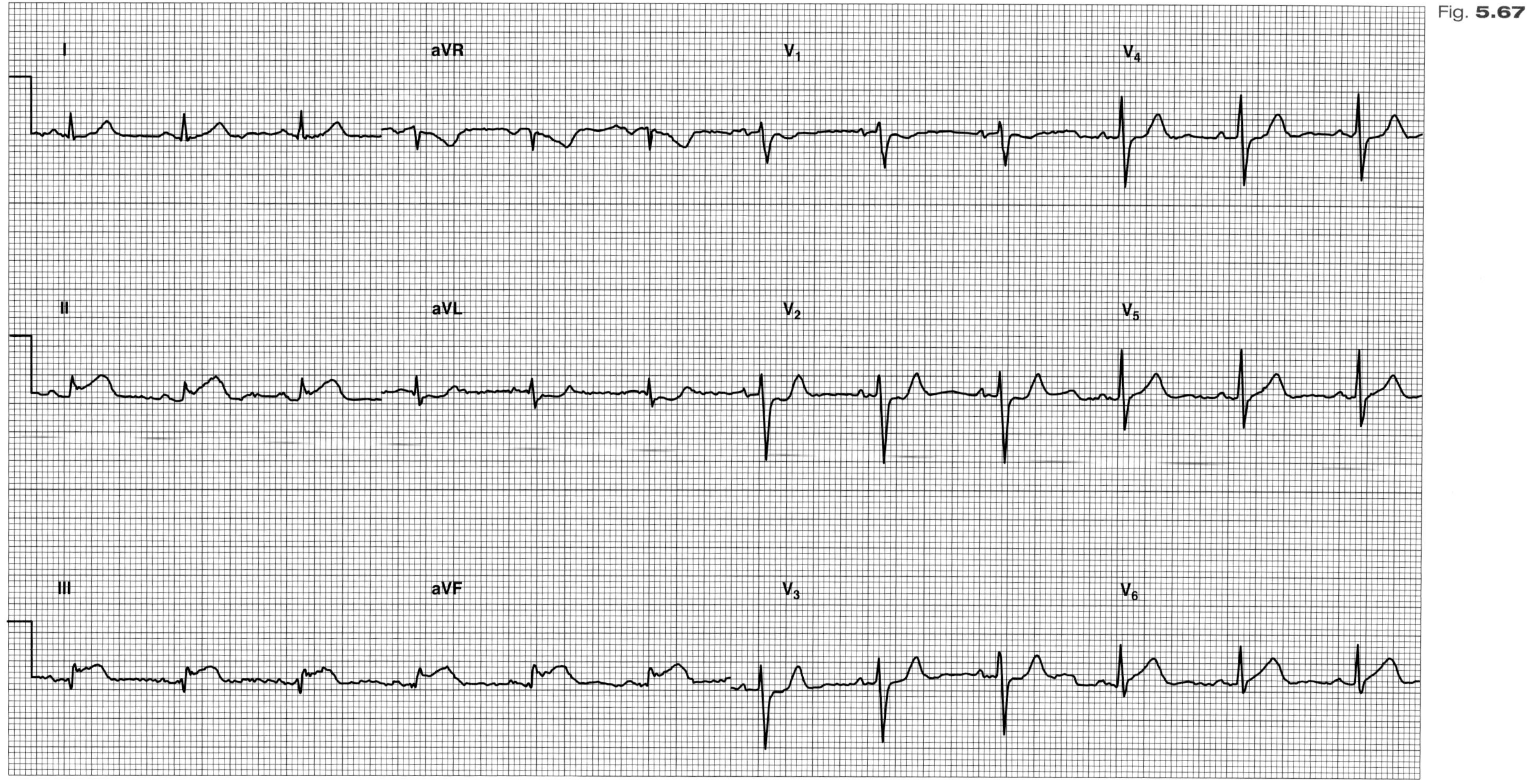

Fig. **5.67**

Rate and rhythm? ______________________ Pathologic Q waves? ______________________

STE? ______________________ ST depression? ______________________ T-wave changes? ______________________

Reciprocal changes? ______________________ Imposter present? ______________________ Axis? ______________________

Interpretation: ______________________

Inferior: II, III, aVF | **Septum: V_1, V_2** | **Anterior: V_3, V_4** | **Lateral: I, aVL, V_5, V_6**

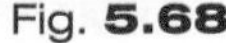
Fig. 5.68

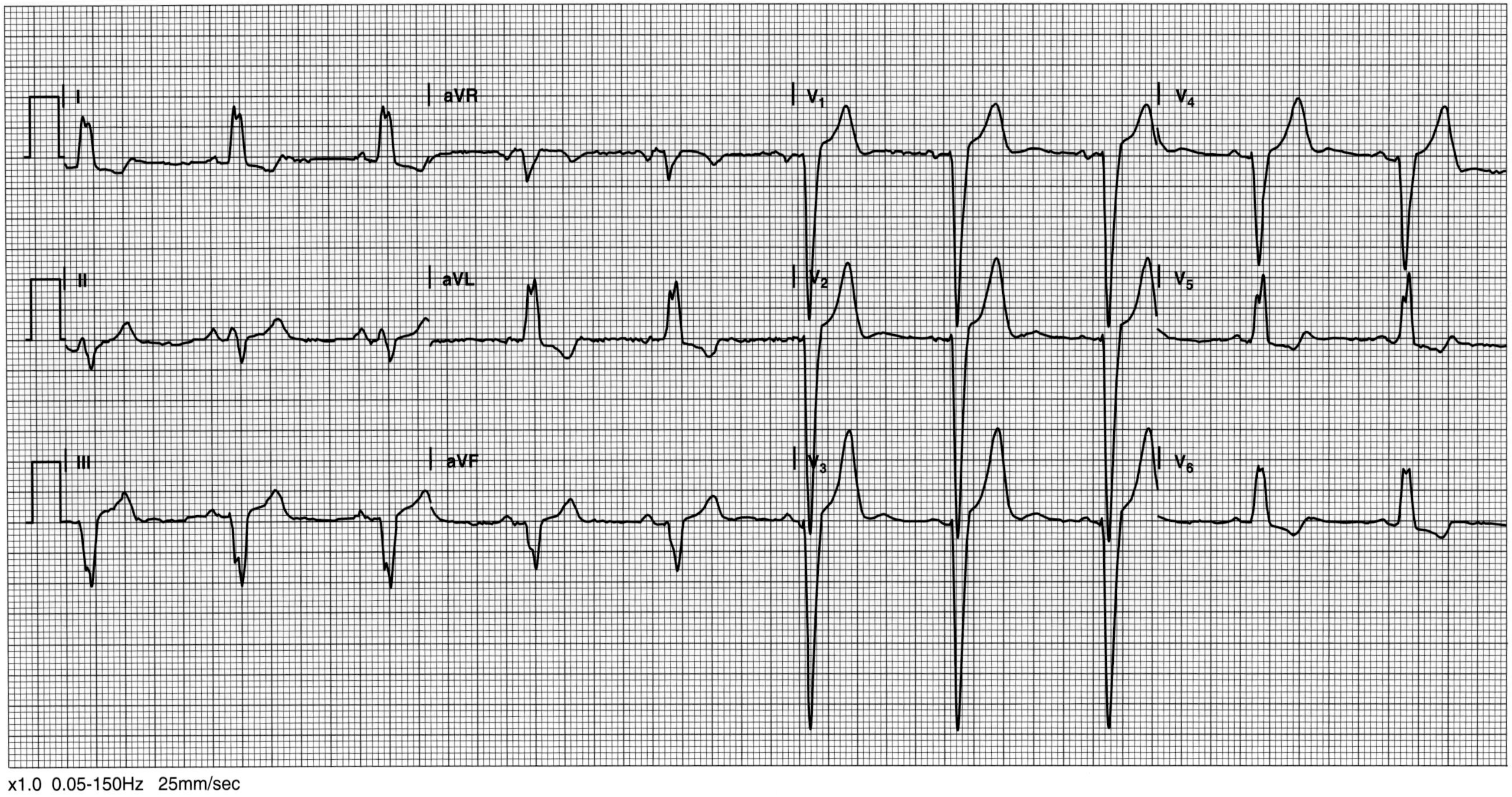

x1.0 0.05-150Hz 25mm/sec

Rate and rhythm? ______ Pathologic Q waves? ______

STE? ______ ST depression? ______ T-wave changes? ______

Reciprocal changes? ______ Imposter present? ______ Axis? ______

Interpretation: ______

Inferior: II, III, aVF | **Septum: V_1, V_2** | **Anterior: V_3, V_4** | **Lateral: I, aVL, V_5, V_6**

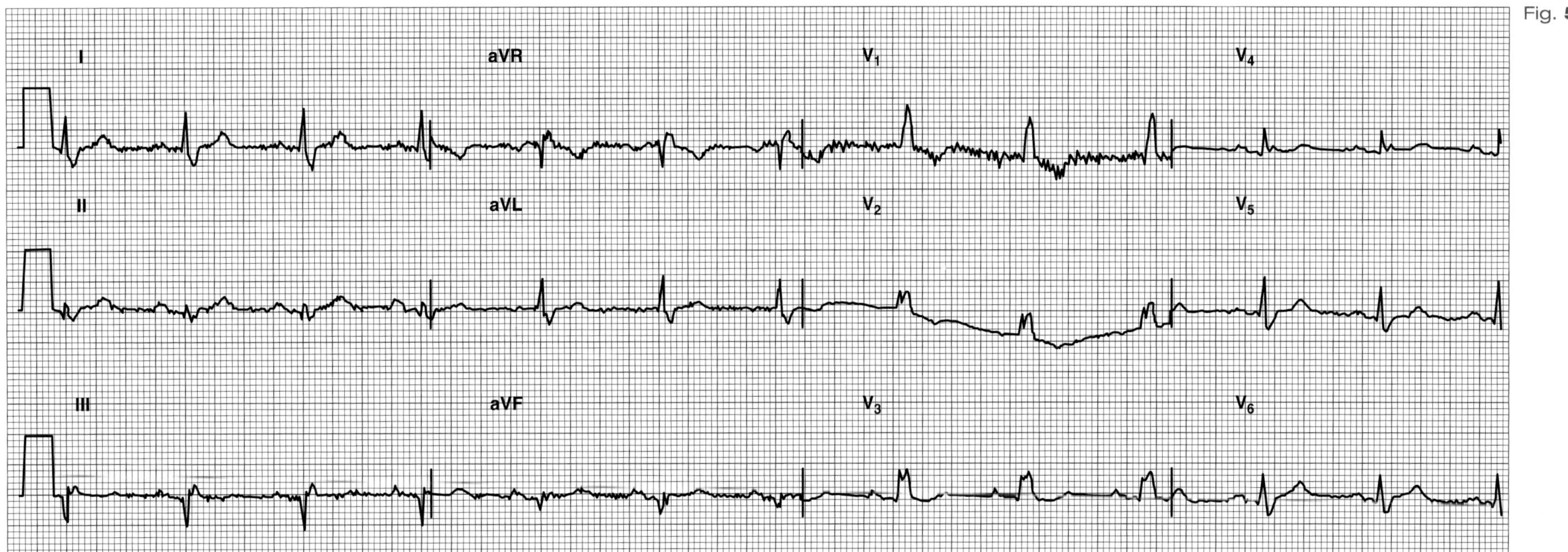

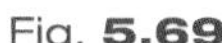
Fig. **5.69**

Rate and rhythm? ______________________ Pathologic Q waves? ______________________

STE? ______________________ ST depression? ______________________ T-wave changes? ______________________

Reciprocal changes? ______________________ Imposter present? ______________________ Axis? ______________________

Interpretation: ____

Inferior: II, III, aVF | **Septum: V_1, V_2** | Anterior: V_3, V_4 | **Lateral: I, aVL, V_5, V_6**

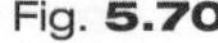

Fig. 5.70

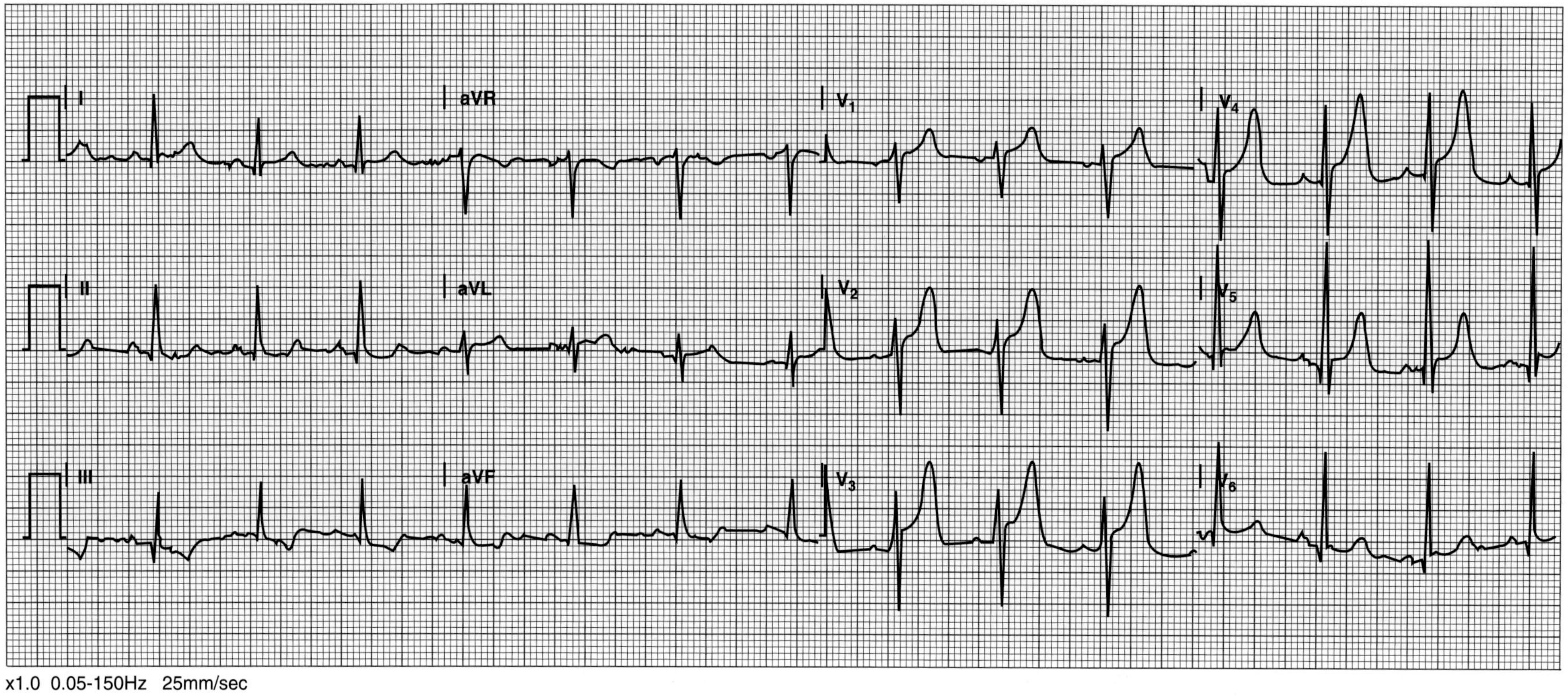

I aVR V_1 V_4

II aVL V_2 V_5

III aVF V_3 V_6

x1.0 0.05-150Hz 25mm/sec

Rate and rhythm? ______ Pathologic Q waves? ______

STE? ______ ST depression? ______ T-wave changes? ______

Reciprocal changes? ______ Imposter present? ______ Axis? ______

Interpretation: ______

Inferior: II, III, aVF | **Septum: V_1, V_2** | **Anterior: V_3, V_4** | **Lateral: I, aVL, V_5, V_6**

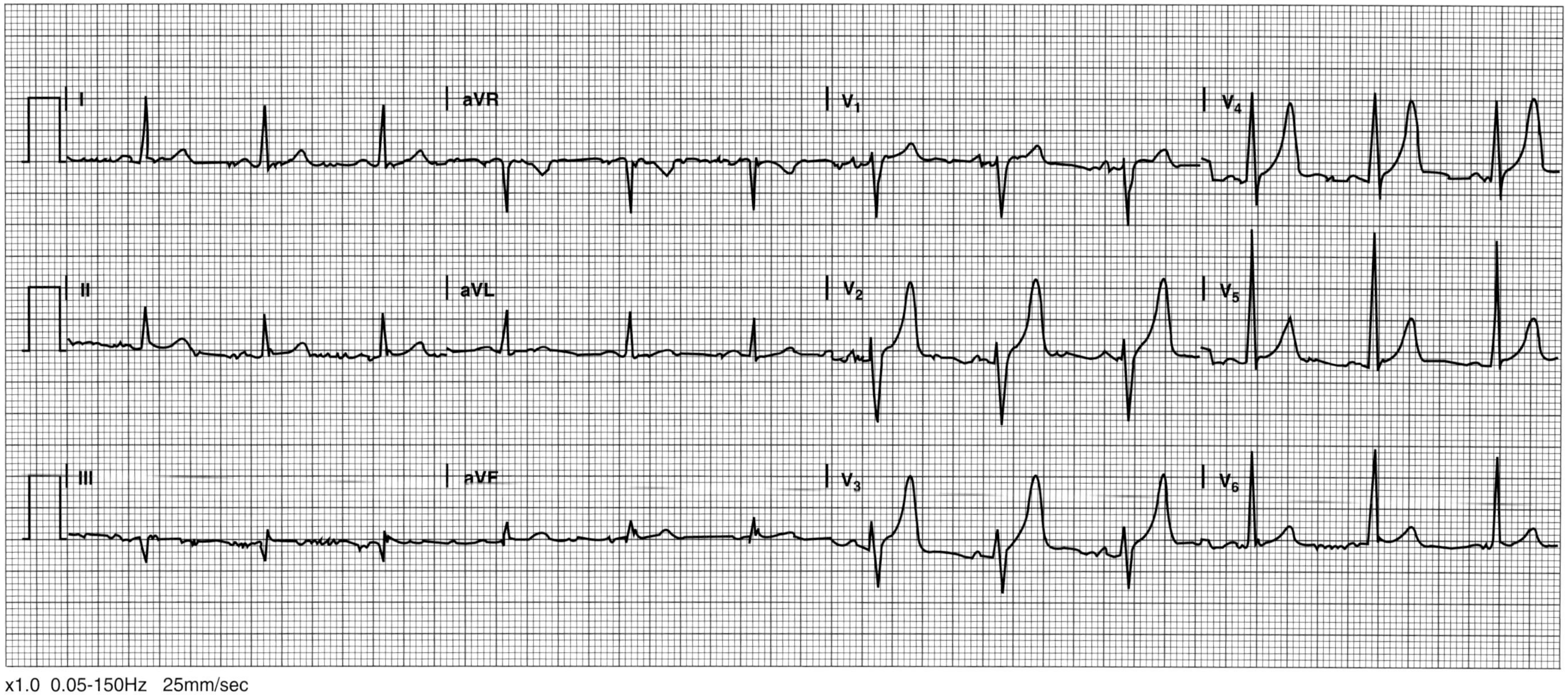

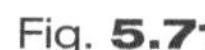

Fig. 5.71

x1.0 0.05-150Hz 25mm/sec

Rate and rhythm? ______________________ Pathologic Q waves? ______________________

STE? ______________________ ST depression? ______________________ T-wave changes?______________________

Reciprocal changes? ______________________ Imposter present? ______________________ Axis? ______________________

Interpretation:____

Inferior: II, III, aVF | **Septum: V_1, V_2** | **Anterior: V_3, V_4** | **Lateral: I, aVL, V_5, V_6**

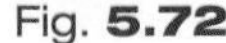

Fig. 5.72

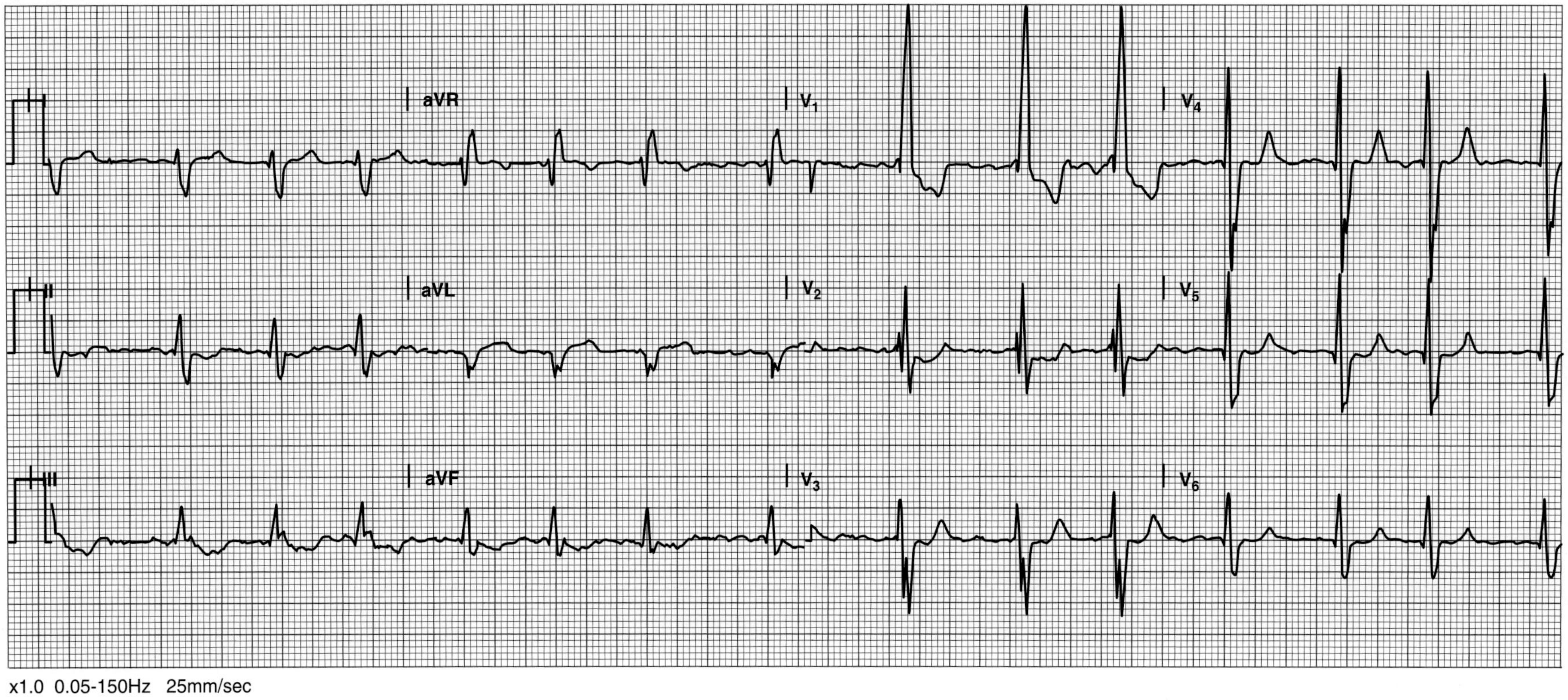

I aVR V_1 V_4

II aVL V_2 V_5

III aVF V_3 V_6

x1.0 0.05-150Hz 25mm/sec

Rate and rhythm? ______________________ Pathologic Q waves? ______________________

STE? ______________________ ST depression? ______________________ T-wave changes? ______________________

Reciprocal changes? ______________________ Imposter present? ______________________ Axis? ______________________

Interpretation: ____

Inferior: II, III, aVF | **Septum: V_1, V_2** | **Anterior: V_3, V_4** | **Lateral: I, aVL, V_5, V_6**

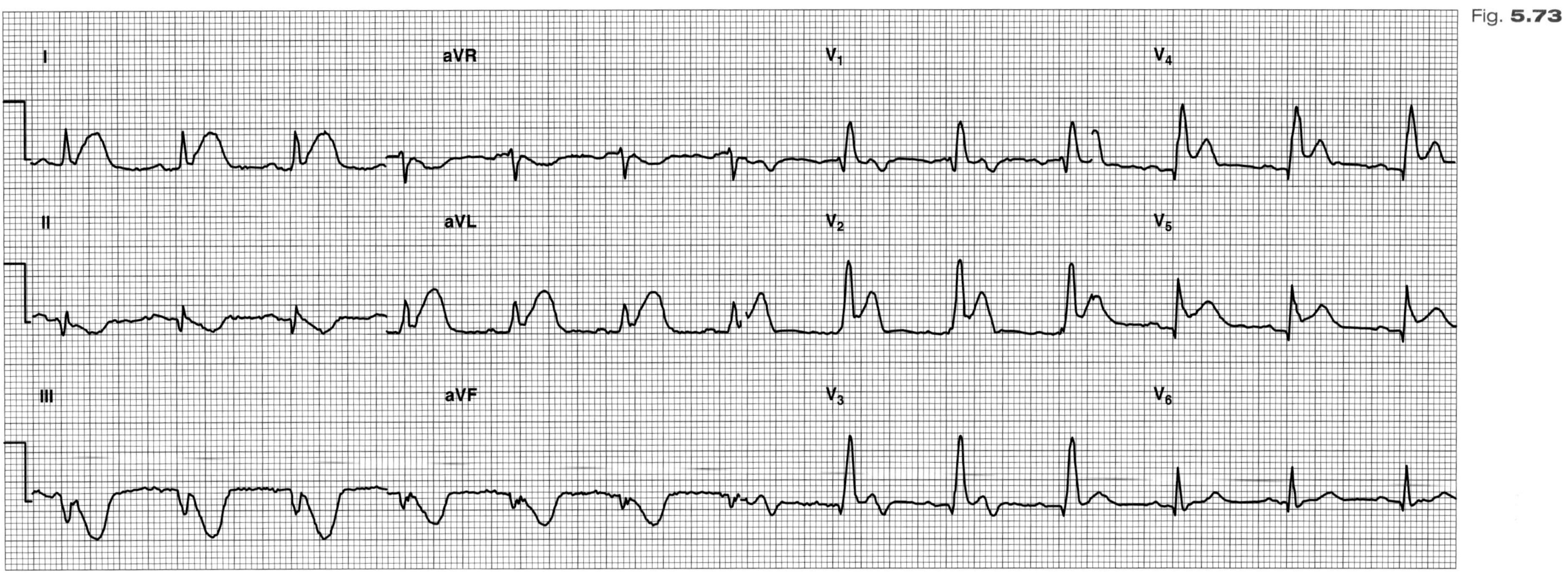

Fig. 5.73

Rate and rhythm? ______ Pathologic Q waves? ______

STE? ______ ST depression? ______ T-wave changes? ______

Reciprocal changes? ______ Imposter present? ______ Axis? ______

Interpretation: ______

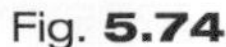
Fig. **5.74**

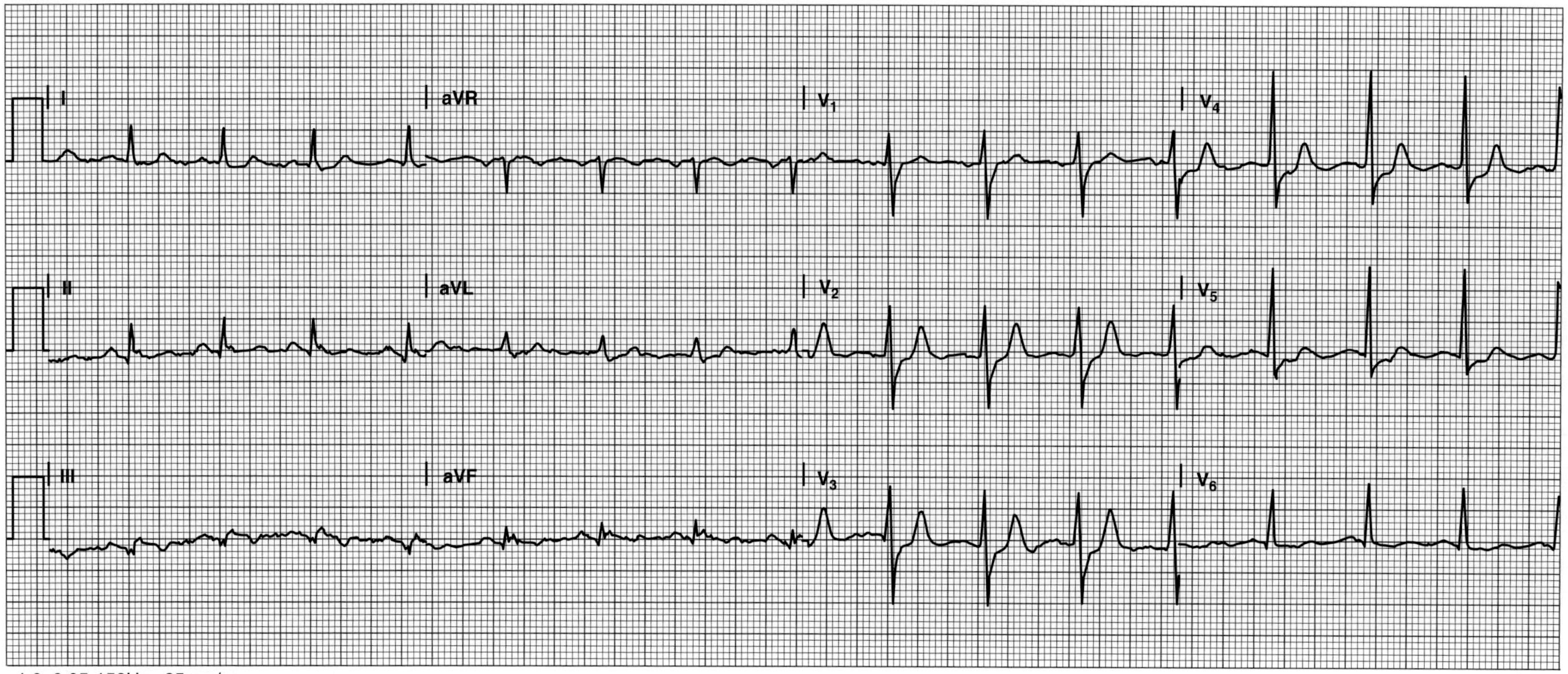

I aVR V_1 V_4
II aVL V_2 V_5
III aVF V_3 V_6

x1.0 0.05-150Hz 25mm/sec

Rate and rhythm? ____________________ Pathologic Q waves? ____________________

STE? ____________________ ST depression? ____________________ T-wave changes? ____________________

Reciprocal changes? ____________________ Imposter present? ____________________ Axis? ____________________

Interpretation: ____

Inferior: II, III, aVF | **Septum: V_1, V_2** | **Anterior: V_3, V_4** | **Lateral: I, aVL, V_5, V_6**

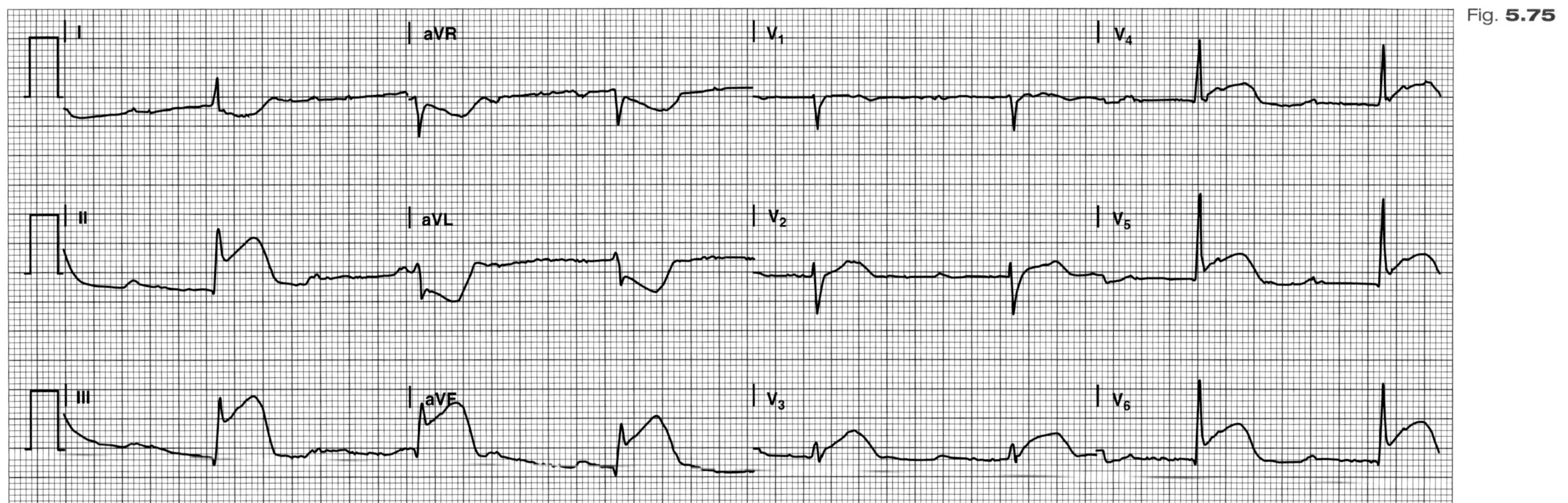

Fig. 5.75

Rate and rhythm? __________ Pathologic Q waves? __________

STE? __________ ST depression? __________ T-wave changes?__________

Reciprocal changes? __________ Imposter present? __________ Axis? __________

Interpretation:__________

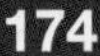

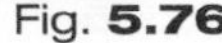

Fig. 5.76

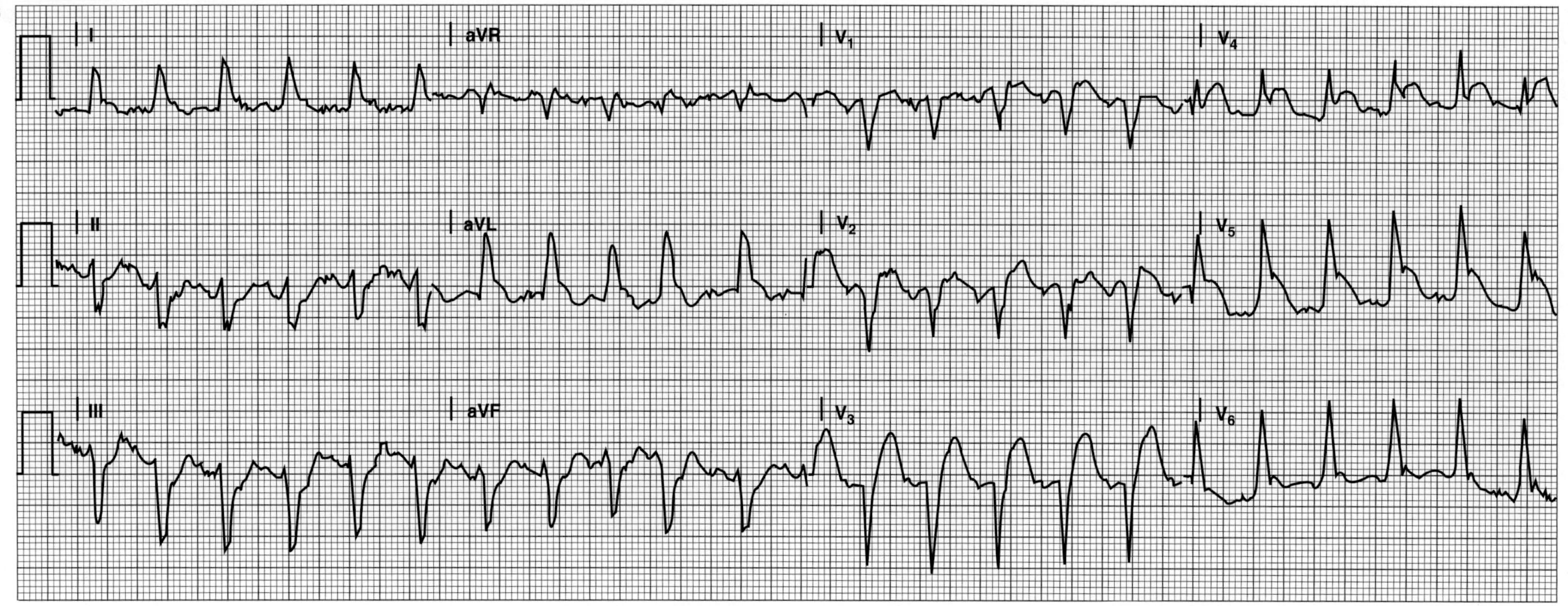

Rate and rhythm? __________ Pathologic Q waves? __________

STE? __________ ST depression? __________ T-wave changes? __________

Reciprocal changes? __________ Imposter present? __________ Axis? __________

Interpretation: __________

Inferior: II, III, aVF | **Septum: V_1, V_2** | **Anterior: V_3, V_4** | **Lateral: I, aVL, V_5, V_6**

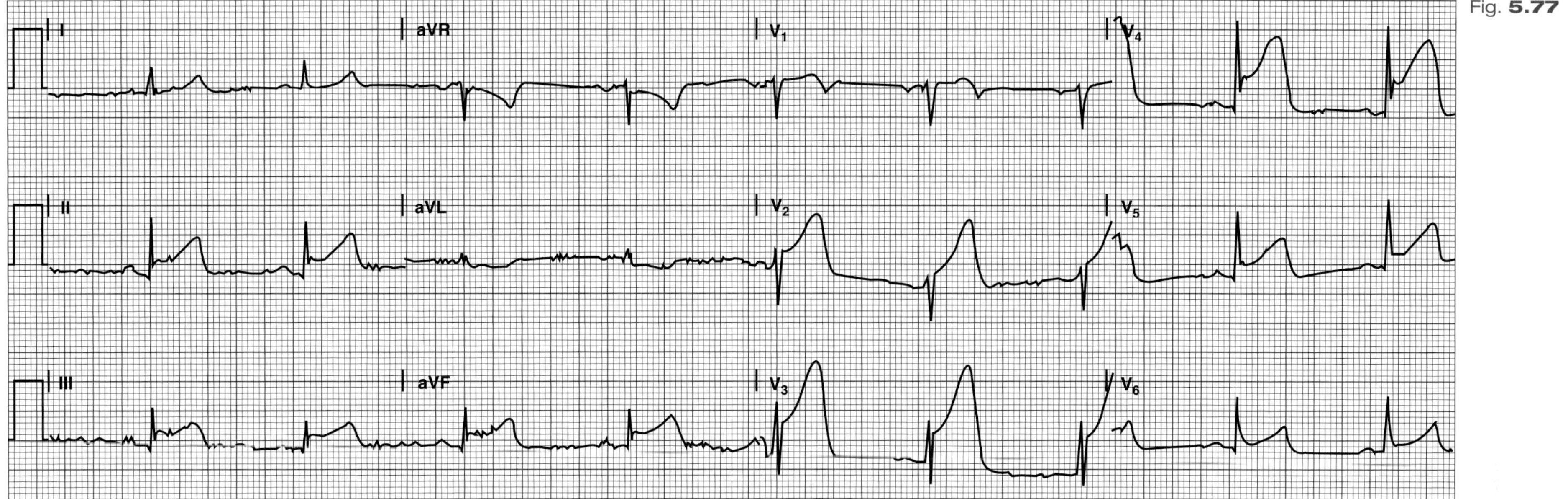

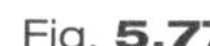
Fig. **5.77**

Rate and rhythm? __________ Pathologic Q waves? __________

STE? __________ ST depression? __________ T-wave changes? __________

Reciprocal changes? __________ Imposter present? __________ Axis? __________

Interpretation: __________

Inferior: II, III, aVF | **Septum: V_1, V_2** | **Anterior: V_3, V_4** | **Lateral: I, aVL, V_5, V_6**

Fig. **5.78**

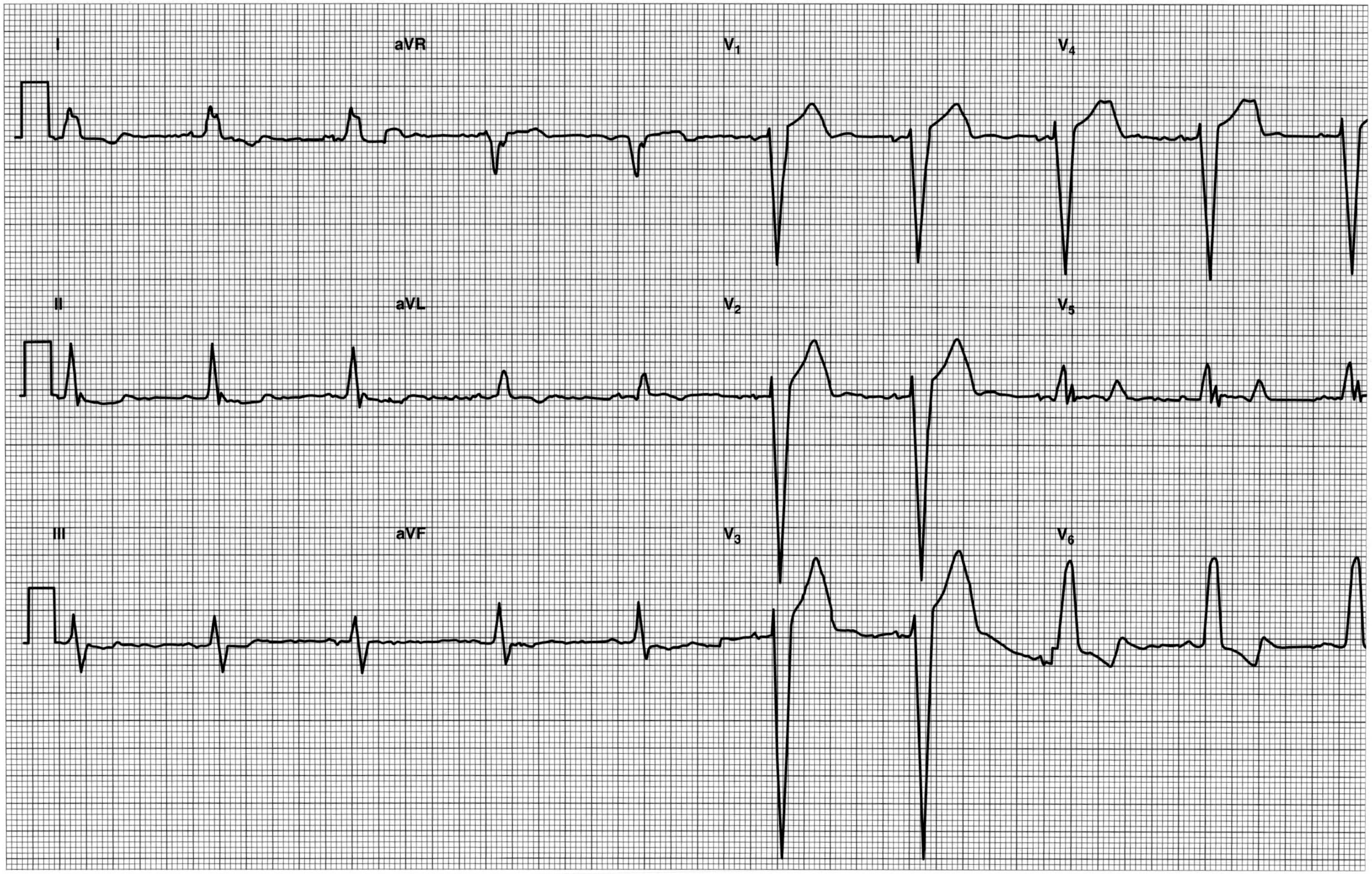

Rate and rhythm? __________ Pathologic Q waves? __________

STE? __________ ST depression? __________ T-wave changes? __________

Reciprocal changes? __________ Imposter present? __________ Axis? __________

Interpretation: __________

Inferior: II, III, aVF | **Septum: V_1, V_2** | Anterior: V_3, V_4 | **Lateral: I, aVL, V_5, V_6**

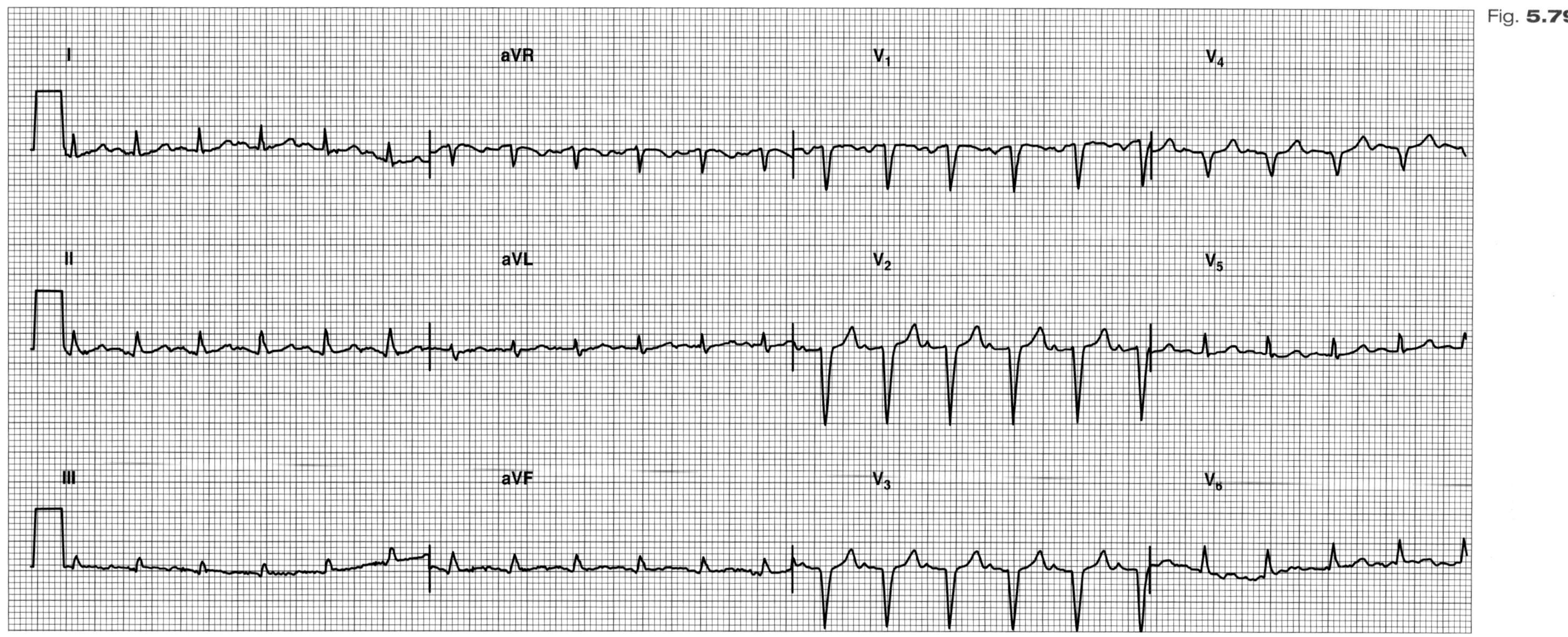

Fig. 5.79

Rate and rhythm? ______ Pathologic Q waves? ______

STE? ______ ST depression? ______ T-wave changes? ______

Reciprocal changes? ______ Imposter present? ______ Axis? ______

Interpretation: ______

Inferior: II, III, aVF | **Septum: V_1, V_2** | **Anterior: V_3, V_4** | **Lateral: I, aVL, V_5, V_6**

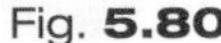

Fig. 5.80

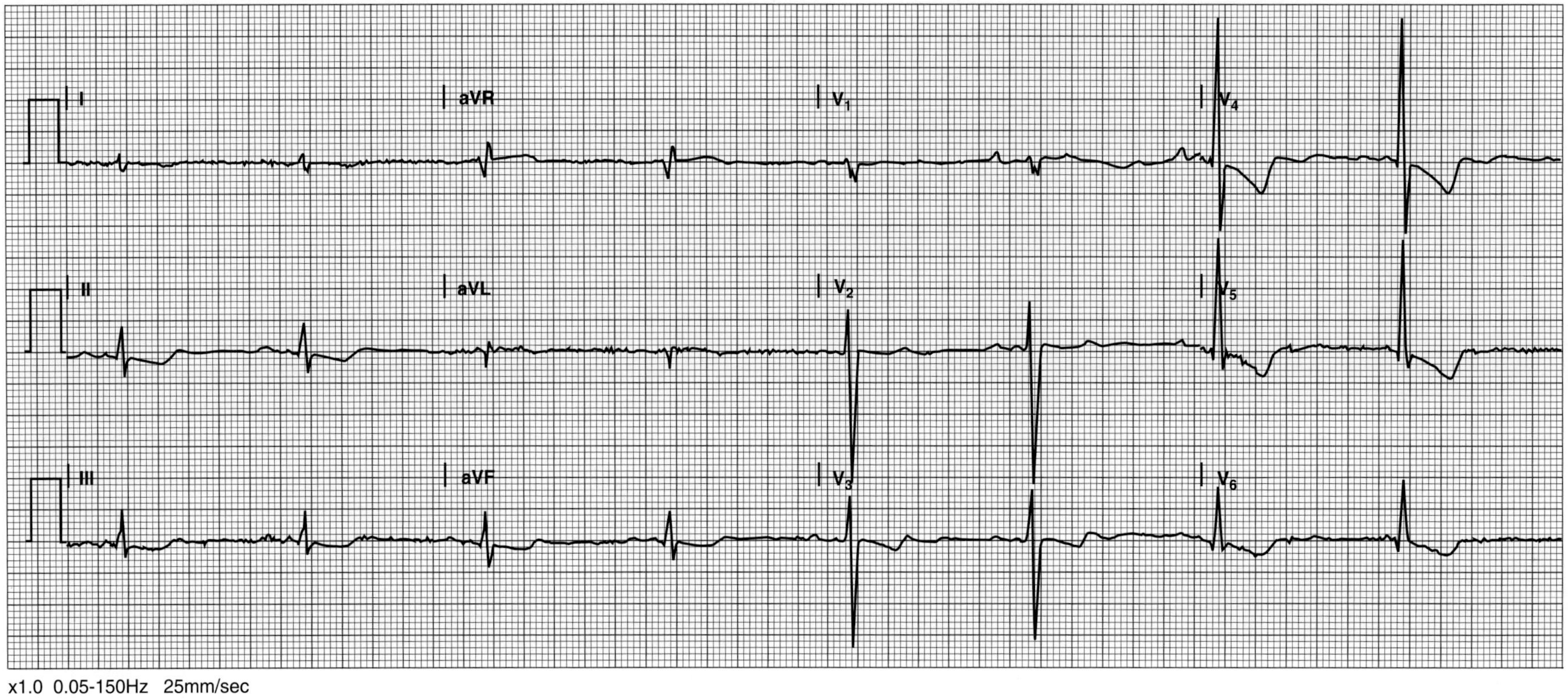

I | aVR | V1 | V4
II | aVL | V2 | V5
III | aVF | V3 | V6

x1.0 0.05-150Hz 25mm/sec

Rate and rhythm? ____________________ Pathologic Q waves? ____________________

STE? ____________________ ST depression? ____________________ T-wave changes? ____________________

Reciprocal changes? ____________________ Imposter present? ____________________ Axis? ____________________

Interpretation: ____________________

Inferior: II, III, aVF | **Septum: V_1, V_2** | **Anterior: V_3, V_4** | **Lateral: I, aVL, V_5, V_6**

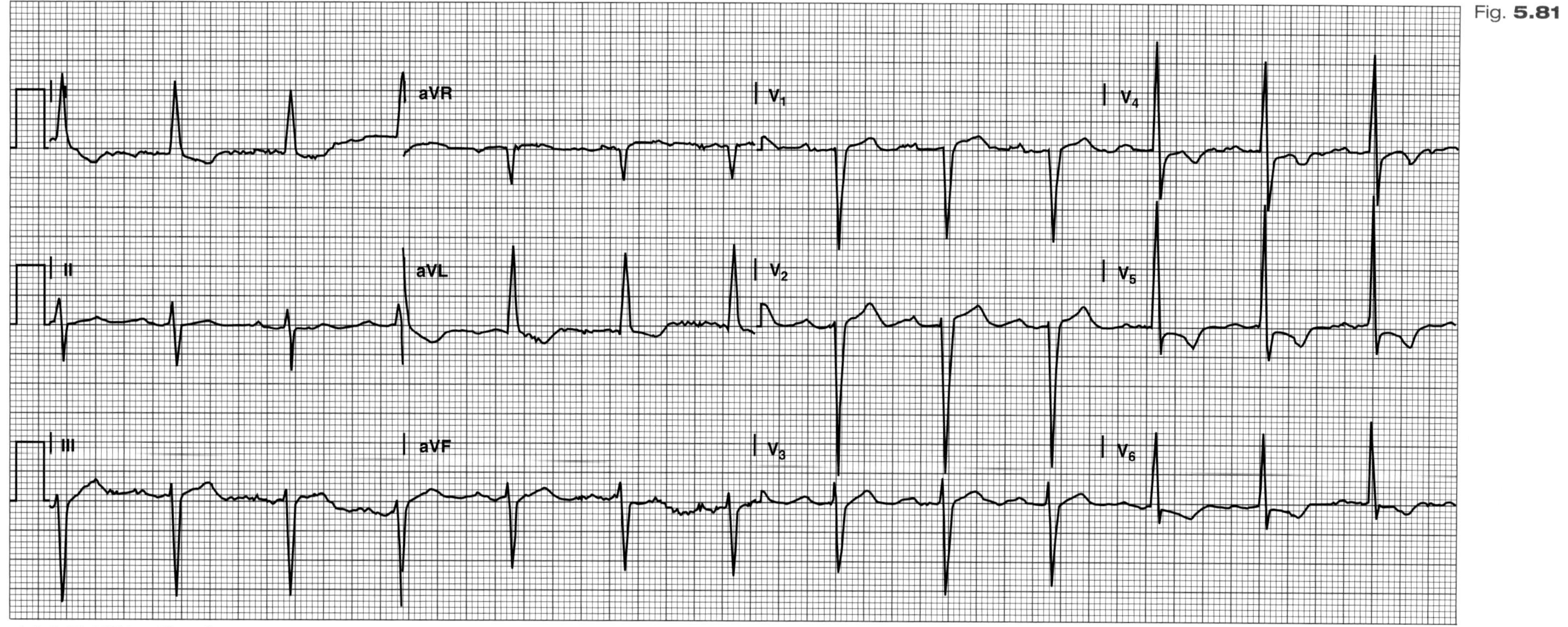

Fig. 5.81

Rate and rhythm? ______ Pathologic Q waves? ______

STE? ______ ST depression? ______ T-wave changes? ______

Reciprocal changes? ______ Imposter present? ______ Axis? ______

Interpretation: ______

Inferior: II, III, aVF | **Septum: V_1, V_2** | **Anterior: V_3, V_4** | **Lateral: I, aVL, V_5, V_6**

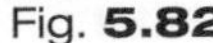
Fig. 5.82

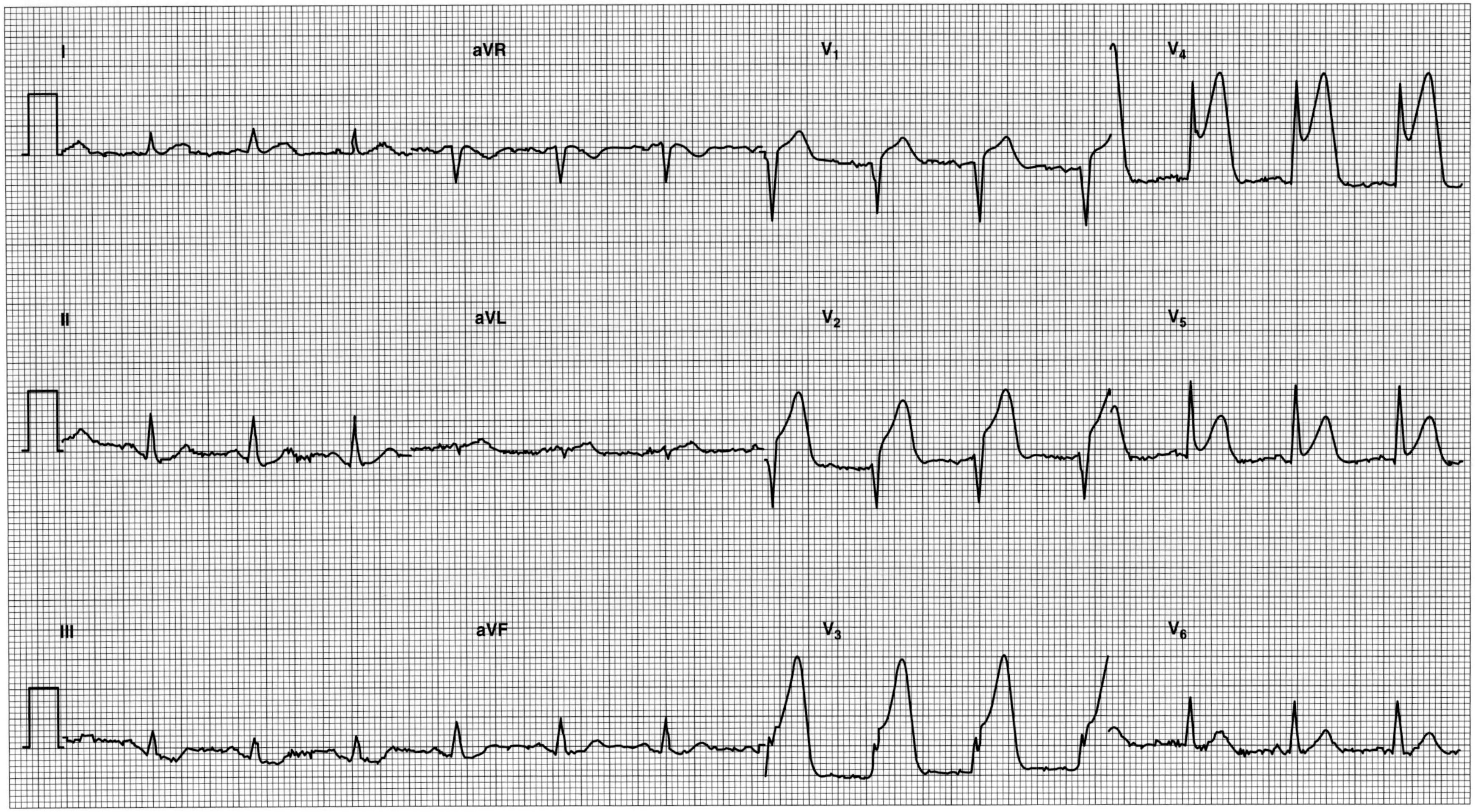

I aVR V_1 V_4

II aVL V_2 V_5

III aVF V_3 V_6

Rate and rhythm? ______________________ Pathologic Q waves? ______________________

STE? ______________________ ST depression? ______________________ T-wave changes? ______________________

Reciprocal changes? ______________________ Imposter present? ______________________ Axis? ______________________

Interpretation: ______________________

Inferior: II, III, aVF | **Septum: V_1, V_2** | **Anterior: V_3, V_4** | **Lateral: I, aVL, V_5, V_6**

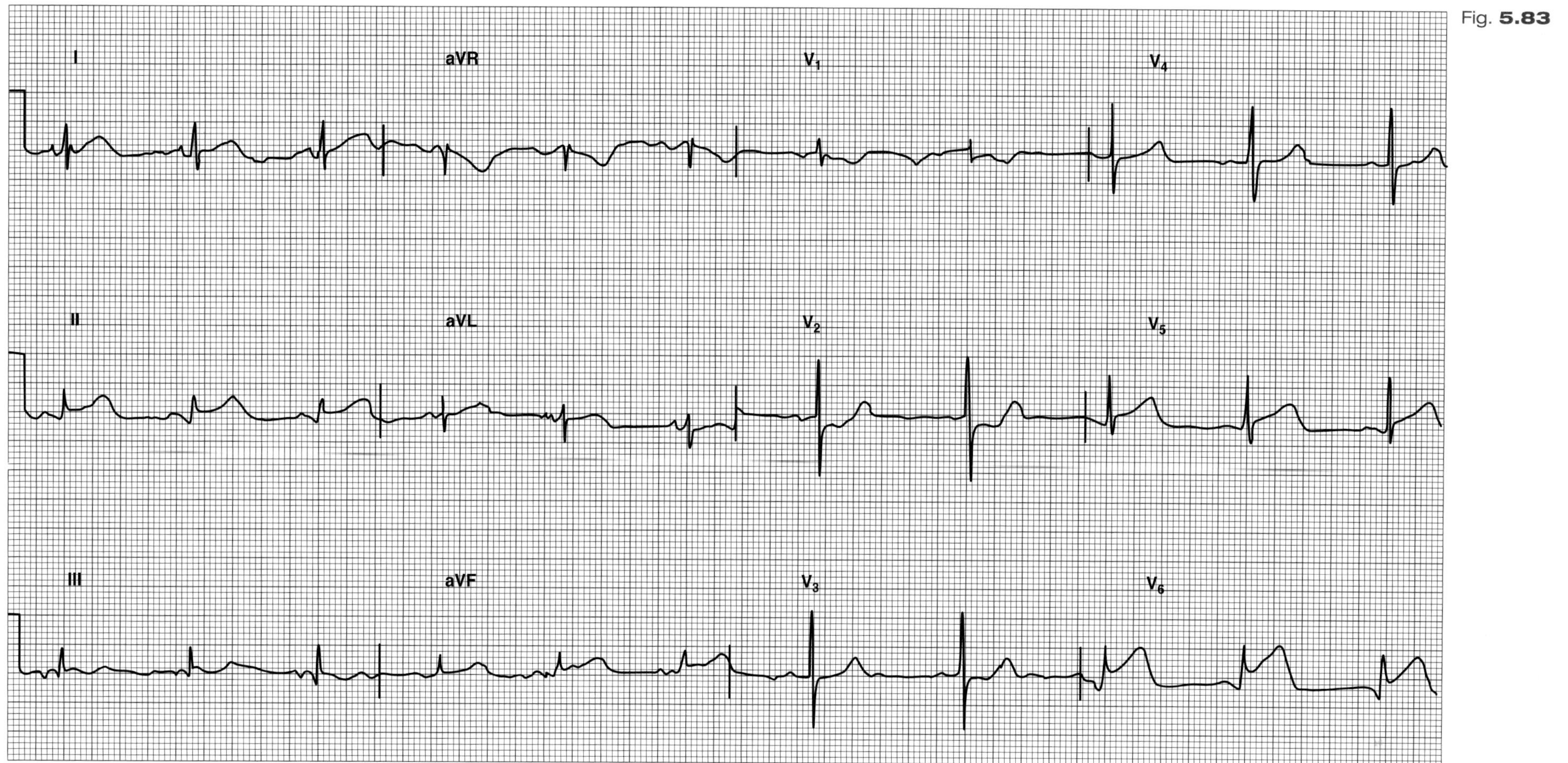

Fig. 5.83

Rate and rhythm? ______ Pathologic Q waves? ______

STE? ______ ST depression? ______ T-wave changes? ______

Reciprocal changes? ______ Imposter present? ______ Axis? ______

Interpretation: ______

Inferior: II, III, aVF | **Septum: V_1, V_2** | Anterior: V_3, V_4 | **Lateral: I, aVL, V_5, V_6**

Fig. **5.84**

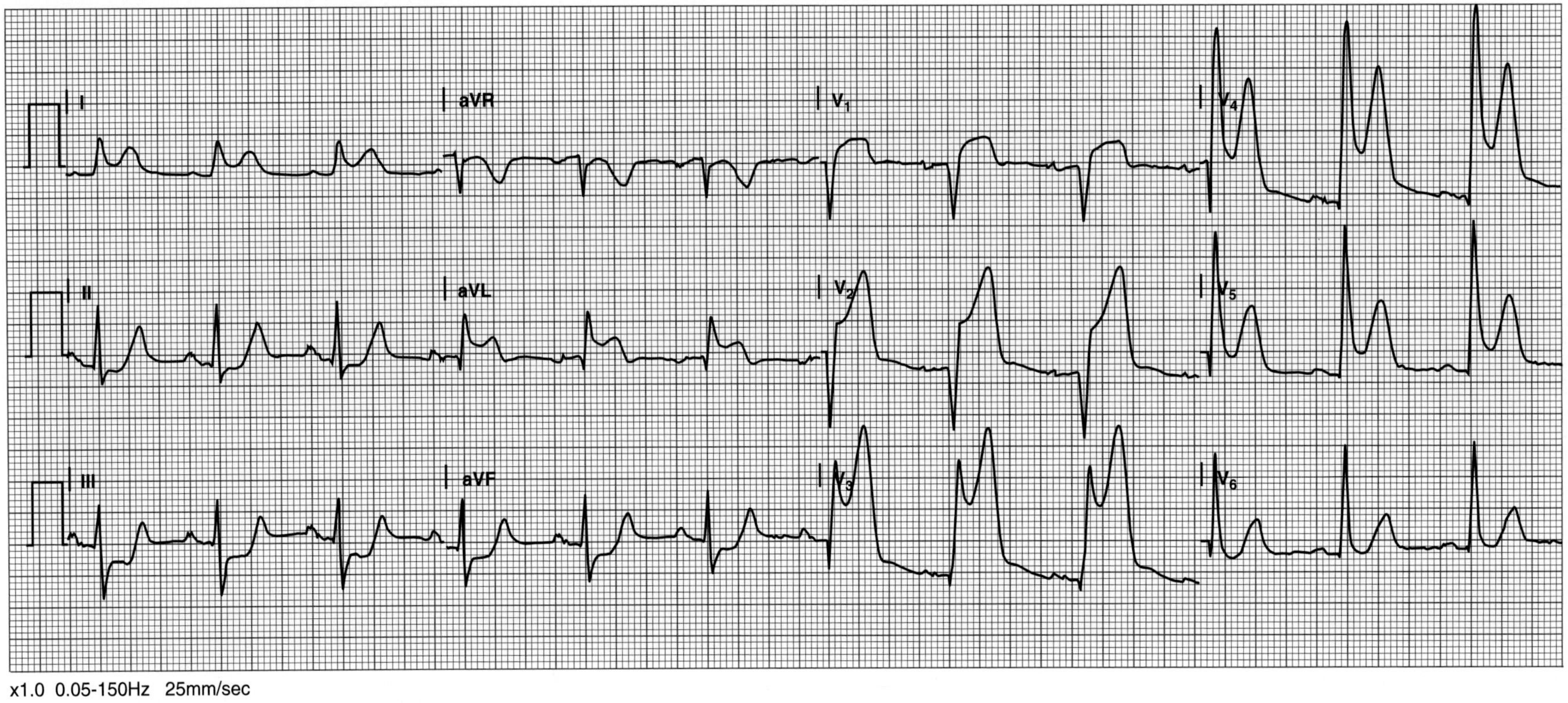

I aVR V_1 V_4
II aVL V_2 V_5
III aVF V_3 V_6

x1.0 0.05-150Hz 25mm/sec

Rate and rhythm? ______ Pathologic Q waves? ______

STE? ______ ST depression? ______ T-wave changes? ______

Reciprocal changes? ______ Imposter present? ______ Axis? ______

Interpretation: ______

Inferior: II, III, aVF | **Septum: V_1, V_2** | **Anterior: V_3, V_4** | **Lateral: I, aVL, V_5, V_6**

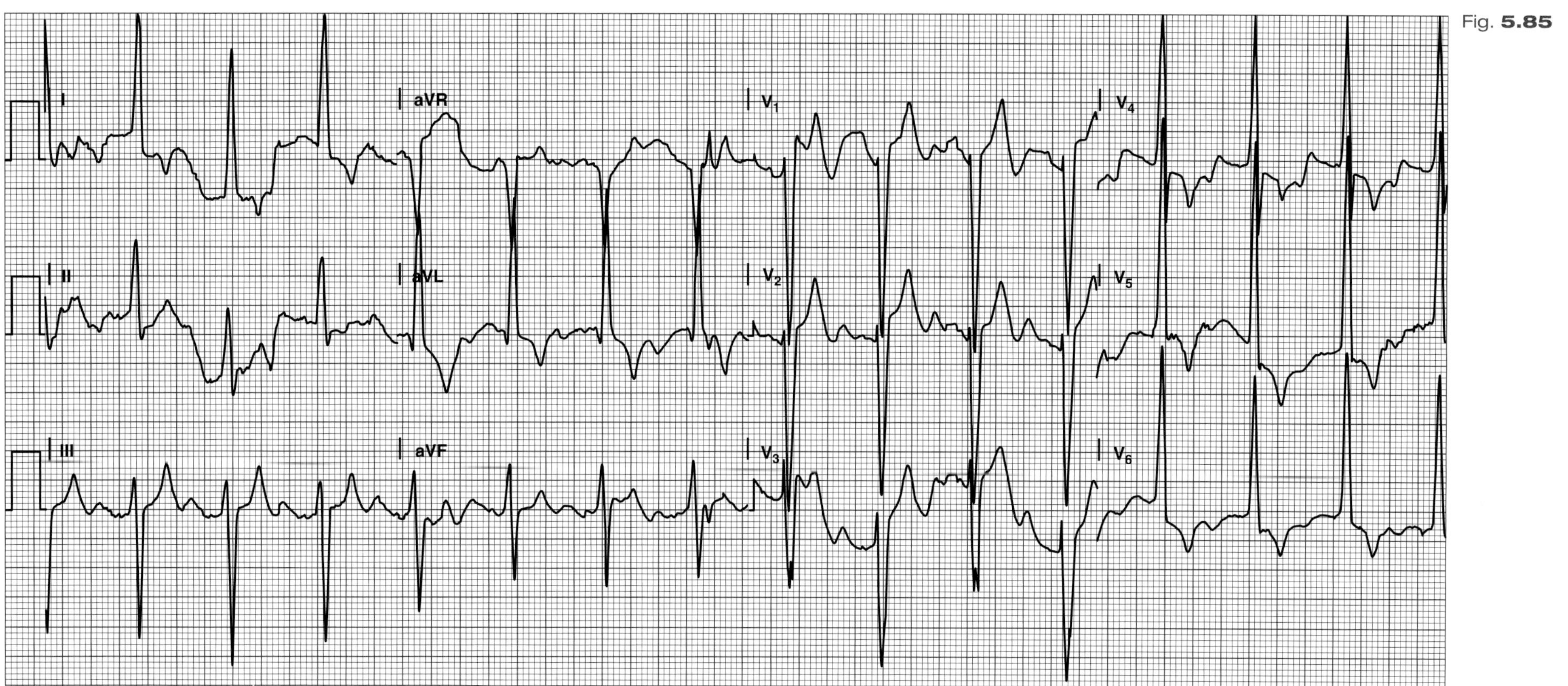

Fig. 5.85

Rate and rhythm? ______________________ Pathologic Q waves? ______________________

STE? ______________________ ST depression? ______________________ T-wave changes?______________________

Reciprocal changes? ______________________ Imposter present? ______________________ Axis? ______________________

Interpretation:______________________

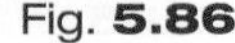
Fig. **5.86**

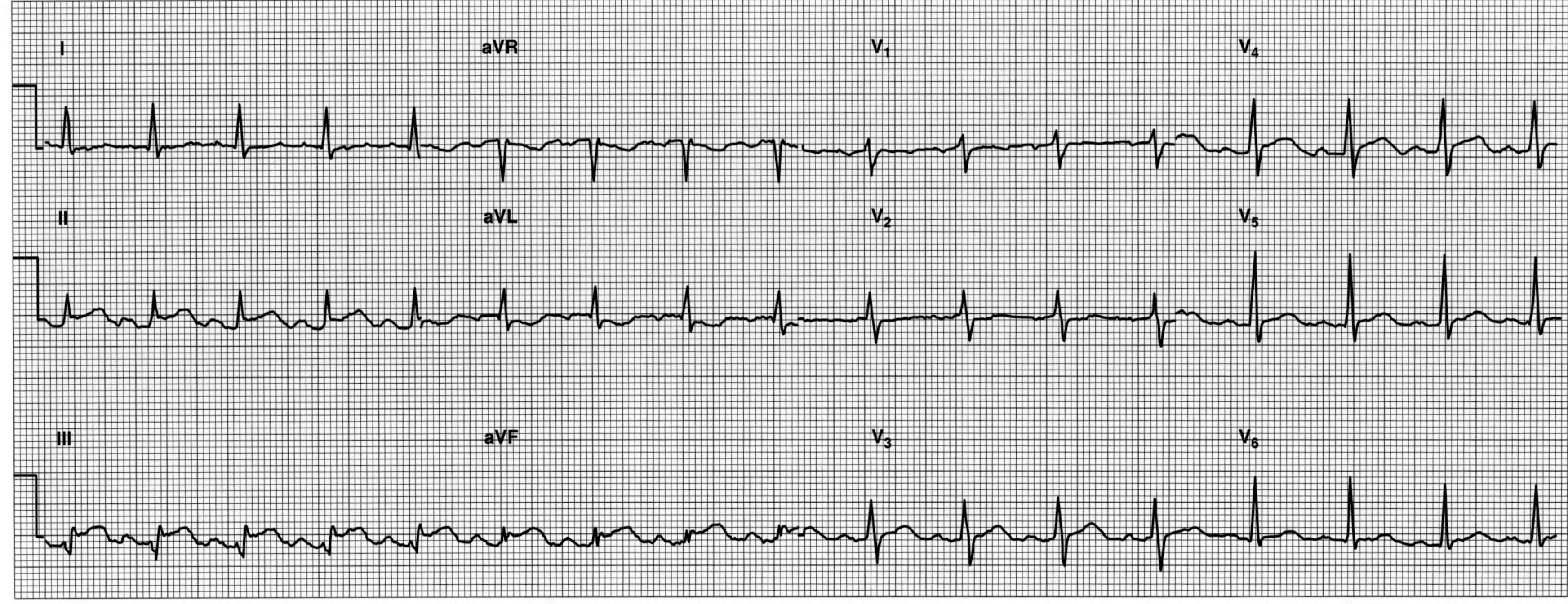

Rate and rhythm? ______ Pathologic Q waves? ______

STE? ______ ST depression? ______ T-wave changes? ______

Reciprocal changes? ______ Imposter present? ______ Axis? ______

Interpretation: ______

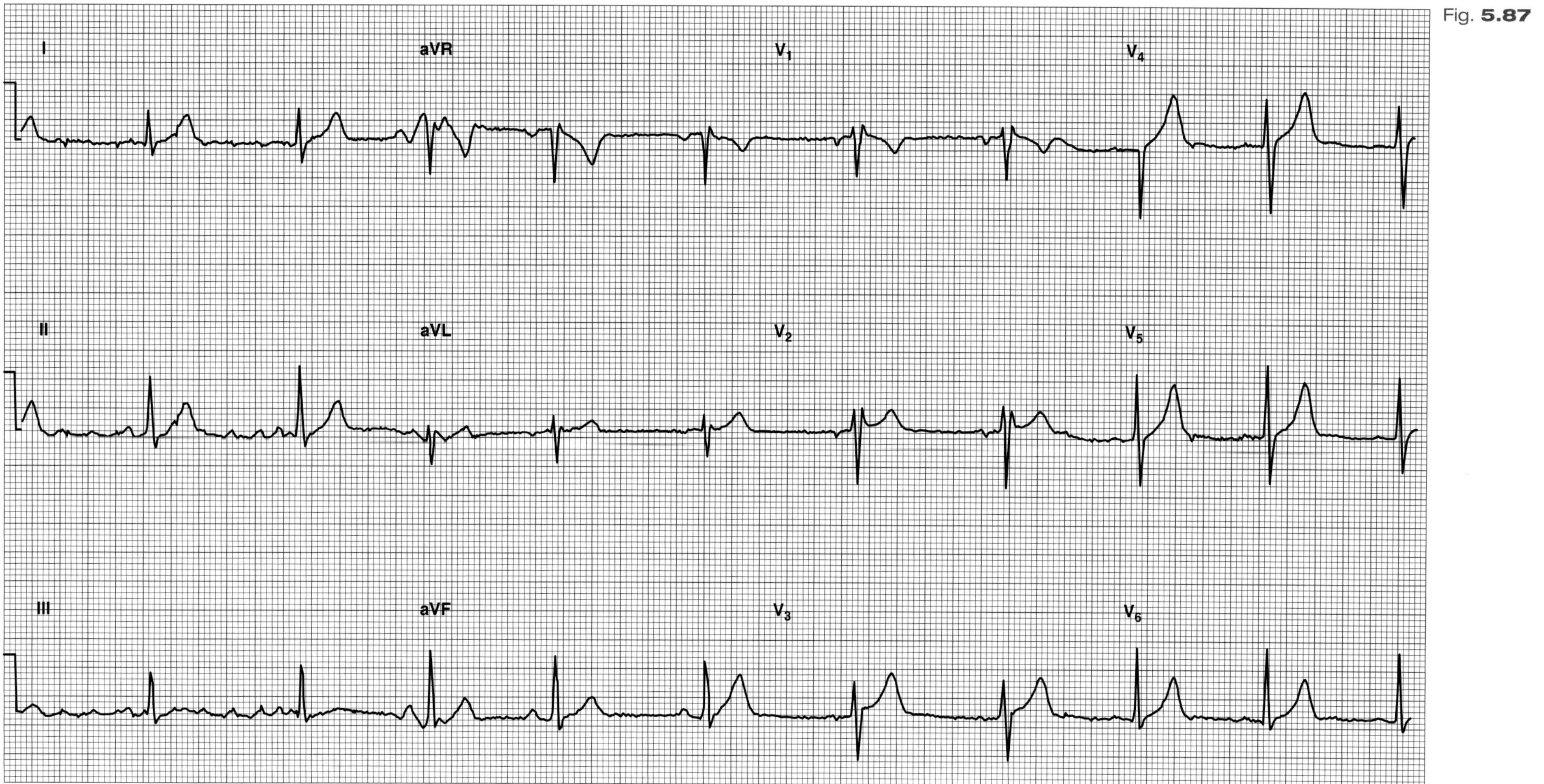

Fig. 5.87

Rate and rhythm? ______ Pathologic Q waves? ______

STE? ______ ST depression? ______ T-wave changes? ______

Reciprocal changes? ______ Imposter present? ______ Axis? ______

Interpretation: ______

Inferior: II, III, aVF | **Septum: V_1, V_2** | Anterior: V_3, V_4 | **Lateral: I, aVL, V_5, V_6**

Fig. **5.88**

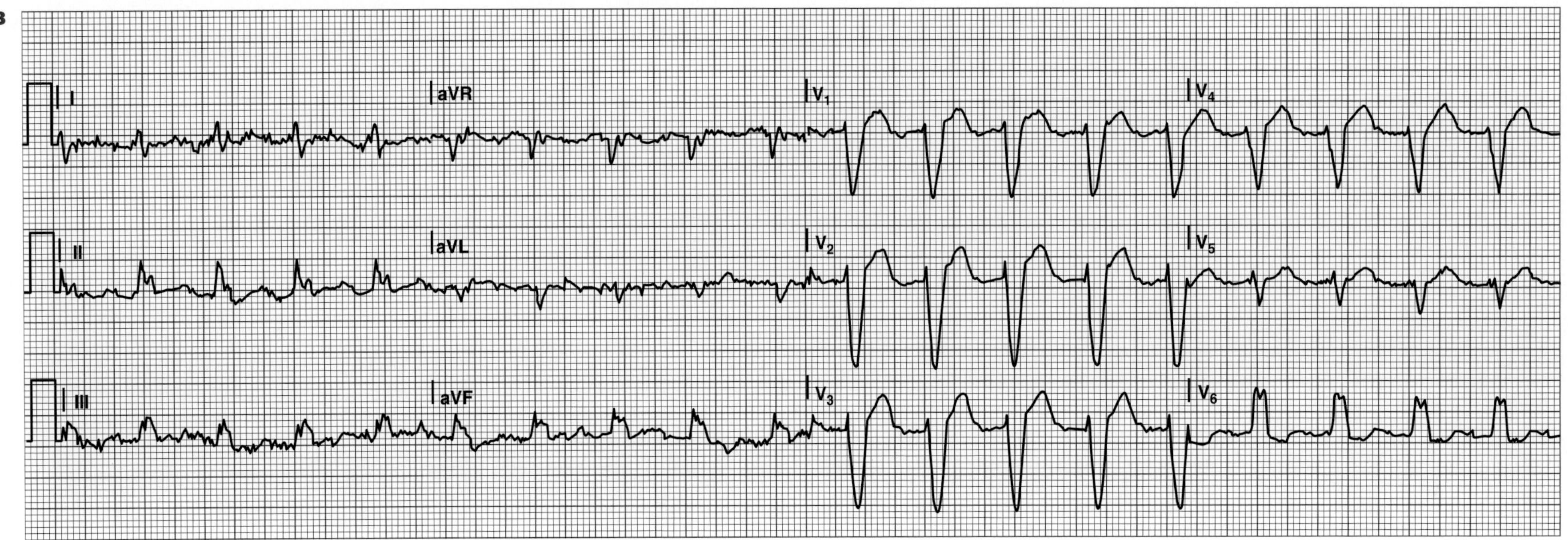

Rate and rhythm? ______ Pathologic Q waves? ______

STE? ______ ST depression? ______ T-wave changes? ______

Reciprocal changes? ______ Imposter present? ______ Axis? ______

Interpretation: ______

Inferior: II, III, aVF | **Septum: V_1, V_2** | **Anterior: V_3, V_4** | **Lateral: I, aVL, V_5, V_6**

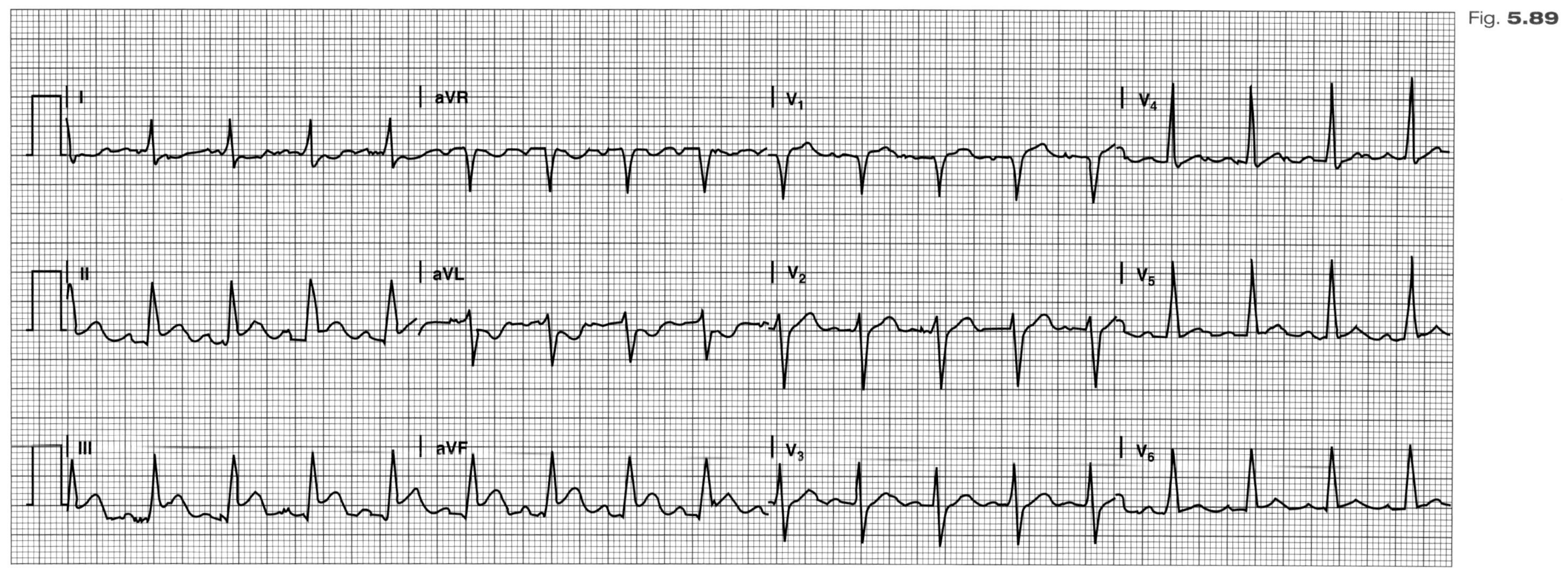

Fig. **5.89**

Rate and rhythm? __________ Pathologic Q waves? __________

STE? __________ ST depression? __________ T-wave changes? __________

Reciprocal changes? __________ Imposter present? __________ Axis? __________

Interpretation: __________

Inferior: II, III, aVF | **Septum: V_1, V_2** | **Anterior: V_3, V_4** | **Lateral: I, aVL, V_5, V_6**

Fig. **5.90**

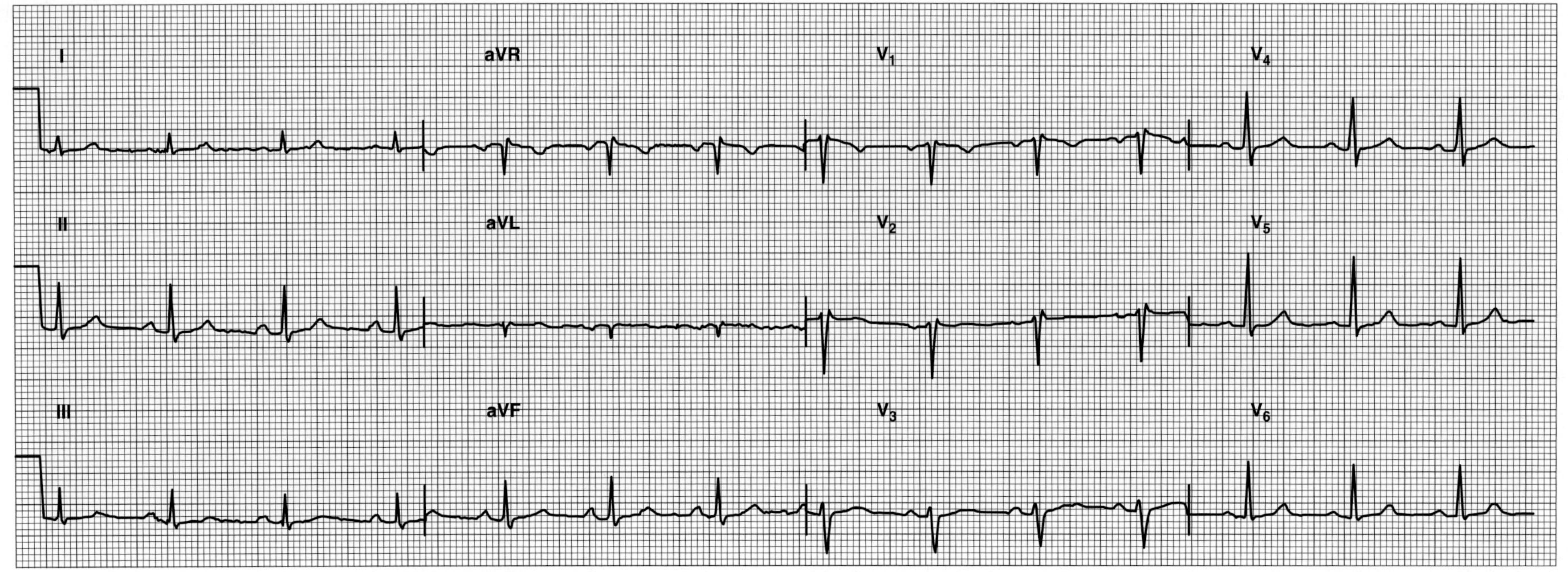

Rate and rhythm? ______ Pathologic Q waves? ______

STE? ______ ST depression? ______ T-wave changes? ______

Reciprocal changes? ______ Imposter present? ______ Axis? ______

Interpretation: ______

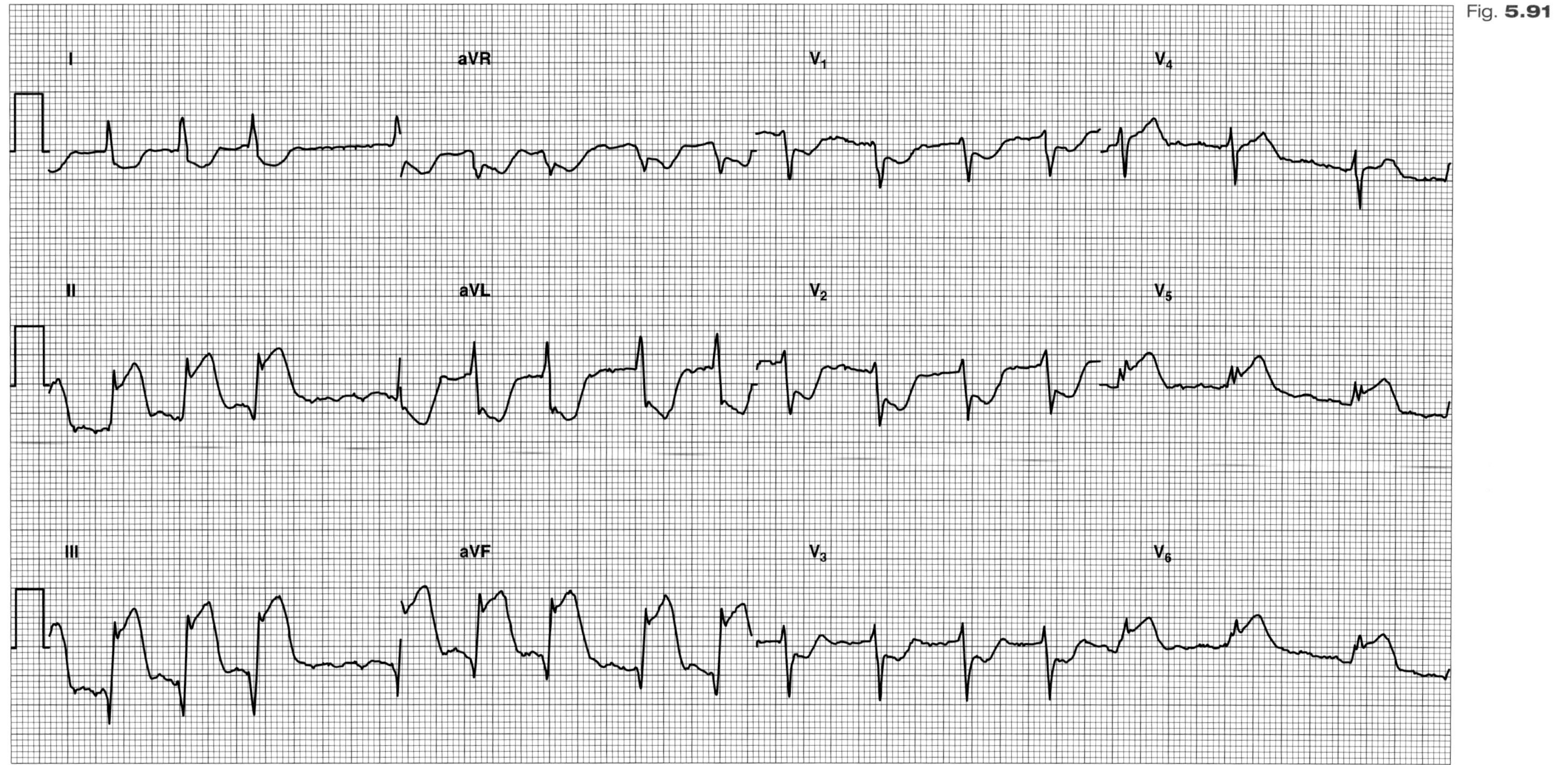

Fig. 5.91

Rate and rhythm? ______ Pathologic Q waves? ______

STE? ______ ST depression? ______ T-wave changes?______

Reciprocal changes? ______ Imposter present? ______ Axis? ______

Interpretation:______

Inferior: II, III, aVF | **Septum: V_1, V_2** | Anterior: V_3, V_4 | **Lateral: I, aVL, V_5, V_6**

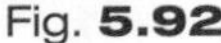
Fig. 5.92

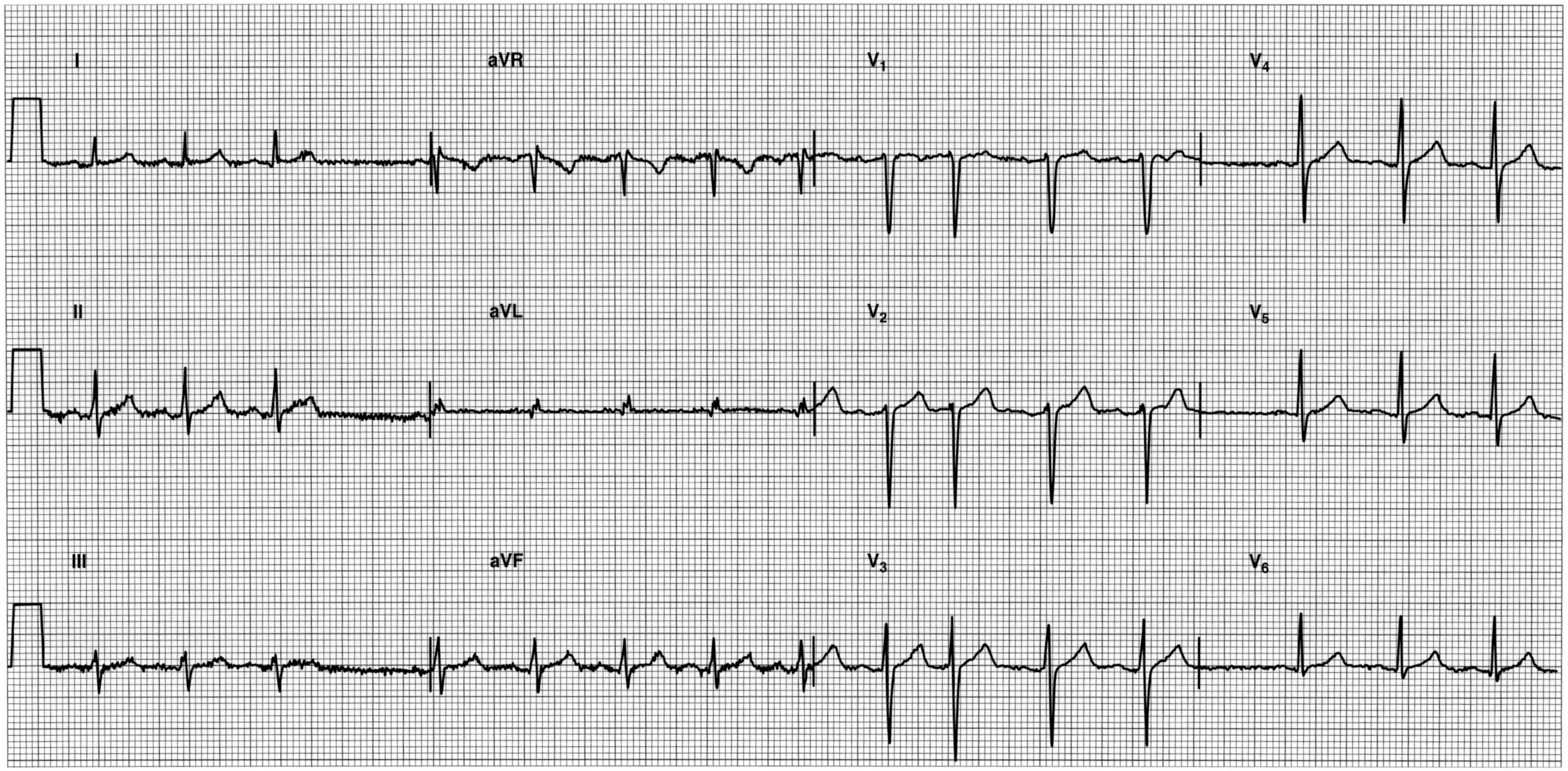

Rate and rhythm? ______________________ Pathologic Q waves? ______________________

STE? ______________________ ST depression? ______________________ T-wave changes? ______________________

Reciprocal changes? ______________________ Imposter present? ______________________ Axis? ______________________

Interpretation: ____

Inferior: II, III, aVF | **Septum: V_1, V_2** | **Anterior: V_3, V_4** | **Lateral: I, aVL, V_5, V_6**

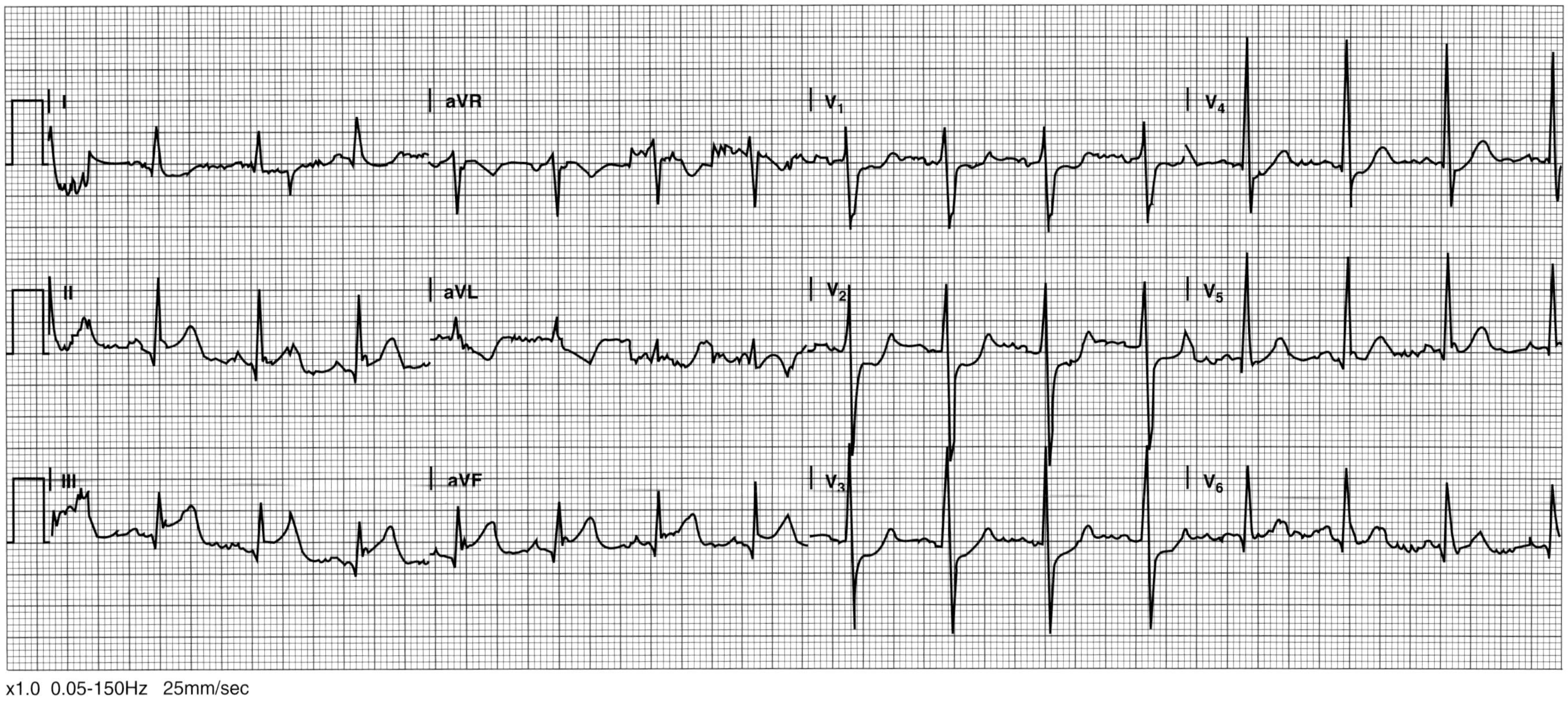

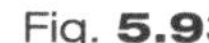

Fig. 5.93

Rate and rhythm? ______ Pathologic Q waves? ______

STE? ______ ST depression? ______ T-wave changes? ______

Reciprocal changes? ______ Imposter present? ______ Axis? ______

Interpretation: ______

Inferior: II, III, aVF | Septum: V_1, V_2 | Anterior: V_3, V_4 | Lateral: I, aVL, V_5, V_6

Fig. **5.94**

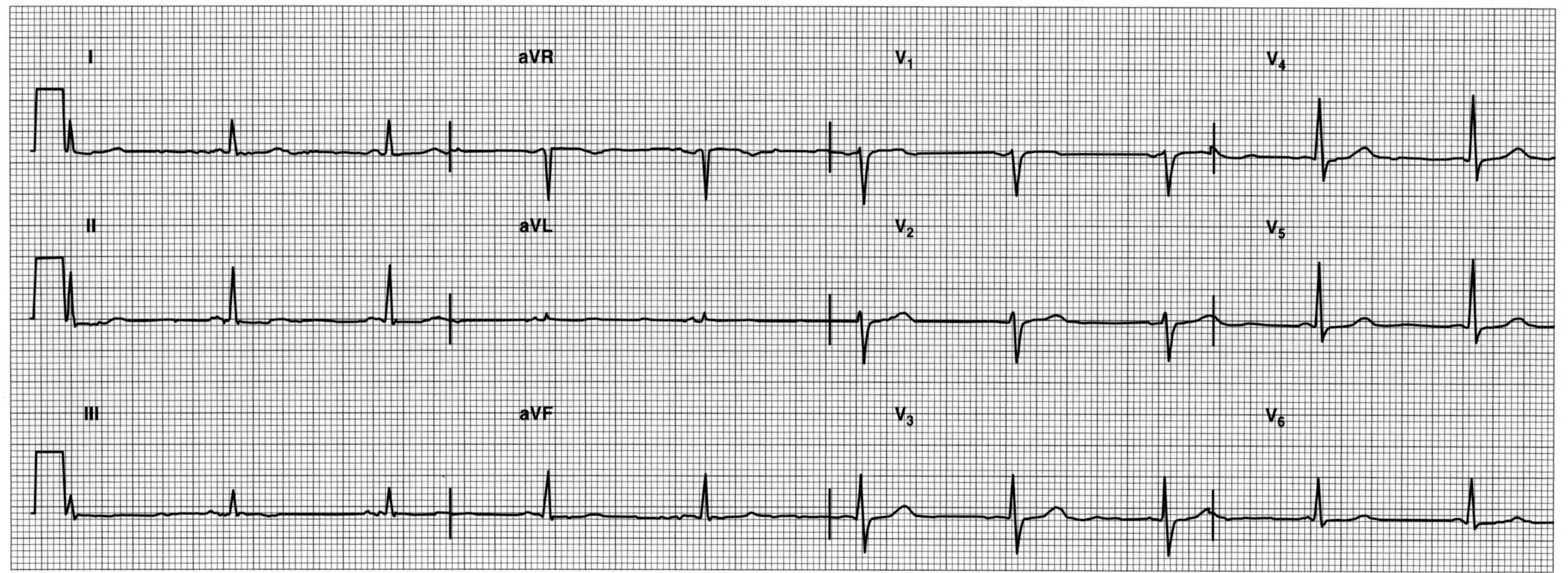

Rate and rhythm? ______________________ Pathologic Q waves? ______________________

STE? ______________________ ST depression? ______________________ T-wave changes? ______________________

Reciprocal changes? ______________________ Imposter present? ______________________ Axis? ______________________

Interpretation: ______________________

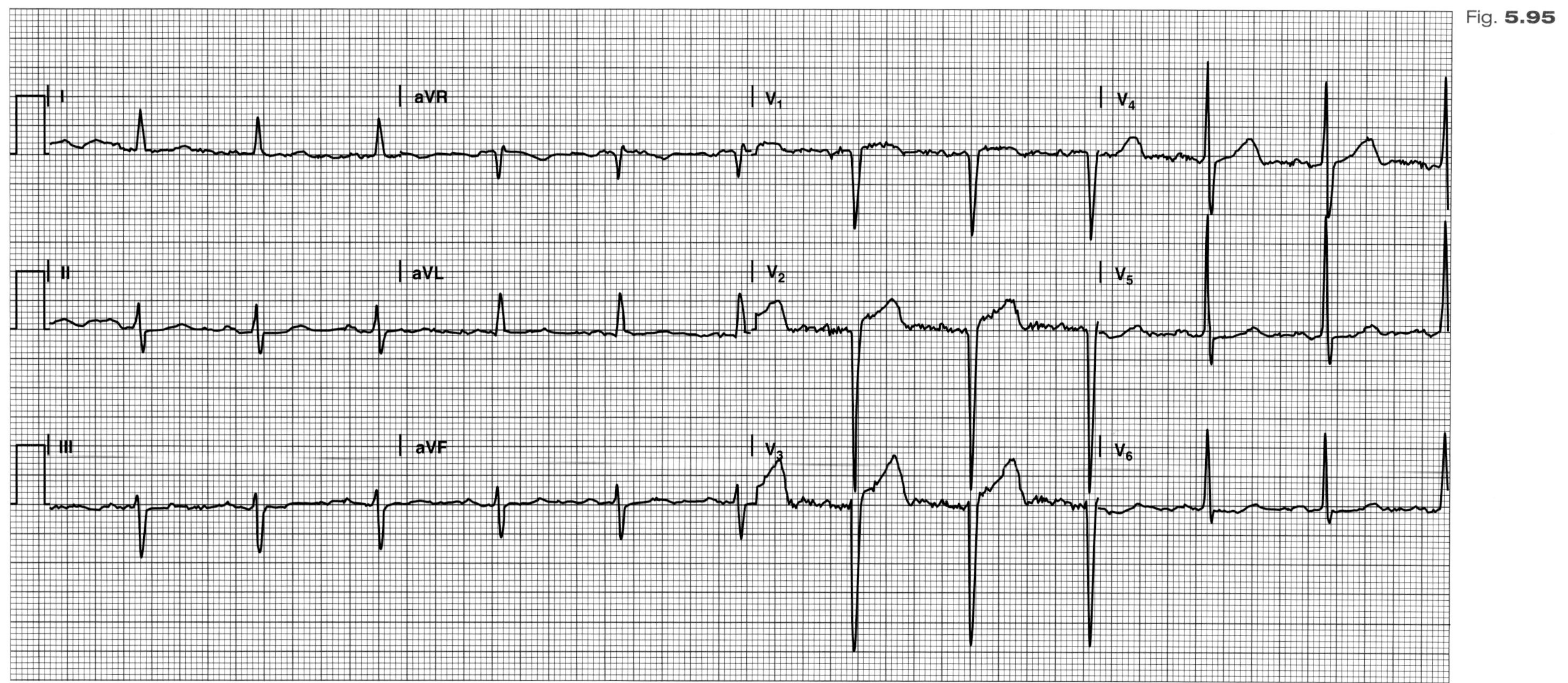

Fig. 5.95

Rate and rhythm? ______ Pathologic Q waves? ______

STE? ______ ST depression? ______ T-wave changes? ______

Reciprocal changes? ______ Imposter present? ______ Axis? ______

Interpretation: ______

Inferior: II, III, aVF | **Septum: V_1, V_2** | Anterior: V_3, V_4 | **Lateral: I, aVL, V_5, V_6**

Fig. **5.96**

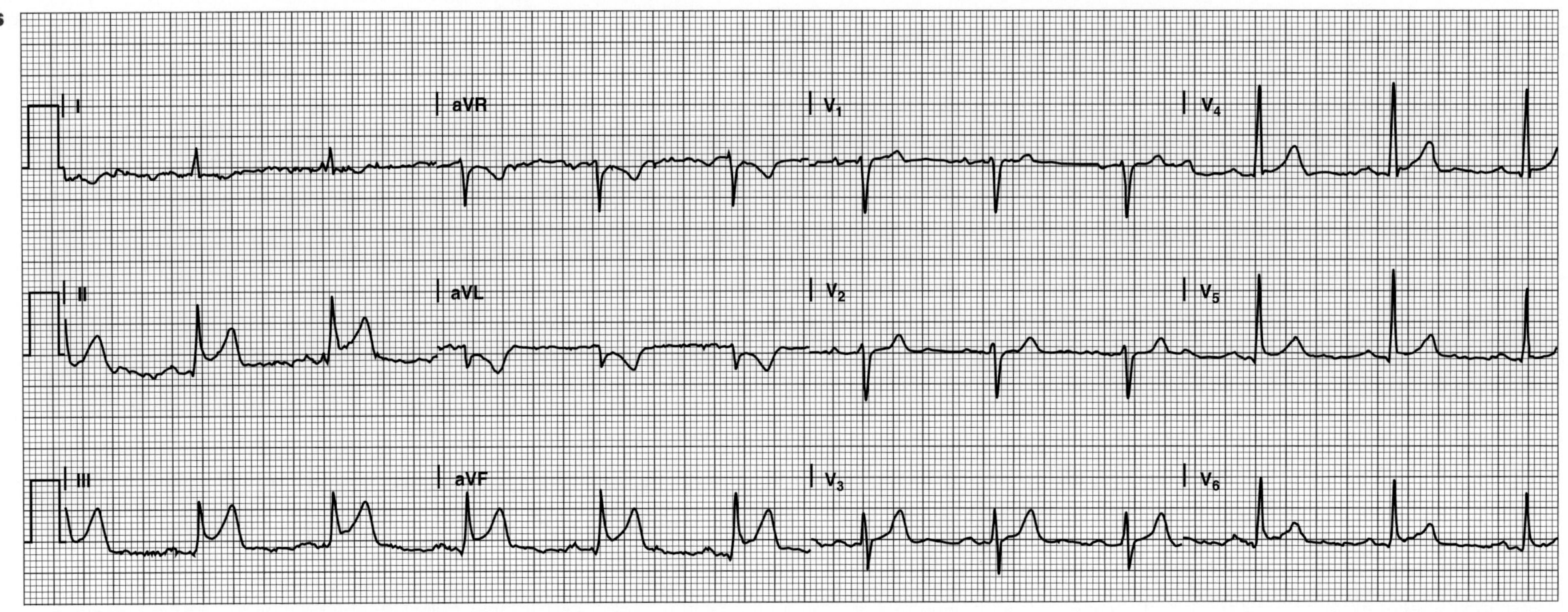

Rate and rhythm? ______ Pathologic Q waves? ______

STE? ______ ST depression? ______ T-wave changes? ______

Reciprocal changes? ______ Imposter present? ______ Axis? ______

Interpretation: ______

Inferior: II, III, aVF | **Septum: V_1, V_2** | **Anterior: V_3, V_4** | **Lateral: I, aVL, V_5, V_6**

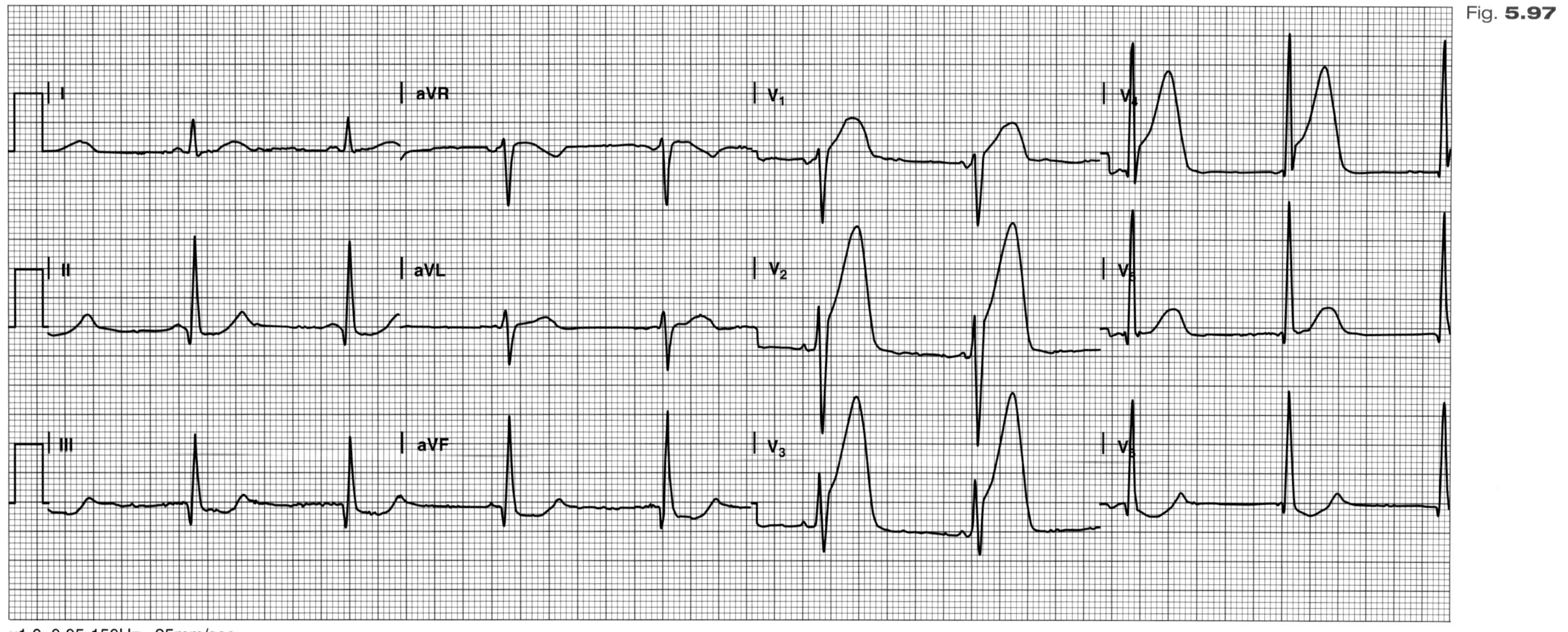

Fig. 5.97

Rate and rhythm? ______ Pathologic Q waves? ______

STE? ______ ST depression? ______ T-wave changes? ______

Reciprocal changes? ______ Imposter present? ______ Axis? ______

Interpretation: ______

Inferior: II, III, aVF | **Septum: V_1, V_2** | Anterior: V_3, V_4 | **Lateral: I, aVL, V_5, V_6**

Fig. **5.98**

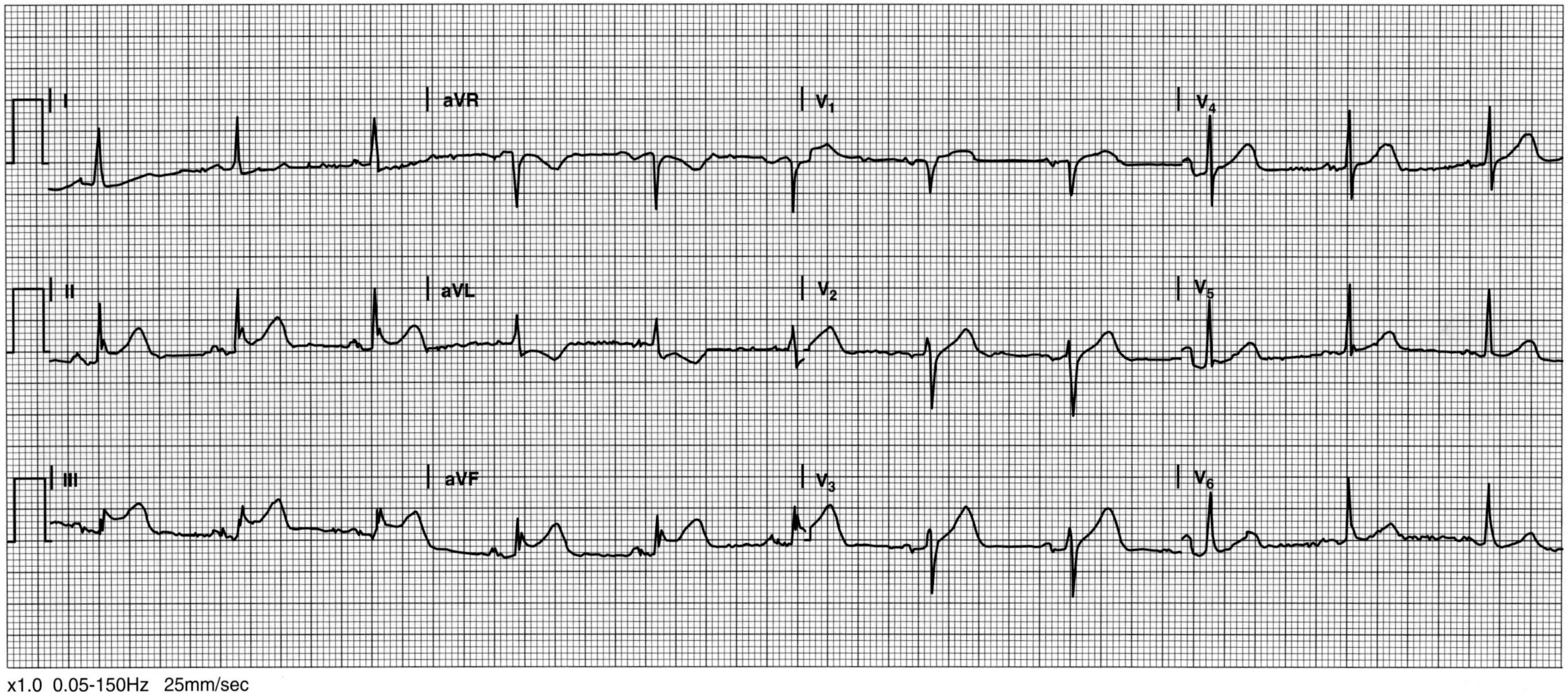

x1.0 0.05-150Hz 25mm/sec

Rate and rhythm? ______________________ Pathologic Q waves? ______________________

STE? ______________________ ST depression? ______________________ T-wave changes? ______________________

Reciprocal changes? ______________________ Imposter present? ______________________ Axis? ______________________

Interpretation: ____

Inferior: II, III, aVF | **Septum: V_1, V_2** | **Anterior: V_3, V_4** | **Lateral: I, aVL, V_5, V_6**

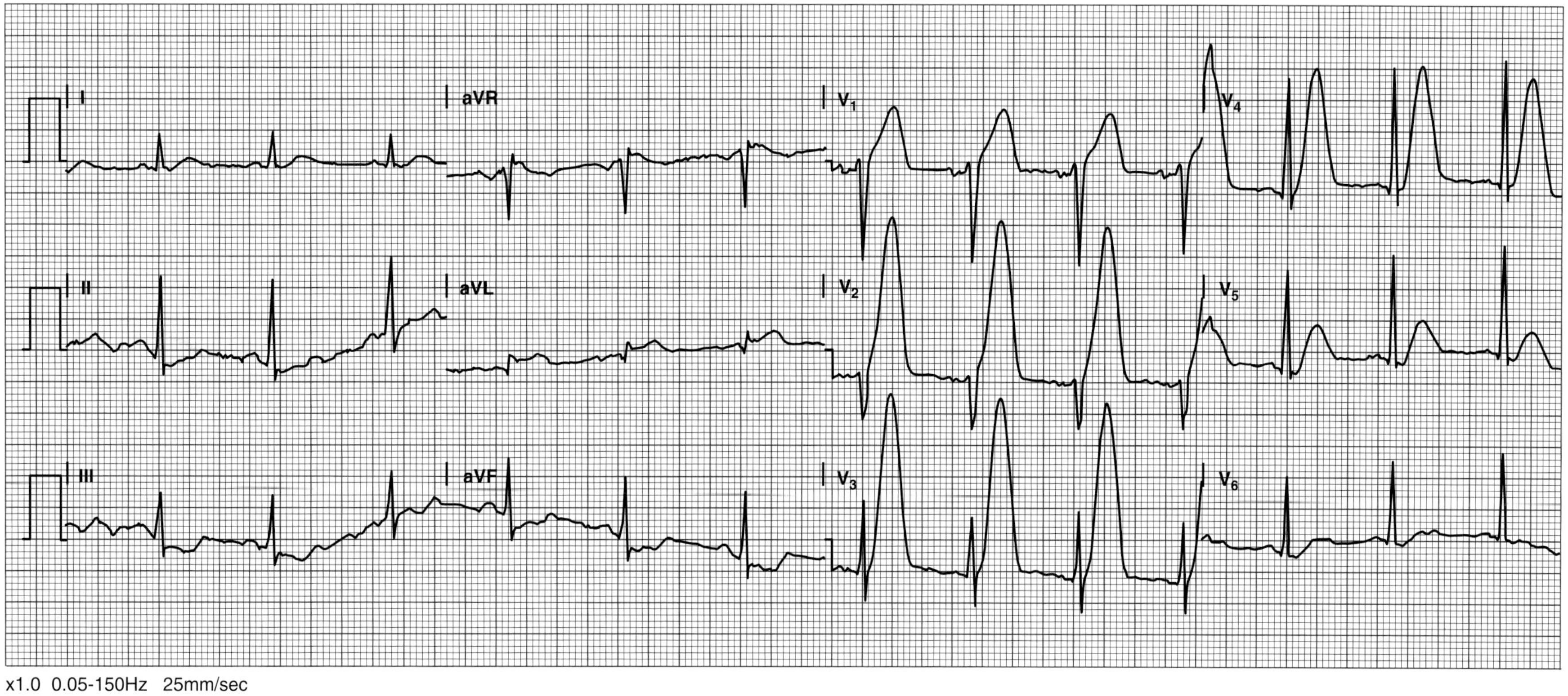

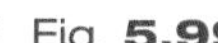

Fig. **5.99**

x1.0 0.05-150Hz 25mm/sec

Rate and rhythm? ______________________ Pathologic Q waves? ______________________

STE? ______________________ ST depression? ______________________ T-wave changes?______________________

Reciprocal changes? ______________________ Imposter present? ______________________ Axis? ______________________

Interpretation:______________________

Inferior: II, III, aVF | **Septum: V_1, V_2** | Anterior: V_3, V_4 | **Lateral: I, aVL, V_5, V_6**

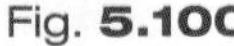
Fig. 5.100

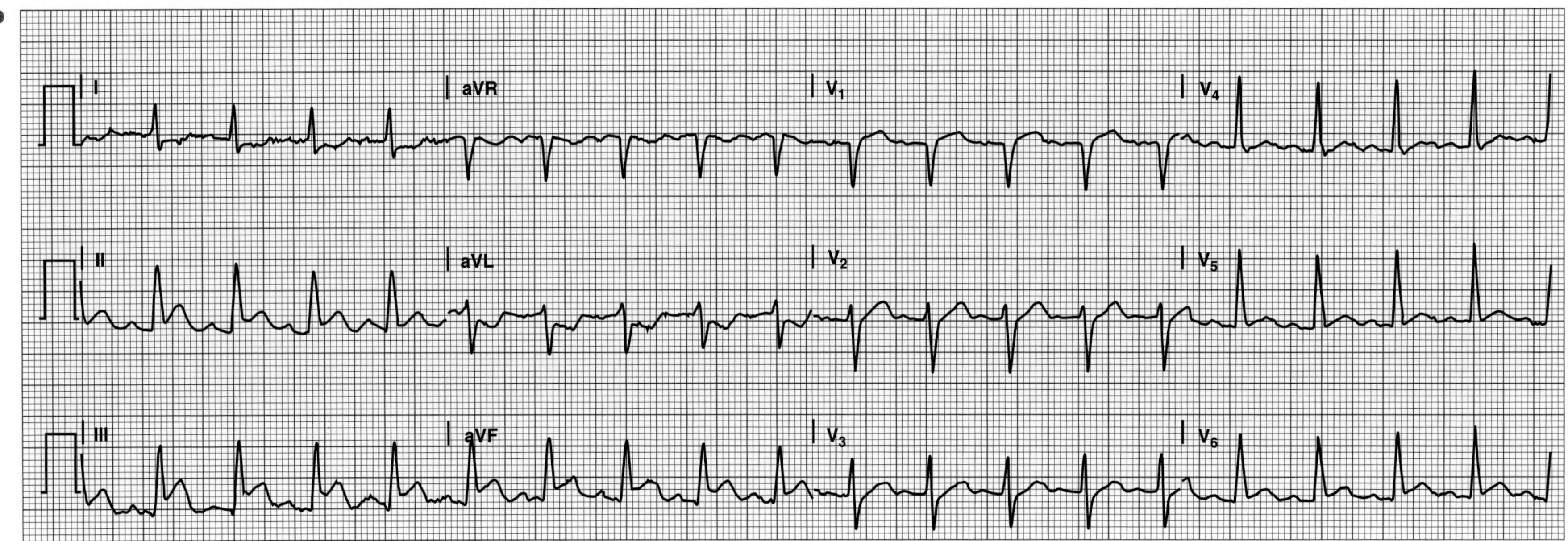

Rate and rhythm? ______ Pathologic Q waves? ______

STE? ______ ST depression? ______ T-wave changes? ______

Reciprocal changes? ______ Imposter present? ______ Axis? ______

Interpretation: ______

Inferior: II, III, aVF | **Septum: V_1, V_2** | Anterior: V_3, V_4 | **Lateral: I, aVL, V_5, V_6**

INTERPRETATION OF PRACTICE ECGS

Fig. 5.1

Rate and rhythm:	Supraventricular bradycardia at 52 beats/min
STE:	II, III, aVF, V_3, V_5, V_6
ST depression:	aVL, V_1, V_2
T-wave changes:	Inverted in aVL, V_1, V_2
Reciprocal changes:	aVL
Axis:	Normal
Interpretation:	Inferolateral STEMI. Second-degree type I AV block present, probably nodal. ST depression and tall R wave in V_1, V_2 suggestive of posterior wall involvement. Obtain right-sided chest leads to assess for right ventricular infarction (RVI) and posterior chest leads to assess for posterior MI. Note: STE in V_3 probably due right coronary artery supplying a portion of the ventricular apex.

Fig. 5.2

Rate and rhythm:	Sinus rhythm at 90 beats/min
STE:	Slight in aVR and V_1
ST depression:	II, III, aVL, aVF, V_3–V_6
Axis:	Normal
Interpretation:	Incomplete LBBB (QRS 112 ms). ST depression in eight or more leads plus slight STE in aVR and V_1 is associated with either three-vessel disease or a left main occlusion.

Fig. 5.3

Rate and rhythm:	Atrial fibrillation at 107 beats/min
ST depression:	V_6
T-wave changes:	Tall in V_2
Axis:	Normal
Interpretation:	Incomplete RBBB pattern (RSR′ pattern in V_1 but QRS is within normal limits [90 ms]). Baseline wander in I and V_4–V_6. Consider clinical presentation and use ST trending or serial ECGs.

Fig. 5.4

Rate and rhythm:	Sinus rhythm at 66 beats/min with first-degree atrioventricular (AV) block (PRI 224 ms)
STE:	V_3
T-wave changes:	Inverted in aVL
STE variant present:	LVH
Axis:	Left
Interpretation:	LVH. Nonspecific intraventricular conduction delay (QRS 126 ms) with left axis deviation.

Fig. 5.5

Rate and rhythm:	Sinus tachycardia at 100 beats/min with ventricular demand pacemaker
Pathologic Q waves:	II, III, aVF, V_1–V_4
STE:	V_1
ST depression:	I, aVL, V_5, V_6
STE variant present:	Ventricular paced rhythm
Axis:	Left
Interpretation:	Ventricular paced rhythm noted. Does not meet Sgarbossa criteria. Pacemaker can diminish STE that may otherwise be present. For that reason, consider STEMI possible. Consider clinical presentation and use ST trending or serial ECGs.

Fig. 5.6

Rate and rhythm:	Sinus bradycardia at 51 beats/min
Pathologic Q waves:	III, V_1
STE:	Slight in aVF, V_2
Axis:	Normal
Interpretation:	Sinus bradycardia. Low voltage in aVF; otherwise normal ECG.

Fig. 5.7

Rate and rhythm: Sinus bradycardia at 51 beats/min
STE: II, III, aVF
ST depression: I, aVL, V_1–V_3
T-wave changes: Inverted in I, aVL, V_1–V_4; tall in II, III, aVF
Reciprocal changes: I, aVL
Axis: Normal
Interpretation: Inferior STEMI with nonspecific intraventricular conduction delay (QRS 112 ms). Reciprocal changes present. ST depression in V_1–V_3, possibly from posterior involvement (poor R-wave progression is present, but posterior STEMI often causes increased R-wave height). Consider obtaining posterior chest leads. Obtain V_4R to assess for RVI.

Fig. 5.8

Rate and rhythm: Sinus rhythm at 71 beats/min
STE: V_1–V_3
ST depression: II
T-wave changes: Tall in V_2–V_4
Axis: Normal
Interpretation: Possible anteroseptal STEMI (baseline wander makes it difficult to confirm).

Fig. 5.9

Rate and rhythm: Sinus rhythm at 75 beats/min
Axis: Left
Interpretation: Low-voltage QRS complexes; poor R-wave progression; left axis deviation; baseline wander in V_5.

Fig. 5.10

Rate and rhythm: Sinus rhythm at 95 beats/min
Pathologic Q waves: I
STE: aVL, V_1–V_4
ST depression: V_5?, V_6
T-wave changes: Peaked in II, III, aVF; inverted in V_2–V_4; not oppositely deflected from QRS in V_5, V_6
STE variant present: LBBB
Axis: Normal
Interpretation: Anteroseptal STEMI with LBBB. In V_4, the J point is elevated and concordant with the QRS, which meets Sgarbossa criteria. Low-voltage QRS complexes in I. Baseline wander I, II, III, aVL. Poor R-wave progression V_2–V_3.

Fig. 5.11

Rate and rhythm: Sinus tachycardia at 109 beats/min with occasional PVCs
STE: II, III, aVF
ST depression: I, aVL, V_2
T-wave changes: Inverted in I, aVL
Reciprocal changes: I, aVL
Axis: Normal
Interpretation: Inferior STEMI with reciprocal changes. Obtain V_4R to assess for RVI. Because of the ST depression in V_2, consider obtaining posterior leads to assess for inferobasal infarction.

Fig. 5.12

Rate and rhythm: Sinus rhythm at 60 beats/min
STE: II, III, aVF
ST depression: aVL
T-wave changes: Tall/peaked in II, III, aVF, V_3–V_5; inverted in aVL
Reciprocal changes: aVL
Axis: Normal
Interpretation: Inferoapical infarct. Obtain V_4R to assess for RVI. Poor R-wave progression V_2–V_3. Artifact I, II, III, aVL, aVF, V_5, V_6.

Fig. 5.13

Rate and rhythm:	Sinus arrhythmia at 62 beats/min with first-degree AV block (PRI 262 ms)
T-wave changes:	Inverted in aVL, V_6
Axis:	Left
Interpretation:	Left anterior fascicular block (LAFB) (left axis deviation, qR pattern in aVL, QRS 116 ms). Low-voltage QRS complexes in V_2. Poor R-wave progression. Nonspecific T wave abnormality.

Fig. 5.14

Rate and rhythm:	Sinus rhythm at 98 beats/min with LBBB
STE:	V_1–V_4
STE variant present:	LBBB
Axis:	Left
Interpretation:	Possible anteroseptal STEMI versus new-onset LBBB (QRS 176 ms). The QRS amplitude is about 40 mV in V_2 and the STE is about 7 mm. The STE of 5 mm or more meets Sgarbossa criteria; however, recall that STE is the least persuasive of the Sgarbossa criteria. The STE would need to equal 10 mm or more to meet the modified Sgarbossa criteria. Therefore, this may very well be a new-onset LBBB. As always, consider clinical presentation and use ST trending or serial ECGs.

Fig. 5.15

Rate and rhythm:	Sinus rhythm at 82 beats/min
STE:	V_1–V_3
STE variant present:	BER? Pericarditis?
Axis:	Normal
Interpretation:	Possible anteroseptal STEMI (STE noted in V_1–V_3). BER and pericarditis are possible explanations for STE. In addition, slight STE in V_1–V_3 can be a normal variant (high take off). Consider clinical presentation and use ST trending or serial ECGs.

Fig. 5.16

Rate and rhythm:	Sinus rhythm at 75 beats/min
STE:	V_2–V_3
ST depression:	II, III, aVF
T-wave changes:	Tall in V_2–V_3
Axis:	Normal
Interpretation:	Anteroseptal STEMI. STE and tall T waves noted in V_2, V_3. With tall T waves, hyperkalemia is a possibility, but in this case, the wide base of the T wave favors the hyperacute T wave of STEMI.

Fig. 5.17

Rate and rhythm:	Sinus rhythm at 85 beats/min
Pathologic Q waves:	V_1–V_3
STE:	Slight in aVL, V_4
ST depression:	II, III, aVF
T-wave changes:	Inverted in II, III, aVF
Axis:	Right
Interpretation:	Slurring of the initial portion of the QRS (i.e., delta wave) seen in leads II, III, aVF, and V_6, and a wide QRS (114 ms) suggests the presence of Wolff-Parkinson-White (WPW) pattern. Consider clinical presentation (WPW vs. inferior ischemia). Poor R-wave progression.

Fig. 5.18

Rate and rhythm:	Atrial fibrillation at 81 beats/min
STE:	I, aVL
ST depression:	II, III, aVF
Reciprocal changes:	II, III, aVF
Axis:	Left
Interpretation:	High lateral STEMI. Reciprocal changes noted in II, III, and aVF.

Fig. 5.19

Rate and rhythm: Electronic atrial pacemaker at 80 pulses/min
Axis: Normal
Interpretation: When the atria are paced with normal conduction in the ventricles, the typical rules for STE are still used. Consider clinical presentation and use ST trending or serial ECGs.

Fig. 5.20

Rate and rhythm: Sinus rhythm at 85 beats/min
STE: II, III, aVF
ST depression: I, aVL, V_2–V_6
T-wave changes: Tall/peaked in II, III, aVF; inverted in aVL, V_1–V_6
Reciprocal changes: I, aVL
Axis: Normal
Interpretation: Inferior STEMI, reciprocal changes present. Possible posterior infarct (ST depression in septal and anterior chest leads). Poor R-wave progression in V_2–V_6. Baseline wander and artifact in I, aVL. Obtain posterior and right-sided chest leads and consider clinical presentation.

Fig. 5.21

Rate and rhythm: Atrial fibrillation with multiform premature ventricular complexes (PVCs); ventricular rate 82 to 117 beats/min
STE: II, V_5
T-wave changes: Inverted in aVL
Axis: Left
Interpretation: RBBB with LAFB (QRS 142 ms). Nearing criteria for LVH (patient is a 74-year-old Caucasian man).

Fig. 5.22

Rate and rhythm: Sinus rhythm at 77 beats/min with first-degree AV block (PRI 224 ms)
STE: II, III, aVF
ST depression: I, aVL, V_1–V_2
T-wave changes: Inverted in I, aVL, subtle in V_1, more prominent in V_2
Reciprocal changes: I, aVL
Axis: Normal
Interpretation: Inferior STEMI, reciprocal changes present. Poor R-wave progression. Obtain right-sided chest leads and consider clinical presentation.

Fig. 5.23

Rate and rhythm: Sinus rhythm at 71 beats/min with first-degree AV block (PRI 212 ms)
Pathologic Q waves: V_1–V_3
STE: V_2, V_3
ST depression: V_5, V_6
Axis: Left
Interpretation: Possible anteroseptal STEMI. Poor R-wave progression. Artifact makes exact identification of the J point and TP segment difficult. QS complexes (counts as a pathologic Q wave) noted in V_1–V_3. Consider STEMI versus normal variant versus previous acute MI with ventricular aneurysm. Consider clinical presentation and use ST trending or serial ECGs.

Fig. 5.24

Rate and rhythm: Sinus rhythm at 91 beats/min with occasional PVCs
STE: Slight in aVR
ST depression: I, II, III, aVF, V_2–V_6
Axis: Normal
Interpretation: Inferior and anterolateral ischemia. Because of the diffuse ST depression in multiple leads and slight STE in aVR, left main or three-vessel disease must be considered. Consider clinical presentation and use ST trending or serial ECGs.

Fig. 5.25

Rate and rhythm:	Sinus bradycardia at 59 beats/min
STE:	I, II, aVL, V_2–V_6
ST depression:	III, aVR, aVF
T-wave changes:	Tall in V_2–V_5
STE variant present:	Pericarditis?
Axis:	Normal
Interpretation:	Suspected global MI. Baseline wander in I, II, III. ECG quality makes interpretation difficult. Low-voltage QRS complexes in the limb leads. Lead V_1 looks mostly normal. If STE is due to STEMI, then the inferior, septal, anterior, and lateral walls are involved (more likely). If an STE variant, then pericarditis would be the only one to account for elevation in these leads (less likely). Consider clinical presentation and use ST trending or serial ECGs.

Fig. 5.26

Rate and rhythm:	Sinus rhythm at 73 beats/min with premature atrial complexes (PACs)
Axis:	Normal
Interpretation:	Normal ECG. Consider clinical presentation.

Fig. 5.27

Rate and rhythm:	Sinus rhythm at 94 beats/min
Pathologic Q waves:	III, aVF
STE:	II, III, aVF, V_1, V_3–V_5
ST depression:	I, aVL
T-wave changes:	Tall in II, III, aVF; peaked in V_2
Reciprocal changes:	I, aVL
Axis:	Normal
Interpretation:	Inferior STEMI, reciprocal changes present. Possible RVI (STE greater in V_1 than V_2). Possible posterior infarction (tall R waves in early chest leads). Possible apical infarction (coving in V_3 and V_4). Artifact in lead I. Obtain posterior and right-sided chest leads and consider clinical presentation.

Fig. 5.28

Rate and rhythm:	Sinus rhythm at 67 beats/min
STE:	V_3
Axis:	Normal
Interpretation:	Incomplete RBBB (QRS 108 ms). This patient is a 16-year-old Caucasian boy who experienced a syncopal episode. Note the rSr′ with STE and an upright T wave in V_2, which creates a saddleback. This pattern may occur if electrodes are placed too high on the chest, it may be a normal variant, and it may be seen in patients with Brugada syndrome. Carefully consider the patient's history and clinical presentation.

Fig. 5.29

Rate and rhythm:	Sinus rhythm at 75 beats/min
STE:	V_2–V_6
T-wave changes:	Inverted in V_1
Axis:	Left
Interpretation:	Anteroseptal STEMI with lateral extension. The artifact present in I, II, III, and aVF makes it difficult to confirm if STE is present in these leads.

Fig. 5.30

Rate and rhythm:	Sinus bradycardia at 54 beats/min
Pathologic Q waves:	II?, III? aVF?
STE:	II, III, aVF
ST depression:	I, aVL
T-wave changes:	Tall/peaked in III, aVF; flattened in V_5, V_6; inverted in I, aVL, V_2–V_4
Reciprocal changes:	I, aVL
Axis:	Normal
Interpretation:	Inferior STEMI, reciprocal changes present. Possible posterior infarct. Possible previous anteroseptal infarct (poor R-wave progression V_2, V_3). Baseline wander in II, III, V_1, V_6. Obtain posterior and right-sided chest leads and consider clinical presentation.

Fig. 5.31

Rate and rhythm:	Sinus rhythm at 74 beats/min with LBBB
Pathologic Q waves:	III, V_1, V_2
STE:	V_1–V_3
ST depression:	V_6
T-wave changes:	Inverted in aVL, tall/peaked in V_2–V_4
STE variant present:	LBBB
Axis:	Left
Interpretation:	LBBB (QRS 138 ms). Does not meet Sgarbossa criteria for infarct-induced LBBB. Consider clinical presentation and use ST trending or serial ECGs.

Fig. 5.32

Rate and rhythm:	Sinus bradycardia at 55 beats/min
STE:	V_5, V_6
T-wave changes:	Inverted in V_1
Axis:	Normal
Interpretation:	Borderline ST changes in V_5 and V_6. Shape of ST segment in II and aVF suspicious as well. Consider clinical presentation and use ST trending or serial ECGs.

Fig. 5.33

Rate and rhythm:	Atrial flutter at 94 beats/min with variable atrioventricular block
ST depression:	V_5, V_6
T-wave changes:	Inverted in I, aVL, V_5, V_6
STE variant present:	LVH
Axis:	Left
Interpretation:	LVH (S in lead III + R in aVL = 21 mm) with repolarization abnormality. This patient is a 77-year-old Caucasian woman.

Fig. 5.34

Rate and rhythm:	Sinus rhythm at 78 beats/min with occasional ectopic premature complexes
STE:	V_1–V_4
ST depression:	II, III, aVF
T-wave changes:	Tall/peaked in V_2–V_5
Axis:	Normal
Interpretation:	Anteroseptal STEMI.

Fig. 5.35

Rate and rhythm:	Sinus tachycardia at 107 beats/min
T-wave changes:	Inverted in I, aVL; tall/peaked in V_2
Axis:	Normal
Interpretation:	Nonspecific T-wave abnormality. Artifact present in most leads. Consider clinical presentation.

Fig. 5.36

Rate and rhythm:	Sinus arrhythmia at 92 beats/min
STE:	II, III, aVF
ST depression:	I, aVL, V_2, V_4–V_6
T-wave changes:	Tall in II, III, aVF; inverted in I, aVL, V_1, V_2
Reciprocal changes:	I, aVL
Axis:	Normal
Interpretation:	Inferior STEMI, reciprocal changes present. Obtain right-sided chest leads to assess for RVI and consider clinical presentation.

Fig. 5.37

Rate and rhythm:	Sinus rhythm at 75 beats/min with LBBB
STE:	V_1–V_3
ST depression:	V_5, V_6
STE variant present:	LBBB
Axis:	Left
Interpretation:	Possible anteroseptal STEMI versus new-onset LBBB (QRS 144 ms). Does not meet Sgarbossa criteria for infarct-induced LBBB but cannot rule out that possibility. Consider clinical presentation and use ST trending or serial ECGs.

Fig. 5.38

Rate and rhythm:	Sinus rhythm at 83 beats/min with RBBB and LAFB
Pathologic Q waves:	I, aVL, V_3–V_6
ST depression:	V_1–V_4
T-wave changes:	Inverted in V_1–V_4
Axis:	Left
Interpretation:	Bifascicular block (RBBB and LAFB). RBBB pattern (RSR′ in V_1, QRS 152 ms); LAFB (left axis deviation, QR pattern in aVL). Consider clinical presentation.

Fig. 5.39

Rate and rhythm:	Sinus rhythm at 62 beats/min
STE:	I, aVL, V_2–V_6
ST depression:	III, aVF
T-wave changes:	Tall in V_2–V_5
Reciprocal changes:	III, aVF
Axis:	Left
Interpretation:	Extensive anterolateral STEMI, reciprocal changes present. Consider clinical presentation and use ST trending or serial ECGs.

Fig. 5.40

Rate and rhythm:	Sinus arrhythmia at 61 beats/min with LBBB
STE:	V_1, V_2
ST depression:	V_4–V_6
T-wave changes:	Inverted in I, aVL
STE variant present:	LBBB
Axis:	Left
Interpretation:	LBBB pattern present (QRS 142 ms). Consider clinical presentation and use ST trending or serial ECGs.

Fig. 5.41

Rate and rhythm:	Sinus rhythm at 95 beats/min
Pathologic Q waves:	V_2
STE:	V_1–V_3
T-wave changes:	Inverted in aVL
Axis:	Left
Interpretation:	Anteroseptal STEMI (if clinical picture suggests acute MI). Baseline wander in V_5, V_6. STE in V_1–V_3 and T-wave inversion suggest possible STEMI. However, QS complex in V_2 and poor R-wave progression through V_4 make previous MI with persistent STE a distinct possibility. Consider clinical presentation and use ST trending or serial ECGs.

Fig. 5.42

Rate and rhythm:	Sinus rhythm at 91 beats/min
Pathologic Q waves:	III, aVF
Axis:	Left
Interpretation:	QS complexes noted in III and aVF, possible previous inferior MI. Consider clinical presentation.

Fig. 5.43

Rate and rhythm:	Sinus rhythm at 79 beats/min
STE:	V_2–V_6
T-wave changes:	Inverted in III, V_1
STE variant present:	BER?
Axis:	Normal
Interpretation:	Artifact in V_1. Probable J-point elevation of 1 mm in V_2. STE in V_3–V_6. This patient is a 33-year-old Caucasian man. BER is a possible cause of STE (STE with normally inflected T wave). Consider clinical presentation.

Fig. 5.44

Rate and rhythm:	Sinus bradycardia at 58 beats/min
STE:	V_1–V_3
ST depression:	III, aVF
T-wave changes:	Inverted in III, tall in V_2–V_4
Axis:	Left
Interpretation:	Anteroseptal STEMI. Consider clinical presentation and use ST trending or serial ECGs.

Fig. 5.45

Rate and rhythm:	Sinus rhythm at 65 beats/min
STE:	II, III, aVF
ST depression:	I, aVL
T-wave changes:	Tall/peaked in II, III, aVF, V_3–V_6; inverted in I, aVL
Reciprocal changes:	I, aVL
Axis:	Normal
Interpretation:	Inferior STEMI, reciprocal changes present. Obtain right-sided chest leads to assess for RVI and consider clinical presentation.

Fig. 5.46

Rate and rhythm:	Sinus rhythm at 68 beats/min
Pathologic Q waves:	III, aVF
STE:	II, III, aVF, V_5, V_6
ST depression:	I, aVL, V_1–V_4
T-wave changes:	Tall/peaked in II, III, aVF; inverted in I, aVL, V_2, V_3
Reciprocal changes:	I, aVL
Axis:	Normal
Interpretation:	Inferolateral STEMI, reciprocal changes present. Possible posterior infarct (ST depression V_1–V_4). Poor R-wave progression in V_4, V_5. Artifact in I, II. Obtain posterior and right-sided chest leads and consider clinical presentation.

Fig. 5.47

Rate and rhythm:	Sinus rhythm at 75 beats/min
Axis:	Normal
Interpretation:	Normal ECG. Artifact in V_1.

Fig. 5.48

Rate and rhythm:	Sinus rhythm at 76 beats/min with LBBB
STE:	V_1–V_4
T-wave changes:	Inverted in I, aVL, V_5, V_6
STE variant present:	LBBB
Axis:	Left
Interpretation:	Possible anteroseptal STEMI versus new-onset LBBB (QRS 144 ms). Does not meet Sgarbossa criteria for infarct-induced LBBB but cannot rule out that possibility. Consider clinical presentation and use ST trending or serial ECGs.

Fig. 5.49

Rate and rhythm:	Sinus tachycardia at 136 beats/min with short PRI (116 ms), short QT interval (228 ms)
STE:	Borderline in II, III, aVF
ST depression:	aVL
T-wave changes:	Inverted in aVL
Reciprocal changes:	aVL
STE variant present:	Pericarditis?
Axis:	Normal
Interpretation:	Possible inferior STEMI. Artifact makes determination of J point and baseline difficult. ECG not typical for BER, but pericarditis is a possibility given the less than obvious reciprocal changes in aVL and PR-segment elevation in aVR. Obtain right-sided chest leads to assess for RVI, consider clinical presentation, and use ST trending or serial ECGs.

Fig. 5.50

Rate and rhythm: Sinus rhythm at 83 beats/min with first-degree AV block and RBBB (PRI 228 ms, QRS 156 ms)
STE: III, aVF
ST depression: I, aVL, V_3–V_6
T-wave changes: Inverted in I, V_1, V_4–V_6
Reciprocal changes: I, aVL
Axis: Right
Interpretation: Possible inferior STEMI versus RBBB. STE noted in III and minimal amount in aVF. RBBB pattern noted. RBB can cause STE. The concordant STE in III suggests STEMI. Obtain right-sided chest leads, consider clinical presentation, and use ST trending or serial ECGs.

Fig. 5.51

Rate and rhythm: Sinus arrhythmia at 67 beats/min
T-wave changes: Inverted in V_1
Axis: Normal
Interpretation: Normal ECG; ST depression is present in one complex in lead III but it is not present in the others.

Fig. 5.52

Rate and rhythm: Sinus rhythm at 61 beats/min with occasional premature supraventricular beats
STE: II, III; slight in V_5, V_6
ST depression: I, aVL, V_1, V_2
T-wave changes: Inverted in I, aVL, V_1, V_2
Reciprocal changes: I, aVL
Axis: Normal
Interpretation: Inferior STEMI; reciprocal changes present. Obtain right-sided chest leads, consider clinical presentation, and use ST trending or serial ECGs.

Fig. 5.53

Rate and rhythm: Atrial fibrillation at 153 beats/min with a premature aberrantly conducted complex
ST depression: I, II, aVL, V_6
Axis: Left
Interpretation: Nonspecific ST abnormality. Consider clinical presentation and use ST trending or serial ECGs.

Fig. 5.54

Rate and rhythm: Sinus rhythm at 86 beats/min
STE: V_2–V_5
T-wave changes: Tall in V_2–V_5; inverted in III
STE variant present: BER?
Axis: Normal
Interpretation: Possible anteroseptal STEMI versus BER. Probably BER (STE with normally inflected T wave). This patient is a 21-year-old Caucasian man. Consider clinical presentation and use ST trending or serial ECGs.

Fig. 5.55

Rate and rhythm: Wide QRS tachycardia at 181 beats/min (QRS 252 ms)
STE variant present: Ventricular rhythm; LBBB
Axis: Left
Interpretation: Wide QRS tachycardia (probably atrial fibrillation with LBBB). Both supraventricular tachycardia (SVT) with aberrant conduction and ventricular tachycardia (VT) are capable of producing STE. Consider clinical presentation and use ST trending or serial ECGs.

Fig. 5.56

Rate and rhythm: Junctional rhythm at 55 beats/min
STE: II, III, aVF
ST depression: I, aVL, V_1–V_4
T-wave changes: Inverted in aVL, V_1
Reciprocal changes: aVL
Axis: Normal
Interpretation: Inferior STEMI; probable posterior as well. Obtain right-sided and posterior chest leads and consider clinical presentation.

Fig. 5.57

Rate and rhythm: Sinus rhythm at 93 beats/min
STE: II, III, aVF, V_4–V_6
ST depression: aVL, V_1–V_3
T-wave changes: Inverted in V_1, V_2
Reciprocal changes: aVL
Axis: Normal
Interpretation: Inferolateral STEMI. ST depression in V_1–V_3 suggestive of posterior wall involvement. Obtain right-sided and posterior chest leads and consider clinical presentation.

Fig. 5.58

Rate and rhythm: Sinus tachycardia at 153 beats/min with LAFB
Pathologic Q waves: II, V_1–V_3
STE: III, aVF, V_3, V_4
ST depression: aVL, V_5, V_6
T-wave changes: Inverted in V_5, V_6
Reciprocal changes: aVL
Axis: Left
Interpretation: Possible inferior STEMI. LAFB. Anteroseptal infarct, age undetermined. Artifact in most leads. Approaching criteria for LVH. Obtain right-sided chest leads, consider clinical presentation, and use ST trending or serial ECGs.

Fig. 5.59

Rate and rhythm: Sinus rhythm at 73 beats/min with LBBB
STE: V_1, V_2
ST depression: I, II, aVL, aVF, V_5, V_6
STE variant present: LBBB
Axis: Left
Interpretation: Possible septal STEMI versus new-onset LBBB (QRS 144 ms). Does not meet Sgarbossa criteria for infarct-induced LBBB but cannot rule out that possibility. Consider clinical presentation and use ST trending or serial ECGs.

Fig. 5.60

Rate and rhythm: Sinus rhythm at 74 beats/min
STE: V_5, V_6
T-wave changes: Inverted in aVL
Axis: Normal
Interpretation: Possible lateral STEMI. STE of 1 mm in V_6 but borderline in V_5. ECG quality makes it difficult to be certain about V_5. Consider clinical presentation and use ST trending or serial ECGs.

Fig. 5.61

Rate and rhythm: Ventricular paced rhythm at 91 pulses/min
STE: II, III, aVF
ST depression: I, aVL, V_2–V_4
T-wave changes: Tall in II, III, aVF; inverted in I, aVL
Reciprocal changes: I, aVL
STE variant present: Ventricular paced rhythm
Axis: Left
Interpretation: Possible inferior STEMI. Wide QRS (QRS 164 ms) and ventricular pacemaker noted. A ventricular pacemaker can account for STE; however, the presence of a paced rhythm does not rule out STEMI. In the presence of a paced rhythm, 5 mm or more of STE is suggestive of STEMI. In leads II and III, that criteria may be met. A steadier baseline would add more certainty to the measurement. The concordant ST depression is also suggestive of STEMI. Obtain right-sided chest leads, consider clinical presentation, and use ST trending or serial ECGs.

Fig. 5.62

Rate and rhythm: Sinus rhythm at 89 beats/min
Axis: Normal
Interpretation: Nonspecific T-wave abnormality; baseline wander in V_5, V_6. Artifact in most limb leads. Consider clinical presentation.

Fig. 5.63

Rate and rhythm: Sinus rhythm at 82 beats/min
STE: V_1–V_3
T-wave changes: Inverted in III, tall in V_2, V_3
Axis: Normal
Interpretation: Borderline STE in V_1–V_3, especially in V_2. Close but does not appear to meet STE criteria at this time. Consider clinical presentation and use ST trending or serial ECGs.

Fig. 5.64

Rate and rhythm: Sinus rhythm at 99 beats/min
STE: aVR
ST depression: I, II, aVL, V_4–V_6
Axis: Normal
Interpretation: Widespread ST depression noted. Baseline wander in I, III. Artifact in most limb leads. Consider clinical presentation.

Fig. 5.65

Rate and rhythm: Sinus bradycardia at 58 beats/min
STE: I, aVL, V_2–V_6
ST depression: II, III, aVF
Reciprocal changes: II, III, aVF
Axis: Normal
Interpretation: Extensive anterolateral STEMI. Consider clinical presentation and use ST trending or serial ECGs.

Fig. 5.66

Rate and rhythm: Sinus bradycardia at 56 beats/min
T-wave changes: Inverted in V_1
Axis: Normal
Interpretation: Sinus bradycardia, otherwise normal ECG. Consider clinical presentation.

Fig. 5.67

Rate and rhythm: Sinus rhythm at 71 beats/min
STE: II, III, aVF
ST depression: V_2–V_4
T-wave changes: Inverted in V_1
Reciprocal changes: aVL
Axis: Normal
Interpretation: Inferior STEMI. Low QRS voltage in limb leads. ST depression in V_2–V_4 suggestive of posterior wall involvement. Obtain right-sided and posterior chest leads and consider clinical presentation.

Fig. 5.68

Rate and rhythm: Sinus rhythm at 60 beats/min with LBBB
STE: V_1–V_4
ST depression: I, aVL, V_5, V_6
T-wave changes: Inverted in I, aVL, V_5, V_6
STE variant present: LBBB
Axis: Left
Interpretation: Possible anteroseptal STEMI versus new-onset LBBB (QRS 136 ms). Does not meet Sgarbossa criteria for infarct-induced LBBB but cannot rule out that possibility. Consider clinical presentation and use ST trending or serial ECGs.

Fig. 5.69

Rate and rhythm: Sinus rhythm at 74 beats/min with RBBB
Pathologic Q waves: III, aVF
T-wave changes: Inverted in V_1, V_2
Axis: Left
Interpretation: RBBB pattern noted (QRS 130 ms). While no ECG evidence exists to suspect STEMI, the RBBB is capable of diminishing STE that might otherwise be present. Consider clinical presentation. Artifact in limb leads and V_1; baseline wander in V_1, V_2.

Fig. 5.70

Rate and rhythm:	Sinus rhythm at 86 beats/min
STE:	V_1–V_4
T-wave changes:	Inverted in III; tall/peaked in V_2–V_4
Axis:	Normal
Interpretation:	Anteroseptal STEMI. Baseline wander in V_6. Consider clinical presentation and use ST trending or serial ECGs.

Fig. 5.71

Rate and rhythm:	Sinus rhythm at 74 beats/min
T-wave changes:	Tall in V_1–V_4
Axis:	Normal
Interpretation:	Although this ECG does not meet the STE criteria for STEMI, there are tall T waves in V_1–V_4, which makes it very possible that this is the hyperacute phase of a STEMI. Consider clinical presentation and use ST trending or serial ECGs.

Fig. 5.72

Rate and rhythm:	Atrial fibrillation at 87 beats/min with RBBB
Axis:	Right
Interpretation:	RBBB pattern present (QRS 136 ms). RVH present (tall R waves in V_1, deeper-than-normal S waves in V_5, V_6). Consider clinical presentation.

Fig. 5.73

Rate and rhythm:	Sinus rhythm at 78 beats/min
Pathologic Q waves:	II, III, aVF
STE:	I, aVL, V_2–V_5
ST depression:	II, III, aVF
T-wave changes:	Inverted in II, III, aVF
Reciprocal changes:	II, III, aVF
Axis:	Left
Interpretation:	Suspected extensive anterolateral STEMI. RSR (QR) in V_1/V_2 consistent with right ventricular conduction delay (QRS 128 ms). Consider clinical presentation and use ST trending or serial ECGs.

Fig. 5.74

Rate and rhythm:	Sinus rhythm at 95 beats/min
ST depression:	V_2–V_5
T-wave changes:	Inverted in III
Axis:	Normal
Interpretation:	Consider isolated posterior infarction; obtain additional leads. Nonspecific intraventricular conduction delay (QRS 112 ms). Consider clinical presentation.

Fig. 5.75

Rate and rhythm:	Supraventricular bradycardia at 42 beats/min
STE:	II, III, aVF, V_2–V_6
ST depression:	I, aVL
Reciprocal changes:	I, aVL
Axis:	Normal
Interpretation:	Inferolateral STEMI with reciprocal changes. Baseline wander in the limb leads. Obtain right-sided chest leads. Consider clinical presentation and use ST trending or serial ECGs.

Fig. 5.76

Rate and rhythm:	Sinus tachycardia at 140 beats/min with occasional ectopic premature complexes and LBBB
STE:	I, aVL, V_4–V_6
ST depression:	II, III, aVF
Reciprocal changes:	II, III, aVF
STE variant present:	LBBB
Axis:	Left
Interpretation:	Lateral STEMI, concordant STE in V_4–V_6 in the presence of LBBB (QRS 124 ms). Meets Sgarbossa criteria (concordant STE in at least one lead). Possible left atrial enlargement. Looking at the P waves that are discernible, it is possible that atrial flutter is present and another flutter wave is not being conducted. This could cause alteration of the J point because of the nonconducted flutter wave. However, we believe that despite this possibility, genuine STE exists in V_4 and V_5 and in I and aVL (just not as clear-cut). Baseline wander in most leads. Consider clinical presentation and use ST trending or serial ECGs.

Fig. 5.77

Rate and rhythm:	Sinus bradycardia at 55 beats/min
STE:	II, III, aVF, V_2–V_6
ST depression:	aVL
T-wave changes:	Tall in II, aVF, V_2–V_4
Reciprocal changes:	aVL
STE variant present:	Pericarditis?
Axis:	Normal
Interpretation:	Global STEMI. With such widespread STE, pericarditis is a consideration. However, the ST depression in aVL (the lead most likely to show a reciprocal change with inferior STEMI) suggests STEMI. Artifact present in most limb leads; baseline wander in most chest leads. Consider clinical presentation and use ST trending or serial ECGs.

Fig. 5.78

Rate and rhythm:	Sinus bradycardia at 54 beats/min
STE:	V_1–V_4
T-wave changes:	Inverted in I, aVL, V_6
STE variant present:	LBBB
Axis:	Normal
Interpretation:	LBBB (QRS 160 ms) STE in the presence of LBBB is generally seen in leads V_1–V_3 but sometimes extends to V_4 and beyond. This ECG demonstrates this pattern. Artifact present in III, aVL, V_4–V_6. Consider clinical presentation.

Fig. 5.79

Rate and rhythm:	Sinus tachycardia at 136 beats/min
Pathologic Q waves:	V_1–V_4
Axis:	Normal
Interpretation:	Low-voltage QRS. Baseline wander in I, III, V_6. Consider clinical presentation.

Fig. 5.80

Rate and rhythm:	Sinus bradycardia at 50 beats/min with short (104 ms) PRI
ST depression:	II, III, aVF, V_4–V_6
T-wave changes:	Biphasic in V_3, inverted in V_4–V_6
Axis:	Right
Interpretation:	Anterolateral ischemia. Consider clinical presentation and use ST trending or serial ECGs.

Fig. 5.81

Rate and rhythm:	Sinus rhythm with at 78 beats/min with first-degree AV block (PRI 220 ms)
STE:	V_2
ST depression:	I, aVL, V_4–V_6
T-wave changes:	Inverted in I, aVL, V_4–V_6
STE variant present:	LVH
Axis:	Left
Interpretation:	Possible lateral ischemia. Criteria met for LVH. Consider clinical presentation and use ST trending or serial ECGs.

Fig. 5.82

Rate and rhythm:	Sinus rhythm at 81 beats/min
Pathologic Q waves:	V_1, V_2
STE:	V_1–V_4
ST depression:	II, III, aVF
T-wave changes:	Tall in V_2–V_4
Axis:	Normal
Interpretation:	Anteroseptal STEMI. Consider clinical presentation and use ST trending or serial ECGs.

Fig. 5.83

Rate and rhythm:	Sinus arrhythmia at 64 beats/min
STE:	II, aVF, V_5, V_6
ST depression:	V_2
T-wave changes:	Inverted in V_1
STE variant present:	Pericarditis?
Axis:	Normal
Interpretation:	Inferolateral STEMI. No obvious reciprocal changes noted so pericarditis is a possibility but unlikely because of localized elevation. Obtain right-sided chest leads. Consider clinical presentation and use ST trending or serial ECGs.

Fig. 5.84

Rate and rhythm:	Sinus rhythm at 73 beats/min
Pathologic Q waves:	V_2, V_4
STE:	I, aVL, V_1–V_5
ST depression:	II, III, aVF
T-wave changes:	Tall in V_2–V_5
Reciprocal changes	II, III, aVF
Axis:	Normal
Interpretation:	Extensive anterolateral STEMI. Consider clinical presentation and use ST trending or serial ECGs.

Fig. 5.85

Rate and rhythm:	Supraventricular rhythm at 91 beats/min
STE:	V_1–V_3
ST depression:	I, II, aVL, V_4–V_6
T-wave changes:	Inverted in I, aVL, V_4–V_6
STE variant present:	LVH
Axis:	Left
Interpretation:	Poor ECG quality. Possible anteroseptal STEMI. Voltage criteria for LVH met. Consider clinical presentation and use ST trending or serial ECGs.

Fig. 5.86

Rate and rhythm:	Sinus rhythm at 100 beats/min
Pathologic Q waves:	III
STE:	III, aVF; borderline in II
ST depression:	aVL
T-wave changes:	aVL
Reciprocal changes:	aVL
Axis:	Normal
Interpretation:	Inferior STEMI with reciprocal changes. Obtain right-sided chest leads, consider clinical presentation, and use ST trending or serial ECGs.

Fig. 5.87

Rate and rhythm:	Sinus rhythm at 69 beats/min with occasional premature complexes
T-wave changes:	Tall in V_4, V_5
Axis:	Normal
Interpretation:	RSR′ (QR) in V_1/V_2 consistent with right ventricular conduction delay (QRS 110 ms). Consider clinical presentation.

Fig. 5.88

Rate and rhythm:	Sinus tachycardia at 113 beats/min with first-degree AV block (PRI 332 ms) and LBBB
STE:	V_1–V_3
ST depression:	V_6
STE variant present:	LBBB
Axis:	Normal
Interpretation:	Possible anteroseptal STEMI; however, wide QRS (QRS 146 ms) and LBBB pattern also present. Artifact in limb leads. Consider clinical presentation and use ST trending or serial ECGs.

Fig. 5.89

Rate and rhythm: Sinus tachycardia at 107 beats/min
STE: II, III, aVF
ST depression: I, aVL
T-wave changes: Inverted in I, aVL
Reciprocal changes: I, aVL
Axis: Normal
Interpretation: Inferior STEMI with reciprocal changes. Obtain right-sided chest leads, consider clinical presentation, and use ST trending or serial ECGs.

Fig. 5.90

Rate and rhythm: Sinus rhythm at 84 beats/min
Axis: Normal
Interpretation: Normal ECG. Consider clinical presentation.

Fig. 5.91

Rate and rhythm: Atrial fibrillation at 115 beats/min
Pathologic Q waves: III, aVF
STE: II, III, aVF, V_5, V_6
ST depression: I, aVL, aVF, V_1–V_3
T-wave changes: Inverted in V_1, V_2
Reciprocal changes: I, aVL
Axis: Right
Interpretation: Inferolateral STEMI with reciprocal changes. ST depression in V_1–V_3 suggests possible posterior involvement. Obtain right-sided and posterior chest leads, consider clinical presentation, and use ST trending or serial ECGs.

Fig. 5.92

Rate and rhythm: Sinus rhythm at 92 beats/min with nonconducted PACs
Axis: Normal
Interpretation: Sinus rhythm with nonconducted PACs; otherwise, normal ECG. Artifact present in the limb leads. Consider clinical presentation.

Fig. 5.93

Rate and rhythm: Sinus rhythm at 92 beats/min
Pathologic Q waves: II, III, aVF
STE: II, III, aVF
ST depression: I, aVL, V_1–V_4
Reciprocal changes: I, aVL
Axis: Normal
Interpretation: Inferior STEMI with reciprocal changes. ST depression in V_1–V_4 suggests possible posterior involvement. Baseline wander in I, II, III. Obtain right-sided and posterior chest leads, consider clinical presentation, and use ST trending or serial ECGs.

Fig. 5.94

Rate and rhythm: Sinus rhythm at 84 beats/min
Axis: Normal
Interpretation: Normal ECG. Consider clinical presentation.

Fig. 5.95

Rate and rhythm: Sinus rhythm at 71 beats/min with first-degree AV block (PRI 212 ms)
Pathologic Q waves: V_1, V_2
STE: V_2, V_3
Axis: Left
Interpretation: Anteroseptal STEMI. Meets STE criteria in V_2, V_3. Poor R-wave progression noted through V_3. Slight STE may be a normal variant in the range of V_1–V_3. Borderline criteria for LVH. Although STEMI ECG criteria are met, integration of clinical picture is particularly important with this ECG. Use ST trending or serial ECGs.

Fig. 5.96

Rate and rhythm:	Sinus rhythm at 69 beats/min
STE:	II, III, aVF
ST depression:	aVL
T-wave changes:	Inverted in I, aVL
Reciprocal changes:	I, aVL
Axis:	Normal
Interpretation:	Inferior STEMI with reciprocal changes. Obtain right-sided chest leads, consider clinical presentation, and use ST trending or serial ECGs.

Fig. 5.97

Rate and rhythm:	Sinus bradycardia at 56 beats/min with short (116 ms) PRI
STE:	V_1–V_4
ST depression:	II, III, aVF
T-wave changes:	Tall in V_2–V_4
Axis:	Normal
Interpretation:	Anteroseptal STEMI. Consider clinical presentation and use ST trending or serial ECGs.

Fig. 5.98

Rate and rhythm:	Sinus rhythm at 65 beats/min
STE:	II, III, aVF
ST depression:	aVL
T-wave changes:	Inverted in aVL
Reciprocal changes:	aVL
Axis:	Normal
Interpretation:	Inferior STEMI with reciprocal changes. Baseline wander in I, III. Obtain right-sided chest leads, consider clinical presentation, and use ST trending or serial ECGs.

Fig. 5.99

Rate and rhythm:	Sinus rhythm at 81 beats/min
STE:	aVL, V_1–V_2
ST depression:	II, III, aVF
T-wave changes:	Inverted in III; tall/peaked in V_1–V_4
Axis:	Normal
Interpretation:	Septal STEMI. STE noted in V_1–V_2 (aVL suspicious but ECG quality makes it difficult to be certain). Baseline wander in most limb leads. Consider clinical presentation and use ST trending or serial ECGs.

Fig. 5.100

Rate and rhythm:	Sinus tachycardia at 114 beats/min
STE:	II, III, aVF
ST depression:	I, aVL
Reciprocal changes:	I, aVL
Axis:	Normal
Interpretation:	Inferior STEMI with reciprocal changes. Subtle ST changes noted in V_5 and V_6 but do not meet criteria. Artifact present in I, III. Obtain right-sided chest leads, consider clinical presentation, and use ST trending or serial ECGs.

Index

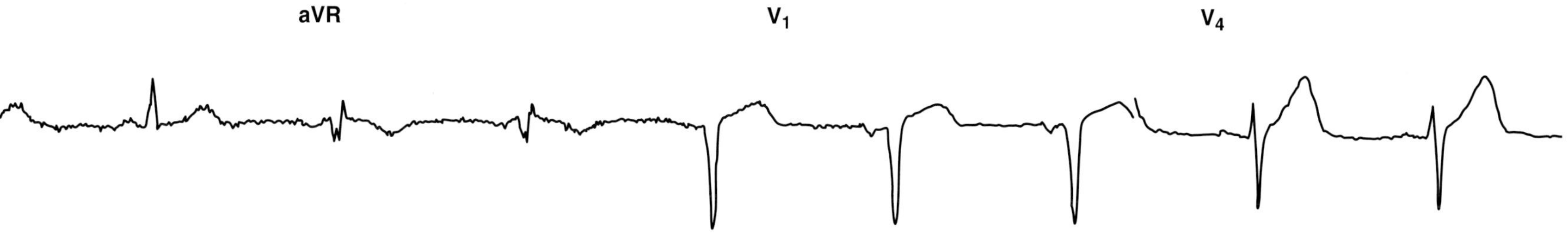

Note: Page numbers followed by *f* indicate figures, *t* indicate tables and *b* indicate boxes.

A

E

F

G

H

I

J

L

M

N

P

Q

R